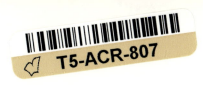

The Archaeology of Childhood

THE INSTITUTE FOR EUROPEAN AND MEDITERRANEAN ARCHAEOLOGY

DISTINGUISHED MONOGRAPH SERIES

Peter F. Biehl, Sarunas Milisauskas, and Stephen L. Dyson, editors

The Magdalenian Household: Unraveling Domesticity
Ezra Zubrow, Françoise Audouze, and James G. Enloe, editors

Eventful Archaeologies: New Approaches to Social Transformation in the Archaeological Record
Douglas J. Bolender, editor

The Archaeology of Violence: Interdisciplinary Approaches
Sarah Ralph, editor

Approaching Monumentality in Archaeology
James. F. Osborne, editor

The Archaeology of Childhood
Güner Coşkunsu, editor

THE
ARCHAEOLOGY OF
CHILDHOOD

Interdisciplinary
Perspectives
on an
Archaeological
Enigma

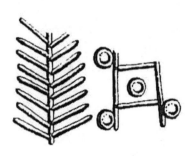

IEMA Proceedings,
Volume 4

EDITED BY
Güner Coşkunsu

STATE UNIVERSITY OF
NEW YORK PRESS

Logo and cover/interior art: A vessel with wagon motifs from Bronocice, Poland, 3400 B.C. Courtesy of Sarunas Milisauskas and Janusz Kruk, 1982, Die Wagendarstellung auf einem Trichterbecher au Bronocice, Polen, *Archäologisches Korrespondenzblatt* 12: 141–144

Published by
State University of New York Press, Albany

© 2015 State University of New York

All rights reserved

Printed in the United States of America

No part of this book may be used or reproduced in any manner whatsoever without written permission. No part of this book may be stored in a retrieval system or transmitted in any form or by any means including electronic, electrostatic, magnetic tape, mechanical, photocopying, recording, or otherwise without the prior permission in writing of the publisher.

For information, contact
State University of New York Press, Albany, NY
www.sunypress.edu

Production, Eileen Nizer
Marketing, Michael Campochiaro

Library of Congress Cataloging-in-Publication Data

The archaeology of childhood : interdisciplinary perspectives on
an archaeological enigma / edited by Güner Coşkunsu.
        pages cm. — (SUNY series, The Institute for European and
Mediterranean archaeology distinguished monograph series)
    Includes bibliographical references and index.
    ISBN 978-1-4384-5805-2 (hardcover : alkaline paper)
    ISBN 978-1-4384-5806-9 (e-book)
    1. Children, Prehistoric.   2. Children—History.   3. Infants—
History.   4. Human remains (Archaeology)   5. Social archaeology.
6. Household archaeology.   I. Coşkunsu, Güner.

    GN799.C38A73 2015
    305.2309—dc23   2014044284

                    10 9 8 7 6 5 4 3 2 1

This book is wholeheartedly dedicated to Dr. Saubhagya Shah of Harvard University, a very precious friend and brilliant scholar, whom I lost in very young age.

Contents

PART IV
COMMENTARIES

Illustrations

Tables

Acknowledgments

The IEMA Distinguished Monograph Series Editors would like to thank Thomas Harper, Hannah Quaintance, and Heather Rosch for copyediting and indexing and editorial assistance for the production of this book. We would also like to express our gratitude to the staff at SUNY Press, namely Michael Campochiaro, Rafael Chaiken, Ryan Morris, and Michael Rinella, for their assistance in publishing this volume. And finally, we would like to thank all the authors for their excellent chapters and their patience and support.

Children as Archaeological Enigma

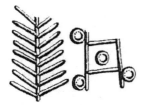

Güner Coşkunsu

The history of childhood is a nightmare from which we have only recently begun to awaken.

—Lloyd De Mause, *The History of Childhood*

The notions of children and childhood are seriously underresearched subjects in archaeology. This is regrettable for several reasons, discussed below. This volume is a modest attempt to redress this imbalance.

I should admit that the theme of this book, children in the archaeological record, is not my specialty but a product of my long-lasting curiosity. My curiosity greatly increased during my PhD research. While my specific interest in the presence of ancient children in archaeological contexts goes back to my first field experience while in college, I became more conscious of these children during my PhD research while, firstly, observing potential knapping marks of children on flint artifacts and secondly, observing current-day rural children's activities and objects, which were sometimes found in a very similar form and context to those in archaeological excavations on which I have worked. Through my graduate course, "Children in Archaeological Context" (Advanced Archaeological Research, APY 736 COS), and the preparation of the Third IEMA Visiting Scholar Spring Conference ("Children as Archaeological Enigma: Are Children Visible or Invisible in the Archaeological Record?"), as well as the preparation of this subsequent volume during and after my postdoctoral fellowship at the Institute for European and Mediterranean Archaeology (IEMA) at SUNY Buffalo, the subject became of great interest to me. Since then I have delved further into this essential subject in order to explore it more deeply and to contribute to a better understanding of the development of childhood from an archaeological perspective. I hope that this volume will open new vistas to archaeologists who have not thought about the children of the past.

Interest in the archaeology of children and childhood is very recent and, for several reasons that will be discussed later, moves forward slowly despite continuing research by some archaeologists (all women!), many of whom are contributors to this volume. These include Kathryn Kamp, Jane Eva Baxter, Joanna Sofaer, and Traci Ardren. These researchers are following in the footsteps of seminal work by Jenny Moore and Eleanor C. Scott in *Invisible People and Processes: Writing Gender and Childhood into European Archaeology*, which appeared in 1997. This, in turn, was followed by Scott's *The Archaeology of Infancy and Infant Death* two years later, Joanna R. Sofaer Derevenski's *Children and Material Culture* in 2000, Jane Eva Baxter's *The Archaeology of Childhood* in 2005, Traci Ardren and Scott Hutson's *The Social Experience of Childhood in Ancient Mesoamerica* in 2006, and by the IEMA Conference organized by me in 2010 and the present volume. The Society for the Study of Childhood in the Past (SSCIP) and this multidisciplinary society's journal, *The Journal of Childhood in the Past*, are certainly worthy of mention in this overview for their effort to promote the study of childhood and children in the past through conferences, lectures, and publications since the late 2000s under the editorial direction of Eileen Murphy and Sally Crawford.

Save for a few early pioneers such as Andrew T. Chamberlain, this newly emerged interest has now started to capture widespread attention among male colleagues, most notably including professors Frank Hole, David Soren, and Jack Meacham, and Paul Bahn, Scott Hutson, and Kyle Sommerville (all in this volume). Until a decade ago, children were almost completely missing from many archaeological discourses despite their various important, active roles in households, workshops, temples, and in various other economic activities, and despite the fact that given the relatively low average lifespan of adults in ancient societies children must have represented a larger demographic component of those societies than they do in the modern world. Yet, children are still largely ignored, not only by archaeologists but also in many cases by ethnographers, historians, social scientists in general, and even scholars in feminist studies (Ardren 2006; Baxter 2005, 2006, 2008; Kamp 2001; Sofaer Derevenski 1997, 2000a, 2000b; in addition to their chapters in this volume).

Despite the importance of studies of children and childhood in antiquity, few studies have been dedicated to children in archaeology (e.g., Ardren and Hutson 2006; Baxter 2005; Crawford 2010; Crawford and Shepherd 2007; Kamp 2002; Moore and Scott 1997). Seeking to help remedy this intellectual gap, in 2009 I organized an interdisciplinary colloquium on this still largely enigmatic subject in order to better understand it, disseminate pertinent available data, and discuss current methodological and theoretical approaches relevant to the subject. Additionally, an important goal of the colloquium was to discover alternative methodologies and theories pertinent to studies of children and childhood in antiquity by promoting intellectual discussion between archaeologists and scholars from varied pertinent disciplines not fully represented in earlier conferences (e.g., developmental psychology, genetics, cognitive studies). To this end, the conference was planned as an open academic platform where both the speakers and the audience could have an opportunity to meet the diverse group of scholars from different disciplines who work on comparable subjects and who would have much to learn from one another in terms of new research strategies and possible new collaborations, resulting in the present volume. Its main goal is to advance research on the archaeology of children and advance our understanding of the evolution of childhood though time.

A Brief Overview

One of most important questions in the emerging field of the archaeology of children and childhood is the definition of "childhood." The notion of childhood in both prehistoric and early historical times is full of controversy. Despite seminal work on childhood conducted from a historical perspective by Philippe Ariès (1962) and Lloyd De Mause (1976), and from an ethnographic perspective by Margaret Mead (1928), a lack of attention to children as agents still generally characterizes much of the work that humanists and social scientists have done on ancient societies. While the reasons for this are varied, I would argue that the subject of the evolution of childhood in antiquity is too complex to be fully understood from a single perspective, due to its time-, history-, region-, culture-, and memory-situated nature. Only with an interdisciplinary approach can we get close to understanding it.

By its very nature, archaeology is a dynamic field and its interests have been dramatically broadened in the last decade by new archaeometric methods and interdisciplinary approaches. Anthropological archaeology in particular has started to focus on the overlapping human agencies that created the archaeological material remains that we study, and much well-deserved attention has been paid to significant issues that before were only marginally studied, such as social identities, ethnicity, gender, and nationalism. Despite these promising developments, however, archaeologists still pay insufficient attention to the role of children, who were active agents in past societies. Only a small group of archaeologists have cared about multivocality in ancient times, or about the marginalized social identities of women and children who are often "invisible" in archaeological publications. Prominent among these scholars are archaeologists and anthropologists studying gender issues who noted the small role of women and children in archaeological interpretations almost twenty years ago (Ardren 2008; Brumfiel and Robin 2008; Conkey and Spector 1984; Conkey and Gero 1991). Their work inspired new theoretical and methodological approaches for considering social identities, including those of children. Recently, for instance, Kathryn Kamp challenges us with questions such as, "Where have all the children gone?" and, "Why are children invisible in the eyes of archaeologists?" (Kamp 2001:1). As a consequence, in the last decade the study of children in archaeology has become an increasingly important avenue used to reconstruct ancient societies with all their diverse agents. This is evidenced most clearly in the work of Kathryn Kamp, Jane Eva Baxter, Joanna Sofaer, Traci Ardren, Grete Lillehammer, Andrew Chamberlain, and, to a smaller degree, in the work of a number of other archaeologists as well (e.g., Baxter 2005, 2006, 2008; Benthall 1992; Bluebond-Langner and Korbin 2007; Cohen and Rutter 2007; Gottlieb 200; Kamp 2001; Lillehammer 1989, 2000, 2008, 2010;

Lorentz 2003; Moore and Scott 1997; Panter-Brick 1998; Park 1998; Scott 1999; Sofaer Derevenski 1994, 1997, 2000a, 2000b; Wileman 2005).

The main focus of study for such archaeologists has involved the consideration of children as social identities and cultural agents and defining the nature of childhood in antiquity (Högberg 2008). Recently, the point of view in the study of childhood has been broadened further by a number of studies focusing on social, cultural, political, economic, behavioral, cognitive, symbolic, religious, artistic, sexual, genetic, medical, and technological issues (e.g., see Baxter 2005; Högberg 2008; Sofaer Derevenski 2000a, 2000b; and all authors in this volume for specific case studies from different regions). Happily, the recent interest in children in antiquity is not limited to archaeology but is mirrored in related disciplines such as: classics and art history, as seen in the publications of Susan Landgon, David Soren, Jeannine Diddle Uzzi (all in this volume), as well as Christian Laes (2011), Ian Jenkins (1980), Stephanie Lynn Budin (2001), and Ada Cohen and Jeremy Rutter (2007); and anthropology (including medical and ethnographic studies), as seen in Nurit Bird-David's studies on the notion of childhood in indigenous studies on hunter-gatherer Nayaka people in India (Bird-David 2005 and in this volume), and the research of Berry S. Hewlett (2005), Robert A. Levine (2007), and Jonathan Benthall (1992). Anthropological archaeology owes thanks to these scholarly pioneers who inspired new theoretical and methodological approaches for considering the social identities of children and women in archaeological contexts. Thus, the previously overlooked women and children of prehistory are now the subject of increasing archaeological debate and research. However, as I mentioned before, the interest in childhood for archaeology has still not been fully established and the process of recognizing children in the archeological record is still in its infancy.

WHY ARE CHILDREN MISSING IN ARCHAEOLOGICAL INTERPRETATIONS?

Archeologists have been neglecting the role of children in antiquity for several probable reasons (see also Ardren, Baxter, Kamp, Sofaer, all in this volume, for a detailed discussion): (1) the supposed intangible nature of childhood in the archaeological record and the a priori assumption that children lack easily recognizable archaeological correlates (yet few archaeologists have made the attempt!); (2) conceptualizations that see children as socioeconomically unimportant; (3) acceptance of a universal/stereotypical view of childhood; (4) gender biases; (5) cultural biases; and (6) the lack of substantial interdisciplinary collaborations on the subject.

Whatever the real reason(s), the field needs to move beyond the present situation by "materializing" children in antiquity, and several of the chapters in this volume discuss how we can address this lacuna (e.g., Baxter, Bahn, Hutson, Kamp, Langdon, Moses). This "materialization" of children in the archaeological record will go far in answering questions about how the concept of childhood has evolved in human societies through time, while setting directions for more detailed archaeological and interdisciplinary studies of children in the future.

WHY DO ARCHAEOLOGISTS NEED TO CARE ABOUT ANCIENT CHILDREN?

As Chamberlain (1997) noted, there is no question that children existed in ancient times and are represented in the archeological record, irrespective of whether we archeologists are careful or competent enough to recognize them. Thus, there is an urgent need to bring archaeologists and scholars from several disciplines to both clarify the problem and establish current definitions about notions of children and childhood. We also need to develop theoretical and methodological approaches to analyze the archeological record in order to explore and understand the role of children in the formation, reproduction, and maintenance of past cultures.

From historical and ethnographic accounts it is known that children are significant actors in social, economic, symbolic, artistic, and political arenas, and they are often very important in the families and societies they lived in, some of which are covered in this volume. Children are visible in a vast array of archaeological remains regardless of whether archaeologists think about them and see them. Past children are evidenced by fingerprints on ceramics and other clay objects as well as on cave walls, as Kathryn Kamp, Paul Bahn, and Scott Hutson demonstrate clearly in this volume (see also Barbour 1975, Kamp et al. 1999; Kamp 2002, Králík and Nejman 2007, Králík, Urbanová, and Hložek 2008; Livingstone 2007, and Van Gelder and Sharpe 2008 for more case studies from North America, Mesoamerica, the Near East and Europe; and Acree 1999, and Åström and Eriksson 1980 for the application of methodology and biases). Children's fossilized behaviors are discernible in the making of stone tools (Coşkunsu 2007; Högberg 2008; Stout 2002) and bead production (Kenoyer et al. 1991; Mackay 1937; Roux and Blasco 2000); as well as in the making of playthings and toys, as Jane Eva Baxter, Kathyrn Kamp, Sharon Moses, Scott Hutson, and Kyle Somerville all highlight in their contributions to this volume (see also Baxter 2005; Casey and Burruss 2010; Kohut 2011; Park 1998; Sillar 1994; Somerville and Barton 2012). Children are also recognizable in data from mortuary, skeletal, DNA, and isotope analyses, presented in this volume by Susan Langdon, David Soren, Eva Rosenstock, and Keri Brown (see also Beck and Sievert 2005; Bentley 2006; Djurić et al. 2011; Finlay 200; Georgiadis 2011; Halcrow and Tayles 2008, 2010; Hamilton 2007; Ingvarsson-Sundström 2003; Lewis 2007; Lorentz 2003; Mays 1997; Oxenham et al. 2008; Perry 2005; Redfern et al. 2011). The behaviors of children can also be detected in architectural features, the spatial distribution and arrangement of domestic material and activities, and microstratigraphy, as Joanna Sofaer, Sharon Moses, and Scott Hutson elaborate in case studies in this volume (see also Hutson 2006; Sofaer 2006). Children are also visible in artistic, iconographic, and textual records of the past, as discussed in the chapters by Paul Bahn, Susan Langdon, and Jeannine Diddle Uzzi (see also Budin 2011; Oppenheim 1967). Finally, information about children can also be inferred from figurines, which can be products of art, magic rituals, or playthings, as argued by Kathryn Kamp, Scott Hutson, Peter Biehl, and Sharon Moses in this volume, who interpret figurines as the material records of children in the context of social identity, representations of body, production, learning, socialization, play, and ritual. Pursuing the psychological reflections of past children and childhoods in the archaeological record seems difficult, at least for now, since archaeologists and anthropologists are usually not well grounded in developmental psychology. However, in an intriguing chapter in this volume Jack Meacham approaches children's development, learning, and social identities through the use of four metaphors (essence, organism, machine, and historical context) that offer much promise for the development of new research questions, theories, and methodologies for archaeologists.

Children's involvement in ceramic, stone tool, and bead production, art (both as subjects in artwork and producers of "art"), sacrifice as victims, hunting, and the fact that they sometimes had special status have been documented in the archaeological literature of both the Old and New Worlds. Culture is not static and is not created only by adults of one gender. Instead, it is constructed by individuals of different ages, gender, class, ethnicity, and occupation. In other words, children are active agents of culture wherever it is present, and therefore children and childhood must be an integral part of archaeological research.

From my own field experience I know well that the role of children varies greatly between urban centers and rural areas. For instance, while the majority of modern urban children do not need to worry about domestic and nondomestic tasks, those who live in rural areas have to take care of their younger siblings, haul water, fish, hunt, spin, tend to small livestock, mine, gather fuel, prepare food, maintain fire, etc. on a daily basis (see Chamberlain 1997 for a discussion of the decrease in the amount of labor and the creation of more leisure time that industrialization and technology have created in Western notions of childhood). Hence, doubtlessly, prehistoric children of nonelite families were also responsible for such crucial tasks (Ardren 2006).

Lillehammer (2000) has argued that children probably took on a greater number of roles when societies shifted from foraging to agriculture, since most likely women had more work to do, which in turn resulted in increased work demand for small children (see Claassen 2002 for a study of early agricultural societies of North America using bioarchaeological data). Algaze (2008) and Yener (2000) emphasized child labor and children's serious involvement in production of ancient Mesopotamia's two major exports, textiles and metal, in early urban economy. One source for the economic importance of children in early urban economies are Mesopotamian texts, which make it clear that children provided a big chunk of the very substantial labor involved in textile production (Algaze 2008). According to Algaze, without children the export economy of Mesopotamia would have been insignificant. Additionally, children provide a big chunk of the labor in mining (e.g., small shafts etc.) and in production of metals, the biggest economic export of the periphery. See also Yener (2000) for the domestication of metals and the ethnographic documentation of how mines are operated in traditional preindustrial societies. In short, without a doubt, child labor was crucial to that trade if the largest part of ancient Near Eastern exchange was textiles from the south and metals from the north.

When adults had a heavy burden of labor outside the domestic sphere, they might not have been able to take good care of their children (Ardren 2006; Vogt 1970). See Bird-David (2005; and in this volume) for more on the notion of childhood from a non-Western point of view, children-parent/adult relations, and children's self-education and maintenance in the Nayaka hunter-gatherer group in South India, which is a situation quite unfamiliar to Western notions of childhood and motherhood identities. Additionally, Somerville presents the case of middle-class Victorian childhood and identities (in this volume). Meacham's and Sofaer's arguments in this volume, respectively, show similarities in the dynamics involved in children's learning and children's reactions toward instructions they are given, but they depict a different picture from Bird-David's arguments for hunting and gathering societies (see Hole for his comments on Meacham's chapter; in this volume). Going back to Lillehammer's point, she argued for the possibility of children assuming a caretaking role for other children while adults shifted to other labor in ancient societies, particularly those societies in which life expectancy was relatively low (Lillehammer 2000:23). In short, like adults, children play important roles in their societies and they help shape, transmit, and maintain their culture, as well as their own lives. Without acknowledging the agency of ancient children in the creation of culture, archaeologists' interpretations of data and reconstructions of past societies must necessarily be incomplete. It is time, therefore, to bring ancient children back into archaeological research. Children were important in the past and at times they were as fundamental to ancient cultures as their mothers, fathers, grandparents, and rulers. We need only think of the reign of some child rulers who had a supreme, political, or spiritual power in history of the world, such as Thutmosis III and Tutankhamen of ancient Egypt, the seven-year-old Norwegian king Magnus Erlingsson, and three-year-old Chinese emperor Henry Pu Yi. Child rulers did not appear only in highly stratified civilization but also in socially less complex civilizations and cultures, such as in nomadic tribes with the son of the leader of a tribe or chief of a village. Wherever children were present, the specifics of their role and influence were no doubt dependent on the religious, political, and social values and practices of the societies they formed a part of. Environmental, biological, and cognitive factors may also be added to this list. However, we should not fall into the trap of thinking that biology and skeletal remains fully capture the importance of past children. This is an important point made by Sofaer both in an earlier publication (2006) and in this volume, and is a point reflected in ongoing debates (mostly in Britain) between socially oriented archaeologists and bioarchaeologists (e.g., Halcrow and Tayles 2008; Hamilton 2007). According to some bioarchaeologists, skeletons cannot provide any information about the social and cultural aspects of childhood and children (see Lally and Ardren 2008; Sofaer 2006 and in this volume for two strong criticisms of this view). Like some scholars, (e.g., Halcrow and Tayles 2008), I favor a cross-disciplinary perspective that bridges both approaches and that, when applicable, brings in other pertinent perspectives to the study of ancient children.

It follows from the preceding that understanding the role that children played in ancient societies, both as active and passive agents, is crucial if we are to reconstruct those societies as a whole. However, we should not create stereotypes based on modern Western conditions in our analysis of the data (Ardren, Bird-David, and Kamp in this volume; Kamp 2001) and we should be aware of cross-cultural studies that alert us about the nonuniversal perceptions of childhood and social identities, as Bird-David's cutting-edge chapter demonstrates (see also Meacham's chapter for how psychological effects related to identity formation can be similar due to cognitive features and heredity, regardless of culture; see also Hole in this volume). By neglecting children in their reconstructions of ancient societies, archaeologists are unwittingly adopting a universal notion of childhood which is unwarranted on theoretical and evidentiary grounds.

Additionally, some current archaeological literature draws potentially wrong conclusions about past societies due to the use of inapplicable methodological and/or theoretical approaches. I strongly believe that the lack of attention to children in archaeological interpretations, the use of unclear definitions of notions of childhood, and the uncritical acceptance of a universal notion of childhood combine to cause a misleading or incomplete reconstruction of past societies (see Bird-David for concrete examples and a thorough discussion). The historian Ariès (1962) was surely correct when he argued that the concept of childhood is constructed both socioeconomically and culturally and that it differs across time and space (see also Ardren, Bird-David, Kamp, and Sofaer in this volume; Kamp 2001; and Sofaer Derevenski 2000 for similar arguments). Often, the age definition of life cycles employed by archaeologists is based on Western perceptions of children, rather than on concepts about the nature of childhood that existed in the past. It should be noted here that some of the most common conflicts among archaeologists regarding the definition of childhood and children in the material record derive from age determinations and terminology in the study of bioarcheology (Perry 2005). Since there is no consensus about these, there is a general tendency in our field to study children as incidental or irrelevant and to insist on seeing children as visible only through burial remains (Baxter, in this volume). There is a lack of harmony in applying different methodologies with interests in the social aspects versus the bioarchaeological aspects of children. Rotshchild (2002) warns us that we cannot expect to find childhood in every society and that the definition of what constitutes childhood is often constructed by Western notions of biological "realities." The definition of childhood is also not clear in religion; a range of symbolic meanings are adduced to childhood. The image of children is represented with a diversity of meanings, and it is full of metaphors. The notion of who is a child changes due to age, condition, lineage, or sources of imagery as well as an author's own point of view (Francis 2006:14, 283). The bottom line is that a universal view of childhood results in inadequate reconstructions of past societies and their cultures. Hence, the definition of childhood has to be discussed further by scholars, and more cross-cultural studies need to done.

An example of biases in current research methodologies and theories in the archaeological study of childhood can be obtained from the mortuary record (i.e., skeleton and dental remains; grave goods; type and location of burial; etc.). The burial rates of children are highly dependent on the nature of preservation (commonly incomplete); the type of burial (single or multiple burials with parents; cremation or inhumation); whether or not child burials are incorporated into adult mortuary areas (spatial segregation); recovery techniques; data analyses; definition of age and sex by experts; and the level of experience of experts (Chamberlain 2000). Due to these factors, information about biometric, population, health, social status as well as the ethnic identity of children in mortuary contexts is often explored incorrectly (Baxter 2005). Archaeologists often assume that special grave goods found in children's graves signal social ranking within a given society (Crawfort 2000; Sofaer Derevenksi 1997). However, from ethnographical and historical documents it is known that health conditions and age at the time of death are not always related with socioeconomic conditions and social status/wealth. The notion of childhood plays an ideological and communicative role in the ancient Andean and Roman worlds. For instance, ancient Andean societies sometimes sacrificed children as part of rituals intended to communicate with saints and deities (Ardren 2011; Sillar 1994). Those selected for sacrifice were from the nonelite class and they were fed well before being sacrificed.

How Do We Rescue Children in Archaeological Records?

The vital question to ask is not whether children are visible or invisible, but how archaeologists can correctly discern the activities, identities, and behavior of children in the archaeological record for a more accurate construction of ancient societies. I argue that we should accept the presence of children, as well as the fact that they played active roles in the past, in order to refine the problem, define the kinds of anthropological questions that can be addressed, establish methodologies for studying children archaeologically, and improve current studies on this subject. This can be done most productively through interdisciplinary exchanges, such as are reflected in both this volume and the conference that gave rise to it.

Perhaps we will never be able to fully reconstruct what childhood was really like in the past, but we can certainly bring abandoned children back into archaeological thinking and research and correct archaeologists' erroneous and gender-biased interpretations.

By its nature, the study of childhood thus stimulates an interdisciplinary dialogue. This is reflected in this volume, which brings together scholars who work on various aspects of this question with experience in different regions, diverse methodological and theoretical approaches, and evidence from sites spanning from the Paleolithic to the historical ages both in Old and New Worlds. What is most attractive about this volume is that it emphasizes linkages between anthropological archaeology, ethnography, and anthropological theory, as well as other disciplines in the social sciences, humanities, and natural sciences. I hope that the interdisciplinary nature of this work will result in further dialogue and widen the range of perspectives that can be applied to the study of childhood in the past. Each of the contributions in this volume expands the field of childhood studies and provides a better understanding of the various meanings of the notion of childhood and its social and cultural context. In addition, the contributions of new dating and laboratory techniques, which are also emphasized by some of the contributors to this volume, expand our comprehension of the subject. In this book we discuss the notion of childhood in the past and the importance of children in social, economic, cultural, psychological, symbolic, artistic, sexual, biological, biometric, and health-related contexts. The volume considers how the notion of childhood is expressed in artifacts and the material record and examines how it is described in the literary and historical sources of people from different regions and cultures.

I hope that the conference and its volume will broaden the perspective of many non-Western archaeologists in a positive way and enhance their appreciation of gender and childhood studies in archaeology, by being a timely addition to a current interest among archaeologists in reexamining our assumptions.

STRUCTURE OF THE BOOK

The articles (sixteen) and commentaries (two) in this volume are revised versions of papers initially presented at the Third Visiting Scholar Conference for the Institute for European and Mediterranean Archaeology (IEMA) of the University of Buffalo, entitled "Children as Archaeological Enigma: Are Children Visible or Invisible in the Archaeological Record?" The conference was held on April 24–25, 2010. It should be noted that three challenging papers by Patricia Wattenmaker, Karen Johnson, Trina Arpin, and one very promising poster presentation by Jessica Coone that were all presented at the conference are unfortunately lacking in the volume. Originally, nineteen papers, one poster, and four commentary speeches were delivered at the conference by scholars from the United States, Europe, and the Middle East. Having speakers and authors trained in different countries and cultures (some of them are even multicultural), provided a very productive dialogue and expanded our collective horizons. Fields represented at the conference included Mediterranean and European archaeology, bioarchaeology, geoarchaeology, physical anthropology, classics, art history, psychology, and genetics. This interdisciplinary approach to the study of ancient childhood and children presented opportunities to question issues, present new studies, highlight what is important, what is not and what type of techniques, theories, methods we need in order to elaborate a broader social and cultural perspective on the evolution of childhood across time and space.

The volume is structured into three main sections that includes more specific subjects and one commentary session:

1. Theorizing (In)Visibility, Legitimacy, and Biases in Archaeological Approaches to Children and Childhood

2. Interdisciplinary and Archaeological Approaches to Studying Children and Childhood in the Past

3. Case Studies in the Archaeology of Childhood.

These sections are followed by commentaries by Frank Hole and Traci Ardren. Steve Dyson and Mehmet Özdoğan also acted as discussants at the conference, but their work schedules prevented them from submitting written comments after the conference.

As a conclusion, I hope that this book will urge new research questions and will be followed by many new publications and conferences to approach a better understanding of the subject through new theories and methodologies. I hope that this book will provide a forum clarifying what the current problems are, and what possible research strategies and collaborations could be used to address those problems. Doubtless, we are still at the very beginning of a long journey to bring back the unintentionally lost children of the past.

ACKNOWLEDGMENTS

I am deeply thankful to the authors of this book for their enthusiasm, patience, kindness, understanding, cooperation, and support during and after the preparation of the conference and this volume, as well as for their arduous efforts involved in traveling to Buffalo when the Eyjafjallajökull Volcano in Iceland interrupted so much air and land travel in Europe. I can never forget the joy I felt when almost all of our speakers finally could make their way to Buffalo, one by one. I would like to express my thanks and appreciation to the authors also for sharing their ideas and helping me both before and after the conference whenever I needed it. I am particularly indebted to Kathryn Kamp, Jane Eva Baxter, and Traci Ardren for their comments and sound advice for structuring the book at various stages of its publication. I am immensely thankful to Guillermo Algaze, Kathryn Kamp, and John Whittaker for their thorough and critical editing of this chapter.

I owe thanks to the former and current members of the IEMA board: Peter Biehl, Ted Pena, Samuel M. Paley, Tim Chevral, Stephen Dyson, Ezra Zubrow, Sarunas Milis-auskas, and Bradley Ault for awarding me with the IEMA Post-doctoral Fellowship and offering me the opportunity to organize this conference, to give my graduate course on children in archaeology at the Department of Anthropology at SUNY Buffalo, and to meet the distinctive speakers and authors of the conference and this volume. I owe many thanks also to Prof. Donald Pollock, chair of the Department of Anthropology, and the administrative staff of the anthropology and classics departments.

I would like to thank and express my appreciation also to my graduate students at SUNY Buffalo who took my seminar course on the archaeology of childhood. Their interest in the subject as well as the stimulating discussions and ideas kept my enthusiasm lively when I was both teaching and organizing the conference. Seeing some of them, such as Kyle Somerville and Jennifer Faux, delving into the subject of childhood archaeology at that time and later, and engaged in internationally recognized symposia and writings in prestigious scholarly books and journals is a source of happiness, satisfaction, and hope for me.

I am very grateful to my colleagues and friends Warren Barbour, Patricia Wattenmaker, and Guillermo Algaze for intellectual and friendly support as well as for their always wise advice; Elizabeth Dundon, Janet Akçakal, Arkadiusz (Arek) Klimowicz, Patrycja (Pati) Klimowicz, Mesut Aygün, Işıl Demirtaş, Sarah Ralph, Aleksander I. Oga-dzhanov, Heather Cahill, Kyle Somerville, and UB Department of Anthropology and Classics students for all their support, friendship, and guidance during the preparation of both the conference and the resulting publication.

A very precious friend and scholar, Dr. Saubhagya Shah of Harvard University, whom I lost at a very young age and to whom this book is dedicated, deserves deepest thanks and appreciation for the many beautiful qualities he added to my professional and private life.

REFERENCES CITED

Acree, M.A. 1999 Is There a Gender Difference in Fingerprint Ridge Density? *Forensic Science International* 102:35–44.

Algaze, G. 2008 *Ancient Mesopotamia at the Dawn of Civilization: The Evolution of an Urban Landscape.* University of Chicago Press, Chicago.

Ardren, T. 2006 Setting the Table: Why Children and Childhood are Important in an Understanding of Ancient Mesoamerica. In *The Social Experience of Childhood in Ancient Mesoamerica*, edited by T. Ardren and S. Hutson, pp. 3–24. University Press of Colorado, Boulder.

Ardren, T. 2008 Studies of Gender in the Prehispanic Americas. *Journal of Archaeological Research* 16:1–35.

Ardren, T. 2011 Empowered Children in Classic Maya Sacrificial Rites. *Childhood in the Past: An International Journal* 4(1):133–145.

Ardren, T., and S. Hutson (editors) 2006 *The Social Experience of Childhood in Ancient Mesoamerica.* University of Colorado Press, Boulder.

Ariès, P. 1962 *Centuries of Childhood.* Vintage Books, London.

Åström, P., and S. A. Eriksson 1980 Fingerprints and Archaeology. *Studies in Mediterranean Archaeology* 28:8.

Barbour, W. D. T. 1975 *The Figurines and Figurine Chronology of Ancient Teotihuacan, Mexico.* Unpublished PhD Dissertation, Department of Anthropology, University of Rochester.

Baxter, J. E. 2005 *The Archaeology of Childhood: Children, Gender, and Material Culture.* Altamira Press, Walnut Creek.

Baxter, J. E. (editor) 2006 *Children in Action: Perspectives on the Archaeology of Childhood.* Archaeological Papers of the American Anthropological Association, Vol. 15. University of California Press, Berkley.

Baxter, J. E. 2008 The Archaeology of Childhood. *Annual Review of Anthropology* 37:159–175.

Beck, L. A., and A. K. Sievert 2005 Mortuary Pathways Leading to the Cenote at Chichen Itza. In *Interacting with the Dead: Perspectives on Mortuary Archaeology for the New Millennium*, edited by G. Rakita, J. Buikstra, L. Beck, and S. Williams, pp. 290–304. University Press of Florida, Gainesville.

Benthall, J. 1992 A Late Developer? The Ethnography of Children. *Anthropology Today* 8(2):1.

Bentley, R. A. 2006 Strontium Isotopes from the Earth to the Archaeological Skeleton: A Review. *Journal of Archaeological Method and Theory* 13:135–187.

Bird-David, N. 2005 Studying Children in "Hunter-Gatherer" Societies. Reflections from a Nayaka Perspective. In *Hunter-Gatherer Childhoods: Evolutionary, Developmental, and Cultural Perspectives*, edited by Barry S. Hewlett, pp. 92–101. Aldine Transactions, New Brunswick, New Jersey.

Bluebond-Langner, M., and J. E. Korbin 2007 Challenges and Opportunities in the Anthropology of Childhoods: An Introduction to "Children, Childhoods, and Childhood Studies." *American Anthropologist* 109(2):241–246.

Brumfiel, E. M., and C. Robin 2008 Gender, Households, and Society: An Introduction. *Archeological Papers of the American Anthropological Association* 18(1):1–16.

Budin, S. L. 2011 *Images of Woman and Child from the Bronze Age: Reconsidering Fertility, Maternity, and Gender in the Ancient World.* Cambridge University Press, New York and Cambridge.

Casey, J., and R. Burruss 2010 Social Expectations and Children's Play Places in Northern Ghana. *Ethnoarchaeology* 2(1):49–72.

Chamberlain, A. T. 1997 Commentary: Missing Stages of Life: Towards the Perception of Children in Archaeology. In *Invisible People and Processes: Writing Gender and Childhood into European Archaeology*, edited by J. Moore and E. Scott, pp. 248–250. Leicester University Press, London.

Chamberlain, A. T. 2000 Minor Concerns: A Demographic Perspective on Children in Past Societies. In *Children and Material Culture*, edited by J. Sofaer-Derevenski, pp. 206–212. Routledge, London.

Claassen, C. 2002 Mother's Workloads and Children's Labor During the Woodland Period. In *Pursuit of Gender: Worldwide Archeological Approaches*, edited by S. M. Nelson and M. Rosen-Ayalon, pp. 225–234. AltaMira Press, Walnut Creek, California.

Cohen, A., and J. B. Rutter (editors) 2007 *Constructions of Childhood in the Ancient World Greece and Italy*. The American School of Classical Studies at Athens, Athens.

Conkey, M., and J. Spector 1984 Archaeology and the Study of Gender. In *Advances in Archaeological Method and Theory*, edited by M. B. Schiffer, pp. 1–38. Academic Press, New York.

Conkey, M. W., and J. M. Gero 1991 Tensions, Pluralities, and Engendering Archaeology: An Introduction to Women and Prehistory. In *Engendering Archaeology: Women and Prehistory*, edited by J. M. Gero and M. W. Conkey, pp. 3–30. Blackwell, Oxford.

Coşkunsu, G. 2007 The End of the Pre-Pottery Neolithic in the Middle Euphrates Valley. The Lithic Assemblages of Mezraa Teleilat, Southeastern Turkey. Unpublished PhD dissertation. Department of Anthropology, Harvard University.

Crawford, S. 2000 Children, Grave Goods, and Social Status in Early Anglo-Saxon England. In *Children and Material Culture*, edited by J. Sofaer Derevenski, pp. 169–179. Routledge, London.

Crawford, S. 2010 "Our Race Had Its Childhood": The Use of Childhood as a Metaphor in Post-Darwinian Explanations for Prehistory. *Childhood in the Past* 3(1):107–122.

Crawford, S., and G. Shepherd (editors) 2007 *Children, Childhood and Society*. BAR International Series 1696. Archaeopress, Oxford.

De Mause, L. (editor) 1976 *The History of Childhood*. Psychohistory Press, New York.

Djurić, M., K. Djukić, P. Milovanović, A. Janović, and P. Milenković 2011 Representing Children in Excavated Cemeteries: The Intrinsic Preservation Factors. *Antiquity* 85(327):250–262.

Finlay, N. 2000 Outside of Life: Traditions of Infant Burial in Ireland from Cillín to Cist. *World Archaeology* 31(3):407–422.

Francis, J. M. M. 2006 *Adults as Children: Images of Childhood in the Ancient World and the New Testament*. Peter Lang, Oxford and Bern.

Georgiadis, M. 2011 Child Burials in Mesolithic and Neolithic Southern Greece: A Synthesis. *Childhood in the Past* 4(1):31–45.

Gottlieb, A. 2000 Where Have All the Babies Gone? Towards an Anthropology of Infants (and Their Caretakers). *Anthropological Quarterly* 73(3):121–132.

Gruen, E. S. (editor) 2010 *Cultural Identity in the Ancient Mediterranean*. Issues & Debates. Getty Research Institute, Los Angeles.

Halcrow, S. E., and N. Tayles 2008 The Bioarchaeological Investigation of Childhood and Social Age: Problems and Prospects. *Journal of Archaeological Method and Theory* 15:190–215.

Halcrow, S. E., and N. Tayles 2010 The Archaeological Infant in Biological and Social Context: A Response to Mike Lally and Traci Ardren 2008. Little Artefacts: Rethinking the Constitution of the Archaeological Infant. *Childhood in the Past* 3(1):123–130.

Hamilton, M. D. 2007 Review of The Body as Material Culture: A Theoretical Osteoarchaeology, by J. R. Sofaer. *American Journal of Physical Anthropology* 132:161–162.

Hewlett, B. S. (editor) 2005 *Hunter-Gatherer Childhoods: Evolutionary, Developmental, and Cultural Perspectives*. Aldine Transactions, New Brunswick, New Jersey.

Högberg, A. 2008 Playing with Flint: Tracing a Child's Imitation of Adult Work in a Lithic Assemblage. *Journal of Archaeological Method and Theory* 15(1):112–131.

Hutson, S. R. 2006 Children not at Chunchcmil: A Relational Approach to Young Subjects. In *The Social Experience of Childhood in Ancient Mesoamerica*, edited by T. Ardren and S. Hutson, pp. 103–131. University Press of Colorado, Boulder.

Ingvarsson-Sundström, A. 2003 *Children Lost and Found: A Bioarchaeological Study of the Middle Helladic Children in Asine with a Comparison to Lerna*. Department of Classical Archaeology and Ancient History, Uppsala University, Uppsala.

Jenkins, I. 1980 *An Athenian Childhood*. Joint Association of Classical Teachers in London, London.

Kamp, K. 2001 Where Have All the Children Gone?: The Archaeology of Childhood. *Journal of Archaeological Method and Theory* 8(1):1–34.

Kamp, K. 2002 *Children in the Prehistoric Puebloan Southwest*. University of Utah Press, Salt Lake City.

Kamp, K. A., N. Timmerman, G. Lind, J. Graybill, and I. Natowsky 1999 Discovering Childhood: Using Fingerprints to Find Children in the Archaeological Record. *American Antiquity* 64(2):309–315.

Kenoyer, J. M., M. Vidale, and K.K. Bhan 1991 Contemporary Stone Beadmaking in Khambhat, India: Patterns of Craft Specialization and Organization of Production as Reflected in the Archaeological Record. *World Archaeology* 23(1): 44–63.

Kohut, B. M. 2011 Buried with Children: Reinterpreting Ancient Maya "Toys." *Childhood in the Past: An International Journal* 4(1):146–161.

Králík, M., and L. Nejman 2007 Fingerprints on Artifacts and Historical items: Examples and Comments. *Journal of Ancient Fingerprints* 1:1–13.

Králík, M., P. Urbanová, and M. Hložek 2008 Finger, Hand and Foot Imprints: The Evidence of Children on Archaeological Artefacts. In *Children Identity and the Past*, edited by L. H. Dommasnes and M. Wrigglesworth, pp. 1–15. Cambridge Scholars Publishing, Newcastle.

Laes, C. 2011 *Children in the Roman Empire: Outsiders Within*. Cambridge University Press, Cambridge.

Lally, M., and T. Ardren 2008 Little Artefacts: Rethinking the Constitution of the Archaeological Infant. *Childhood in the Past* 1(1):62–77.

Levine, R. A. 2007 Ethnographic Studies of Childhood: A Historical Overview. *American Anthropologist* 109(2):247–260.

Lewis, M. E. 2007 The Bioarchaeology of Children: Perspectives from Biological and Forensic Anthropology. Cambridge University Press, Cambridge.

Lillehammer, G. 1989 A Child Is Born. The Child's World in an Archaeological Perspective. *Norwegian Archaeological Review* 22(2):89–105.

Lillehammer, G. 2000 The World of Children. In *Children and Material Culture*, edited by J. Sofaer Derevenski, pp. 17–36. Routledge, London.

Lillehammer, G. 2008 Something about Children. In *Children, Identity, and the Past*, edited by L. II. Dommasnes and M. Wrigglesworth, pp. 96–112. Cambridge Scholars Publishing, Cambridge.

Lillehammer, G. 2010 Archaeology of Children. *Complutum* 21(2):15–45.

Livingstone, A. 2007 The Pitter-Patter of Tiny Feet in Clay: Aspects of the Liminality of Childhood in the Ancient Near East. In *Children, Childhood and Society*, edited by S. Crawford and G. Shepherd, pp. 15–27. BAR International Series 1696. Archaeopress, Oxford.

Lorentz, K. O. 2003 Cultures and Physical Modifications: Child Bodies in Ancient Cyprus. *Stanford Journal of Archaeology* 2:1–17.

Mackay, E. 1937 Bead Making in Ancient Sind. *Journal of the American Oriental Society* 57(1):1–15.

Mays, S. A. 1997 A Perspective on Human Osteoarchaeology in Britain. *International Journal of Osteoarchaeology* 7:600–604.

Mead, M. 1928 *Coming of Age in Samoa: A Psychological Study of Primitive Youth for Western Civilisation*. Blue Ribbon Books, New York.

Moore, J., and E. C. Scott (editors) 1997 *Invisible People and Processes: Writing Gender and Childhood into European Archaeology*. Leicester University Press, London and New York.

Oppenheim, A. L. 1967 *Ancient Mesopotamia: Portrait of a Dead Civilization*. University of Chicago Press, Chicago.

Oxenham, M., H. Matsumura, K. Domett, N. K. Thuy, N. K. Dung, N. L. Cuong, D. Huffer, and S. Muller 2008 Health and the Experience of Childhood in Late Neolithic Viet Nam. *Asian Perspective* 47(2):190–209.

Panter-Brick, C. (editor) 1998 *Biosocial Perspectives on Children*. Cambridge University Press, Cambridge.

Park, R. W. 1998 Size Counts: The Miniature Archaeology of Childhood in Inuit Societies. *Antiquity* 72:269–281.

Perry, M. A. 2005 Redefining Childhood through Bioarchaeology: Towards an Archaeological and Biological Understanding of Children in Antiquity. In *Children in Action: Perspectives on the Archaeology of Childhood*, edited by J. E. Baxter, pp. 89–111. University of California Press, Berkeley.

Redfern, R. C., A. R. Millard, and C. Hamlin 2011 A Regional Investigation of Subadult Dietary Patterns and Health in Late Iron Age and Roman Dorset, England. *Journal of Archaeological Science* 39(5):1249–1259.

Rothschild, N. 2002 Introduction. In *Children in the Prehistoric Puebloan Southwest*, edited by K. Kamp, pp. 1–13. University of Utah Press, Salt Lake City.

Roux, V., and P. Blasco 2000 *Cornaline de l'Inde/Carnelian in India: From Technical Practices in Cambay to the Techno-systems of the Indus*. Editions de la Maison des sciences de l'homme, Paris.

Scott, E. C. 1999 *The Archaeology of Infancy and Infant Death*. British Archaeological Reports Number 819. Archaeopress, Oxford.

Sillar, B. 1994 Playing with God: Cultural Perceptions of Children, Play, and Miniatures in the Andes. *Archaeological Review from Cambridge* 13(2):47–64.

Sofaer, J. R. 2006 *The Body as Material Culture: A Theoretical Osteoarchaeology*. Cambridge University Press, Cambridge.

Sofaer Derevenski, J. R. 1994 Where Are the Children? Accessing Children in the Past. *Archeological Review from Cambridge* 13(2):7–20.

Sofaer Derevenski, J. R. 1997 Engendering Children, Engendering Archaeology. In *Invisible People and Processes: Writing Gender and Childhood into European Archaeology*, edited by J. Moore and E. Scott, pp. 192–202. Leicester University Press, London.

Sofaer Derevenski, J. R. 2000a *Children and Material Culture*. Routledge, London.

Sofaer Derevenski, J. R. 2000b Material Culture Shock: Confronting Expectations in the Material Culture of Children. In *Children and Material Culture*, edited by J. Sofaer Derevenski, pp. 3–16. Routledge, London.

Somerville, K., and C. P. Barton 2012 Play Things: Children's Racialized Mechanical Banks and Toys, 1880–1930. *International Journal and Historical Archaeology* 16:47–85.

Stout, D. 2002 Skill and Cognition in Stone Tool Production: An Ethnographic Case Study from Irian Jaya. *Current Anthropology* 45(3):693–722.

van Gelder, L., and K. Sharpe 2009 Women and Girls as Upper Palaeolithic Cave "Artists": Deciphering the Sexes of Finger Fluters in Rouffignac Cave. *Oxford Journal of Archaeology* 28(4):323–333.

Vogt, E. Z. 1970 *The Zinacantecos of Mexico: A Modern Mayan Way of Life.* Holt, Rinehart and Winston, Forth Worth, Texas.

Wileman, J. 2005 *Hide and Seek: The Archaeology of Childhood.* Tempus, Stroud, Gloucestershire.

Yener, K. A. 2000 *The Domestication of Metals: The Rise of Complex Metal Industries in Anatolia.* Brill, Leiden.

PART I

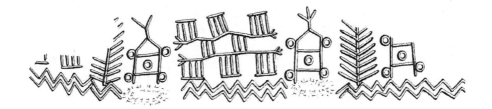

Theorizing (In)visibility, Legitimacy, and Biases in Archaeological Approaches to Children and Childhood

CHAPTER ONE

The Devil's Advocate or Our Worst Case Scenario

The Archaeology of Childhood without Any Children

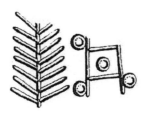

Jane Eva Baxter

Abstract   *The question of the archaeological (in)visibility of children is very much tied to the ways we as scholars choose to situate our understanding of children and childhood in our research. Scholarship on the archaeology of children and childhood has made some of its greatest inroads into archaeological conversations through the broader conduits of gender and identity. Engaging with these broader themes and interests has shaped much of the current research on children and the archaeological record. Research on particular cultural constructions of children and childhood and the resulting material expressions of these identities is a marked departure from some of the earliest work on children and the archaeological record, which emphasized the archaeological visibility of children through material markers of physiological and cognitive development. The purpose of this chapter is not to offer yet another discussion around nature versus nurture, nor is it to rehash critiques of Western perspectives of a universal, biological childhood; rather, it is to explore the varying ways we as archaeologists may move fluidly between multiple understandings of children and childhood to increase the likelihood of their archaeological visibility. The case study of seventeenth century New England will be used to enrich this discussion, as this period is well documented and researched as a period where children and childhood "did not exist" as cultural categories of identity.*

THE ENDURING QUESTION OF THE (IN)VISIBILITY OF CHILDREN

Developing a conference on the theme of the archaeological (in)visibility of children provides us with an opportunity to confront an enduring and evolving question in archaeological theory and method. The issue of the visibility, recoverability, and viability of children as subjects in archaeological research is essentially independent of questions relating to the value of children and childhood as topics of archaeological inquiry. These two concerns of visibility and value have been inextricably intertwined in the literature on the archaeology of childhood, as archaeologists interested in studying children have used these two strains of argument to convince the broader scholarly community of the merits and possibilities of studying children archaeologically (Baxter 2008). The need to constantly sell the idea of childhood studies as an integral part of archaeological inquiry rather than an interesting curiosity or specialization has been a frustration for those who have seen the potential and results that come from using children as a lens to view the past (Baxter 2006).

Here, I'd like to suggest that the (perceived) need to consistently defend the study of children has affected how we have theorized their visibility in the archaeological record, and to challenge us to move beyond this particular rhetoric to consider multiple ways of rendering children visible in the archaeological record, particularly in non-mortuary contexts. I'd like to make a few suggestions about how we can work to disentangle the ideas of value and visibility so that archaeology that is inclusive of children may be situated in ways that are potent and poignant for the discipline as a whole. These suggestions include: (1) making children and childhood a regular consideration when we conduct archaeological research, although accepting that such a line of questioning might not always bear fruit; (2) considering childhood as one of many possible categorizations of person, and looking for ways that categories of age intersect with other categories of identity; and (3) exploring alternative strategies for analyzing archaeological evidence to address identity; particularly, stepping outside traditional modes of analysis that focus on large categories of materials and instead engaging individual objects or constellations of objects that may transcend such categories, but are particularly salient for discussions of identity and personhood in the past.

The Conflation of Value and Visibility: A Brief Historical Perspective

It was not long ago that archaeologists held no concern for the value of children in the past, and archaeological research was undertaken with the unquestioned assumption that children were fundamentally unimportant to archaeological interpretation. Children only appeared in archaeological literature as convenient explanations for artifacts or depositional patterns that otherwise would have been left unexplained (Baxter 2005). Evoking children as actors in the past was a simple answer, not a topic that begged to be questioned.

Despite this disregard for the value of children, the idea of the archaeological visibility of children was not a topic of disinterest. Ethnoarchaeological and experimental studies from the 1970s and early 1980s were used as grounds to define children as archaeologically invisible (Baxter 2000, 2005). These studies observed children's behavior and noted that children moved objects from their places of discard or storage, thereby distorting the archaeological record created by adults. They also noted that children used artifacts for purposes for which they were not intended, or used natural objects as playthings that would not be identified archaeologically as artifacts. This type of attitude toward the invisibility of children can be summed up by a faculty member who explained that my dissertation project would not work because (and I paraphrase), "You know how kids are—you give them a toy and they take the toy out of the box. They just leave the toy sitting there and go play with the box. You'll spend your whole time looking at the toy, when you should have been looking at the box. Children are different and you'll never see that difference in the materials you have." These constructions of archaeologically invisible children were certainly a product of a value system that determined whose actions and ideas held value in archaeological interpretations, as well as the functionalist understandings of artifacts popularized by processualist ways of thinking about material culture. This widespread assumption regarding the invisibility of children also set the stage for the earliest literature on the archaeology of childhood.

When scholarly interest in children and childhood emerged in archaeology, authors had to combat not only assumptions that devalued children but also the perception that they were archaeologically invisible (Baker 1997; Lillehammer 1989; Sofaer Derevenski 1994a). Grete Lillehammer's seminal article that discusses "The Child's World" (1989) is a testament to the archaeological visibility of children, enumerating the many different areas where children were visible in the material record as a way of demonstrating their value as a topic of study. Many scholars went on to develop a theoretical space for children in archaeological inquiry by invoking the lessons learned from the introduction of gender and women's studies into archaeology (Sanchez-Romero 2009) and critiquing the cultural biases that led to a systematic devaluation and disregard of children by contemporary, Western archaeologists (Ardren 2006; Baker 1997; Baxter 2005; Joyce 2000; Kamp 2001a; Rothschild 2002; Sofaer Derevenski 1994b, 1997, 2000). Others provided evidence that children comprised significant demographic portions of all documented social groups, making any interpretation of the past without them incomplete (Ardren 2006; Baxter 2005; Chamberlain 2000). And still others presented ethnographic and historical evidence that children are significant social and economic actors in their own right, and that the organizations of families, communities, and societies often prioritize the care and training of children (Ardren 2006; Baxter 2005, 2006 a; Kamp 2001a; Sofaer Derevenski 1997, 2000a).

These areas of scholarship used thoughtful critiques to adeptly point out that systems of underlying values around children informed "evidence-based" claims of their invisibility. These writings also shared a common tone of advocacy for the archaeological study of children, and authors created compelling cases to defend and promote the archaeology of childhood. It has been through this very process of establishing a niche for and raising the profile of childhood in the broader discipline that the issues of value and visibility have become constant companions in our writing. Just as past assumptions that devalued children informed ideas of children's archaeological invisibility, this perhaps necessary rhetoric around linking and visibility has in turn shaped the way archaeologists have approached the study of children in the archaeological record.

THE VISIBILITY OF CHILDHOOD AT A
TIME OF DISCIPLINARY ADVOCACY

Archaeological scholarship of children has illustrated their visibility using archaeological data as well as historical, ethnographic, and theoretical approaches. It has been noted that children are identifiable in all of the "traditional" categories of evidence archaeologists encounter regularly in their work (Lillehammer 1989; Wilkie 2000), and this revelation has been backed up with numerous studies designed specifically to illustrate the visibility of children in a variety of archaeological contexts. To summarize these efforts, I took note of the primary analytical foci of the works I reviewed for the recent (Baxter 2008) *Annual Review of Anthropology* article on the archaeology of childhood. Clearly, this effort was somewhat subjective as many studies engage multiple lines of evidence, and I had to select the type of material evidence identified by the author(s) as the focal point of their work. This work is also biased in that it was confined to works specifically on the archaeology of children and childhood that have appeared in peer-reviewed journals and edited volumes. No dissertations or masters' theses were used, and these monograph-length sources represent an important new generation of scholarship on childhood. I also did not use studies that address children within broader analyses, although these studies are still relatively quite rare, but represent a significant evolution in scholarship.

A total of 51 articles and papers were identified in the literature as studies using archaeological evidence for the primary purpose of studying children and childhood. The categories of evidence may be broken down thusly: 18 mortuary studies, 11 ethnoarchaeological studies and/or ethnographic and historical studies with a particular application to an archaeological case, 5 studies of iconography, 14 studies of archaeological materials such as lithics and ceramics, and 3 studies of space and place. It is heartening to recognize the abundance of scholarship that has been produced on the archaeology of childhood beyond review articles, and theoretical studies and these evidentiary studies have created collectively a definitive empirical basis for the study of children in archaeology generally. These studies not only demonstrate the archaeological visibility of children, but also have resulted in significant interpretations that extend beyond children themselves and have been used to highlight the value of childhood as a way to shed light on central issues of archaeological inquiry.

I also attempted to categorize these 51 articles and papers into two primary analytical modes: those that emphasized cultural constructions of identity and those which emphasized the physiological, cognitive, and ontological development of young people. This exercise, I will freely admit, was even more subjective than the first. No evidence-based study focuses solely on cultural construction(s) of identity any more than such a study only engages physiological and cognitive development. Generally, however, most studies prioritize the theorizing and development of constructs of identity or the use of physiological and/or cognitive bases as a means of explaining the archaeological signatures of children.

Twenty-one of the 51 studies employed physiological and cognitive development as the primary way of addressing the visibility of children in the archaeological record. Such studies emphasized the opportunities and limitations afforded by the particular onto-logical development of children. Eight of these studies were ethnographic and ethnoar-chaeological studies of hunter-gather children, two of which tended to be geared toward broader understandings of physiology/cognition, work and identity (Bugarin 2006), and six from a particular genre of ethnoarchaeological work on hunter-gatherer children that has a distinct evolutionary focus (Lamb and Hewlett 2005; Bird and Bird 2000). An example of these latter studies is an ethnoarchaeological study of children of the Meriam, Eastern Torres, which has shown that children's foraging behaviors included a series of age-based practices based on physiological development (stride, hand and arm size, etc.) that were archaeologically visible in the composition of shell middens (Bird and Bird 2000). This study pointed to the archaeological visibility of children, but emphasized the physical characteristics of a developing body that resulted in particular behaviors and prey choices that differed from fully grown adults.

Another area of work on children that emphasized physiological and cognitive development is archaeological research on children's involvement in craft production activities, including stone tool production, ceramic manufacture, and weaving (Bagwell 2002; Crown 1999, 2001, 2002; Finlay 1997; Greenfield 2000; Grimm 2000; Kamp et al. 1999; Kamp 2001b; Shea 2006; Smith 2006). These studies focused on the particular contributions of children to communities of crafters (Lave and Wenger 1991; Shea 2006) through the archaeological signatures of individuals who were still learning to be com-petent crafters in their own right as they passed through various stages of physiological and cognitive development.

The other 30 works used in this review placed identity at the forefront of archaeo-logical analyses as well as interpretations. How children were defined, performed certain roles, and held particular places of importance or unimportance in a particular case provided the primary analytic for these works. All of the studies of iconography fell into this rubric, and such studies have been used successfully to identify emic construc-tions of childhood identity through images of individuals found in literary, artistic, and iconographic sources (e.g., Beaumont 2000; Cohen and Rutter 2007; Hays-Gilpin 2002; Joyce 2000; King 2006). Sixteen of the mortuary studies emphasized identity, most likely because this is an area where intersections of the biological and cultural can be explored in an immediate way through skeletal remains (Sofaer Derevenski 2000). These studies investigated the lives of children and the individual identities embodied by young people (Bradley 2002; Crawford 2000; Janik 2000; McCafferty and McCafferty 2006; Meskell 1994; Mizoguchi 2000; Perry 2006; Scott 1999; Sofaer Derevenski 2000; Storey and McAnany 2006), and several cases highlighted how different groups imbue the time of childhood with particular meanings that can make children significant actors in ritual contexts (Berrelleza and Balderas 2006; Bradley 2002; Sillar 1994). The remaining spatial, material, and ethnographic studies all analyze the spaces, places, and objects of children in relationship to the roles, values, and experiences of individuals at a particular stage in the life cycle. They do not engage how parameters of physical and mental development pro-duced these relationships between individuals, objects, and spaces. For example, Lopiparo (2006) presents an elegant analysis for children's involvement in the production of ritual objects and their subsequent observation of those objects in household rituals. Where previous studies on craft production sought direct evidence for children's participation in manufacture, Lopiparo develops an analysis that focuses on how children's identities were being formed through participation in crafting and ritual at a household level.

These different data sources and analytical modes not only demonstrate the variety of ways that children are visible archaeologically, but they speak to trends in how archaeologists studying children are presenting the value of childhood studies to the broader scholarly community. The 21 studies that emphasize physical/cognitive development include six works that are not theoretically engaged with culturally based theories of human culture, but rather find their theoretical basis in biological and evolutionary anthropology. Of the remaining 15 studies, only two contain data that were generated or were published after the year 2000, marking a shift in analytical modes between some of the earlier studies of children in archaeology and those of this most recent decade.

I'd like to suggest that this trend exists not because studies emphasizing biological differences between adults and children have run their course in terms of producing meaningful work, but rather our ways of theorizing the value of children in archaeology have turned our emphasis away from these types of studies and toward analyses that emphasize identity. I believe the reason for this may be twofold. First, archaeologists studying children have critiqued the exportation of Western views of childhood across the globe and into the past. These critiques have rightly identified a particular trend in Western thought that defines childhood in biological and developmental terms (Baxter 2008; Derevenski 1997; Kamp 2001a, Sofaer Derevenski 1997) that, in turn, lead to the assumption that cognitive and physiological development as observed in contemporary Western cultures can be applied to all children. The imperative to critique the tyranny of biology in how we define children theoretically limits archaeological studies that use these same parameters to identify children in the past. Second, archaeological concerns with identity extend well beyond the study of children and unite those scholars with interests in race, ethnicity, gender, and age in a common theoretical dialog and set of broad analytical goals. It is in this scholarly arena where the value of children is most readily accepted by scholars in other branches of archaeology and has been a fruitful place for archaeologists studying children to make inroads into the archaeological mainstream.

I would like to suggest that engaging broader questions of identity is a positive trend, but it is not without its potential pitfalls as we move farther into a more nuanced and contextualized era of studying children. If we limit our constructions of archaeological visibility to the more social and symbolic understandings of identity, we may be limiting our ability to access children in certain cases, or perhaps invoking children as an analytic where it is not appropriate to do so.

OUR WORST CASE SCENARIO?
THE ARCHAEOLOGY OF CHILDHOOD WITHOUT CHILDREN

Amid this abundance of work that has highlighted the visibility and value of children in archaeology was a brief quote in the introductory article to the 2002 volume, *Children in the Prehistoric Puebloan Southwest*. Nan Rothschild admonished archaeologists not to take their own understandings and expectations of childhood, including those that may be scholarly as well as personal, and impose them onto the past. She wrote (Rothschild 2002:3–4):

> In exporting ideas about modern lives to the examination of the past, it is crucial to recognize our own biases and not impose modern expectations on the lives of the past, whether derived from ethnography or history. Specifically, in the lives of past children we must make certain we are not creating a marked stage where none existed.

Rothschild's admonition was geared toward an "old guard" of archaeologists who projected contemporary childhood into the past as a rationale for deeming children unimportant generally. Her warning is also apropos to scholars who are seeking evidence for children and childhood in the past, particularly those who take an advocative stance in their scholarship and writing. Rothschild's assertion highlights that particular constructions of cultural identity lead to the elaboration or elimination of those categories: an idea that is particularly haunting for a group of scholars trying to debunk the idea of the archaeologically invisible child. At a time when archaeologists have acted as advocates for the visibility of children in the past and the viability of childhood as a topic of study, no one has been seeking evidence suggesting there were cultures where childhood and children were not developed categories of personhood.

This tension between the theoretical possibility of there being no cultural elaboration of childhood in a particular time and place with the desire for an inclusive archaeology requires a refinement in our practice of studying children archaeologically. First, it is essential to actively problematize the categories of children and childhood as analytical categories in archaeology, and to be explicit about how the terms are being used in a particular research case. This clarity acknowledges the many potential ways that children may be useful in archaeological studies, and may increase the breadth of these concepts as interpretive avenues and explanatory devices in archaeological research. Second is to realize that a reasonable ideal for the archaeology of childhood is that children and childhood become a regular part of the repertoire of analytical concepts turned toward archaeological evidence by all archaeologists. As with all such concepts, children and childhood may not always be a feasible or appropriate way to engage all archaeological data sets. Demonstrating the unique types of archaeological knowledge that may be generated by specifically engaging children and childhood is an imperative (Joyce 2006) and inherently embeds the value of children in rigorous archaeological research. It relieves us of the demand that we "find" children, and instead includes them in the host of actors and actions that shaped the archaeological record.

Beyond "Miniature Adulthood": Childhood in Seventeenth-Century New England

Children can be a powerful tool in archaeological analyses in the absence of direct archaeological evidence for their presence, and Rothschild's admonition should not be extended to suggest that children did not exist where child-specific evidence is not recovered. Scott Hutson (2006) was able to undertake a relational study between children and the built environment at the site of Chunchucmil as a way to make children visible where no "traditional" forms of evidence for children were present. As Ardren notes, however, Hutson's analysis was feasible because there is a wealth of historical, ethnographic, and archaeological evidence for children in the Mesoamerican past. This contextual evidence for marked stages of identity in youth made Hutson's assumption that children were present at Chunchucmil a sound one (Ardren 2006) even in the absence of direct archaeological evidence for a marked stage of personhood. There are, however, cases where the historical record reveals that children and childhood were not ideas that were subject to cultural elaboration either socially or materially, and leads to our worst case scenario: the archaeology of childhood when there are no children. I'd like to use this case study as a means of bridging the assertion that children do not have to be found to be engaged archaeologically, and some specific ideas from current work in Historical Archaeology that may increase our means for doing so.

Historians have long debated the nature of childhood in seventeenth-century New England, and this debate has focused around what Kamp (2006) has termed as the "dominant discourse" about children. The "dominant discourse" relates to how children are defined by others rather than their own lived experiences, but it is particularly relevant here as evidence from the dominant discourse is generally what is used in archaeological cases to determine the presence and elaboration of stages of childhood (e.g., Joyce 2000).

Original interest in seventeenth-century childhood dates back as far as the nineteenth century when scholars were looking at the origins of the American nation and sought to understand more about the Pilgrims or Puritans who were the first English colonists and widely recognized as the pioneers of the American nation. This earliest scholarship was based largely on the evaluation of portraiture of families of a higher social standing who posed for itinerant artists in the latter half of the seventeenth century. These portraits show children and adults in identical garb, with identical accessories, and in identical postures leading scholars to state that there was no childhood at this time, only "miniature adulthood," and that Puritans did not see life as a series of stages but rather a continuum (Beales 1976). (Nota Bene: While no such portraits exist for publication in the public domain, a simple Google search for the Freake family should produce the iconic example of such portraiture.) Evidence for children at this time is quite sparse and scholarship is consequently quite limited (Benes 1985, 2002). Some scholars have deemed children to be, for all intents and purposes, historically invisible at this time (Benes and Benes 2002).

Ross Beales's (1975) important reevaluation of historical sources regarding seventeenth-century childhood stands as a definitive piece of scholarship. Beales noted that laws of the time made distinctions between adults and children into their teens, that religious conversions generally did not take place until an individual was at least 10 years of age and more typically around age 14, and that systems of apprenticeship suggested that economic independence was not obtained until a male was aged 17 or 18 (Beales 1975). These sources suggested to Beales that a stage of childhood and/or adolescence must have been recognized in the seventeenth century, but it is clear that sources from the time, both historical and material, do not elaborate on the nature of childhood or adolescence and instead seem to define it only by what it was not.

Karin Calvert (1992) rewrites the history of seventeenth-century children from the perspective of material culture, characterizing children not as miniature adults but as inchoate ones. Her review of portraiture, the limited repertoire of childhood artifacts, and historical sources on child care and rearing (mostly from the early eighteenth century) revealed that children were not miniature adults, but were in fact considered to be incomplete human beings. She noted that children lacked two essential characteristics that for Puritans separated humans from the rest of the world: the ability to walk upright and the ability to speak coherently. Children who crawled on all fours and babbled in incomprehensible tones were to be reared out of these vulnerable states and into the ranks of humanity as quickly as possible. The practice of swaddling, or wrapping babies' limbs to make them stiff and rigid, was a regular practice, and the only pieces of furniture designed for young children were cradles and walking stools, which held children in upright positions and encouraged them to stand and walk as soon as they were able. Children were not "miniature adults" but also were not human (and therefore not spiritually redeemable) until they had been raised into an upright form. This emphasis on hastening children's maturation is reflected in portraiture where children are dressed like adults, thereby making clear gender distinctions but not distinctions of age, and are presented with similar accoutrements to those of their parents (later portraits show children with toys, books, and animals in child-specific artistic tropes). Toys and playthings were prohibited for all members of Puritan society, but contemporaneous colonies in the mid-Atlantic did allow toys and games (penny whistles and cup and ball for example), but they were indulged in equally by adults and children. In either case, toys and playthings were not a distinguishing factor of age.

The only child-specific artifact identified by Calvert (1992) for seventeenth-century children is the coral and bells: an instrument that would have resembled a rattle. Coral was thought to protect children from disease and a piece would be mounted onto a metal instrument that would have been adorned with whistles and bells to hold a child's interest so that they would interact with the protective element. Because these artifacts were often bronze or silver, only children of a certain standing would have been afforded the protection of this early medical device.

If children are "historically invisible" in the seventeenth century (Benes and Benes 2002) they are nearly archaeologically invisible as well. Archaeological work at New England's rare seventeenth-century sites has yielded only a single item thought to belong to a child: a silver whistle from a set of coral and bells. The whistle bears the initials, "EW" and most likely belonged to Elizabeth Winslow, who was born in 1630 to a prominent and prosperous family of the early colonies (Beaudry, Goldstein, and Chartier 2003). Children's furniture from the seventeenth century is quite rare and would not survive archaeologically, and neither would the swaddling cloth that bound children into upright poses. Perhaps straight pins used to secure the cloths may survive, but the opportunity to view children directly through material culture is indeed quite limited.

Seventeenth-century childhood was arguably a period where a marked stage of existence was present, but was not subjected to cultural elaboration. Items for children were deliberately few, and children were not a topic of adult (or child) writing outside of legal and formal records that intimate at cultural differences of those before and after their early teenage years. These records are also heavily biased toward a marked stage that may have affected young males and not necessarily females, suggesting (as with portraits) that gender rather than age was a significant marked category of identity. It would be difficult to proceed here with a relational analysis such as that undertaken by Hutson (2006) as there is no historical basis to assume that childhood existed as an elaborated stage of identity. How might we proceed to study seventeenth-century childhood archaeologically when historical sources suggest that childhood "did not exist" (sensu Rothschild 2002)?

BODIES AND IDENTITIES: RECONFIGURING IDEAS OF (IN)VISIBILITY IN THE ARCHAEOLOGICAL STUDY OF CHILDREN

Historical Archaeology provides us not only with a case study where childhood was culturally unelaborated and nearly invisible to present scholarship, but also some fruitful lines of analysis to broaden how we might render children visible even in a scenario such as this. Here, particularly, I'd like to offer that a reconsideration of materiality and embodiment be integrated into our theoretical approaches to childhood in ways that bridge the valuable theoretical links to archaeologies of identity with a continued appreciation for the unique physiological and cognitive realities of immature humans. Ideas of materiality and the body were well introduced some ten years ago into the literature of the archaeology of childhood (Sofaer Derevenski 2000) and to date have informed mortuary studies of Bradley (2002), Crawford (2000), Janik (2000), McCafferty and McCafferty (2006), Meskell (1994), Mizoguchi (2000), Perry (2006), Scott (1999), Sofaer Derevenski (2000), and Storey and McAnany (2006), but have had less influence on studies of children in active contexts of everyday life.

IDENTITY AND PERSONAL OBJECTS

Early scholars of childhood made appeals based on the parallels between gender and childhood in archaeology, and similarly studies of identity in Historical Archaeology can provide useful models to move forward in interpretations of childhood, age, and identity. These models can be usefully employed, as appropriate, in many time periods and geographic regions. Interest in identity in Historical Archaeology stemmed from a desire to illuminate the lives of people traditionally omitted from historical narratives, such as African Americans and women, much as the archaeology of childhood has been an endeavor to redress the absence of children in archaeological ones. Early studies of identity in Historical Archaeology tended to focus on a single aspect of identity (such as race, ethnicity, or gender). This emphasis persisted despite early calls to take an expansive, multistranded approach to identity (Meskell 1994; Scott 1994). Multistranded approaches demand that archaeologists look at the interplay between the many types of identities that can be situationally embodied by an individual, and some work on childhood has begun to link age and gender (Baxter 2005; Joyce 2000; Sanchez-Romero 2009) in more complex ways than studies emphasizing childhood as a singular analytical category of identity. Seeking ways that age-based identity intersects with other types of identity in meaningful ways is a significant strategy for enhancing the visibility of children in the archaeological record.

Recently, White and Beaudry (2009:210) have elegantly summarized the nature of identity thusly:

> The concept of identity is complicated, paradoxical, and culturally situated in time, place, and society. Identity is at once both imposed by others and self imposed, and is continuously asserted and reasserted in ways that are fluid and fixed. Identity can lie at the individual level and at the broadest of imaginable scales as it defines a person both as part of a group and as an individual.

This construction of identity is a prelude to looking at artifacts of personal identity in the archaeological record. Rather than looking at large functional categories of material culture that group objects together in large numbers, this approach allows archaeologists to select an object or a constellation of objects that were engaged on a personal level by individuals as they negotiated identity in daily life through objects, practice, and embodiment (White and Beaudry 2009). The conceptualization of personal artifacts benefits from the theoretically robust area of materiality that emphasizes the situated experiences of material life and the reciprocal shaping of objects and human experiences (Meskell 2004, 2005; Miller 2005). Personal artifacts or artifacts of individual identity have significance because of their rarity: they are artifacts that would have been recognized as unique or special in the material and social worlds of the past as well as in archaeological assemblages in the present. Personal artifacts have further significance because of their direct associations with individual bodies, as adornment, as objects of personal practice, or through other individual actions.

The idea of artifacts of the individual can be a powerful force in the archaeological study of children and childhood. Objects that are often identified as child-specific (whether toys, artifacts of child rearing, or other such objects) are generally rare, not easily grouped into larger categories, and are very small percentages of archaeological assemblages. These reasons have been used to discount the study of children using objects as approaches, which rely on the analysis of large numbers of artifacts grouped into categories or typologies that do not translate to such categories of evidence (Beaudry 2009; Beaudry and White 2009). There is no reason, however, that archaeological interpretations need to be bound to these traditional approaches.

The single whistle from a coral and bells from the entire known assemblage of seventeenth-century archaeological materials from multiple domestic sites offers a way to consider such analytical possibilities (Beaudry et al. 2003). In her analysis of seventeenth-century bodkins from early English and Dutch sites in America, Beaudry (2009) makes a compelling case for the writing of artifact biographies and biography through artifact. This approach celebrates the rarity and individuality of personal artifacts, and through a contextual study using archaeological materials and historical sources presents bodkins as a defining object of class and gender for seventeenth-century women. Similar analyses of individual, personal objects may serve as loci to understand how childhood was one of many identities worn by children in a particular time and place (e.g, Spector 1991; Wilkie 2000). A young child, E. W., was not only an incomplete adult who needed to be reared into human form in good health and in haste, but also a member of a wealthy family who could afford a silver whistle, and a girl who would grow into a woman in a particular station of domestic comfort. These identities were not only referential to other colonial families, but also to the Native Americans who were a significant part of the seventeenth-century cultural landscape. These examples and contemporary theory highlight the possibility of using artifacts from history and prehistory to tell the stories of individual lives and the role of objects and bodies in presenting and enacting multistranded identities.

IDENTITY AND BIOGRAPHICAL OBJECTS

Child-specific artifacts are rare, but it may also be argued that all objects in a household are a part of the material world of children who engage these artifacts and spaces at different ages, sizes, and levels of understanding and knowledge (Crawford 2009; Wood 2009). The notion that artifacts as well as individuals have their own ontogeny compels us to view *all artifacts as artifacts of childhood*. Much as Hutson (2006) offered a relational view that suggested children were engaging with the entire material world around them, it is important to imagine how artifacts and spaces changed along with individuals as they transformed physiologically, cognitively, and socially. The idea of object biographies, or approaches that emphasize accumulated meanings imbued in and imparted to objects (Gosden and Marshall 1999; Loren and Beaudry 2006) may help bridge transformations in identity that occur over an individual lifetime. Some archaeologists have argued that iconographic images of children are imbued with particular meanings for the adults who created and viewed such images, including invoking a sense of memory (Lillehammer 2000) and nostalgia (Joyce 2006) for their own childhoods. The same may be said of everyday objects that form the material surroundings of individuals as they learned to experience the world through physical, social, and symbolic lenses that changed over time.

The idea of objects being experienced by actors in the past links materiality to ideas of embodiment (Fischer and Loren 2003). Changing constructions of the body as a node of identity can be a powerful lens to understand childhood. Physiological changes that relate to important changes in identity may be elaborated in ways that alter understandings of self (Perry 2006) much as changing social and cultural milieu can transform understandings and practices of how identity is embodied. Loren (2007) has shown that the cultural contact of the seventeenth century produced significant if not radical changes in practices of personal adornment among Native Americans of the Eastern woodlands. Confronted by new individuals and new expressions of identity, new objects and configurations of objects were selected for personal adornment and were used as a means of retaining a sense of identity in a shifting cultural landscape. This kind of transformation in strategies of embodiment corresponded to shifts in understandings of gender, age, and otherness in many forms. It is likely that reciprocal understandings of identity reinforced decisions about how seventeenth-century colonists embodied their self-perceived roles as moral and social superiors to local natives—decisions that undoubtedly affected how they viewed and raised their children.

Certainly, archaeologists studying childhood already embrace many of these ideas about identity, materiality, and embodiment in current work on children. These ideas are most clearly reflected in the most abundant form of archaeological research on children: studies of burials and mortuary treatment. These contexts enable archaeologists to directly engage ideas of materiality and embodiment as skeletal remains and material culture are displayed in ritual presentation and in configurations that facilitate multiscalar analyses. These studies have resulted in more complex and nuanced understandings of individual identities that consider age-based identity as only one constituent element of how individuals saw themselves and were seen by others.

Less clear is the acknowledgment of the physicality of childhood as individuals pursued their daily lives and created the archaeological record of non-mortuary contexts. These analyses tend to focus more on the identity of children as a singular category, and offer a way to intersect studies of childhood with broader disciplinary concerns while distancing contemporary scholarship on children with the Western emphases on biology and development. Ideas of materiality and embodiment offer archaeologists opportunities to address both the unique physical and cognitive aspects of young humans and the ways that those characteristics came to have meaning in particular contexts. Personal artifacts that were designed for and used by children offer a way to explore not only meanings of childhood but also the ways that individual children were embedded in other systems of social and symbolic meaning that shaped identities. Simultaneously, recognizing that all artifacts were once the domain of children unlocks the possibility of imagining how spaces and objects transformed in meaning over the course of individual lives and life cycles.

REFERENCES CITED

Ardren, T. 2006 Setting the Table: Why Children and Childhood Are Important in an Understanding of Ancient Mesoamerica. In *The Social Experience of Childhood in Ancient Mesoamerica*, edited by T. Ardren and S. Hutson, pp. 3–24. University of Colorado Press, Boulder.

Bagwell, E. 2002 Ceramic Form and Skill: Attempting to Identify Child Producers at Pecos Pueblo, New Mexico. In *Children in the Prehistoric Puebloan Southwest*, edited by K. Kamp, pp. 90–107. University of Utah Press, Salt Lake City.

Baker, M. 1997 Invisibility as a Symptom of Gender Categories in Archaeology. In *Invisible People and Processes: Writing Gender and Childhood into European Archaeology*, edited by J. Moore and E. Scott, pp. 183–191. Leicester University Press, London.

Baxter, J. E. 2000 An Archaeology of Childhood: Children, Gender, and Material Culture in Nineteenth Century America. Unpublished PhD dissertation, Department of Anthropology, University of Michigan, Ann Arbor.

Baxter, J. E. 2005 *The Archaeology of Childhood: Children, Gender, and Material Culture*. Alta Mira Press, Walnut Creek, California.

Baxter, J. E. 2006 Introduction: The Archaeology of Childhood in Context. In *Children in Action: Perspectives on the Archaeology of Childhood*, edited by J. E. Baxter, pp. 1–12. Archeological Papers of the American Anthropological Association, Number 15. University of California Press, Berkeley.

Baxter, J. E. 2008 The Archaeology of Childhood. *Annual Review of Anthropology* 37:159–175.

Beales, R. 1975 In Search of the Historical Child: Miniature Adulthood and Youth in Colonial New England. *American Quarterly* 27(4):379–398.

Beaudry, M. 2009 Bodkin Biographies. In *The Materiality of Individuality: Archaeological Studies of Individual Lives*, edited by C. L. White, pp. 95–108. Springer, New York.

Beaudry, M., K. J. Goldstein, and C. Chartier 2003 Archaeology of the Plymouth Colony in Massachusetts. In *The English in America 1497–1696*, edited by J. A. Tuck and B. Gaulton, pp. 155–185. Avalon Chronicles Volume 8. Memorial University, St. Johns, Newfoundland.

Beaumont, L. 2000 The Social Status and Artistic Presentation of "Adolescence" in Fifth Century Athens. In *Children and Material Culture*, edited by J. Sofaer Derevenski, pp. 39–50. Routledge, New York.

Benes, P. (editor) 1985 *Families and Children*. The Dublin Seminar for New England Folklife Annual Proceedings Volume 10. Boston University, Boston.

Benes, P. (editor) 2002 *The Worlds of Children, 1620–1920*. The Dublin Seminar for New England Folklife Annual Proceedings Volume 27. Boston University, Boston.

Benes, P., and J. M. Benes 2002 Introduction. In *The Worlds of Children, 1620–1920*, edited by P. Benes, pp. 5–8. The Dublin Seminar for New England Folklife Annual Proceedings Volume 27. Boston University, Boston.

Berrelleza, A. J. R, and X. Chavez Balderas 2006 The Role of Children in the Ritual Practices of the Great Temple of Tenochtitland and the Great Temple of Tlateloco. In *The Social Experience of Childhood in Ancient Mesoamerica*, edited by T. Ardren and S. Hutson, pp. 233–248. University Press of Colorado, Boulder.

Bird, D., and R. B. Bird 2000 The Ethnoarchaeology of Juvenile Foragers: Shellfishing Strategies among Meriam Children. *Journal of Anthropological Archaeology* 19:461–476.

Bradley, C. 2002 Thoughts Count: Ideology and the Children of Sand Canyon Pueblo. In *Children in the Prehistoric Puebloan Southwest*, edited by K. Kamp, pp. 169–195. University of Utah Press, Salt Lake City.

Bugarin, F. 2006 Constructing an Archaeology of Children: Studying Children and Child Material Culture from the African Past, In *Children in Action: Perspectives on the Archaeology of Childhood*, edited by J. E. Baxter, pp. 13–26. Archaeological Papers of the American Anthropological Association Volume 15. University of California Press, Berkeley.

Calvert, K. 1992 *Children in the House: The Material Culture of Early Childhood, 1600–1900*. Northeastern University Press, Boston.

Chamberlain, A. T. 2000 Minor Concerns: A Demographic Perspective on Children in Past Societies. In *Children and Material Culture*, edited by J. Sofaer Derevenski, pp. 206–212. Routledge, New York.

Cohen, A., and J. Rutter (editors) 2007 *Constructions of Childhood in Ancient Greece and Italy*. American School of Classical Studies at Athens, Athens.

Crawford, S. 2000 Children, Grave Goods, and Social Status in Early Anglo-Saxon England. In *Children and Material Culture*, edited by J. Sofaer Derevenski, pp. 169–179. Routledge, New York.

Crawford, S. 2009 The Archaeology of Playthings: Theorising a Toy Stage in the "Biography" of Objects. *Childhood in the Past* 1(2):55–70.

Crown, P. 1999 Socialization in American Southwest Pottery Decoration. In *Pottery and People: A Dynamic Interaction*, edited by J. Skibo and G. Feinman, pp. 25–43. University of Utah Press, Salt Lake City.

Crown, P. 2001 Learning to Make Pottery in the Prehispanic American Southwest. *Journal of Anthropological Research* 57:451–469.

Crown, P. 2002 Learning and Teaching in the Prehispanic American Southwest. In *Children in the Prehistoric Puebloan Southwest*, edited by, K. Kamp, pp. 108–124. University of Utah Press, Salt Lake City.

Finlay, N. 1997 Kid Knapping: The Missing Children in Lithic Analysis. In *Invisible People and Processes: Writing Gender and Childhood into European Archaeology*, edited by J. Moore and E. Scott, pp. 203–212. Leicester University Press, London.

Fisher, G., and D. D. Loren 2003 Embodying Identity in Archaeology. *Cambridge Archaeological Journal* 13(2):225–230.

Gosden, C., and Y. Marshall 1999 The Cultural Biography of Objects. *World Archaeology* 31(2):169–178.

Greenfield, P. 2000 Children, Material Culture, and Weaving: Historical Change and Developmental Change. In *Children and Material Culture*, edited by J. Sofaer Derevenski, pp. 72–86. Routledge, New York.

Grimm, L. 2000 Apprentice Flintknapping: Relating Material Culture and Social Practice in the Upper Paleolithic. In *Children and Material Culture*, edited by J. Sofaer Derevenski, pp. 53–71. Routledge, New York.

Hays-Gilpin, K. 2002 Wearing a Butterfly, Coming of Age: A 1,500 Year Old Pueblo Tradition. In *Children in the Prehistoric Puebloan Southwest*, edited by K. Kamp, pp. 196–210. University of Utah Press, Salt Lake City.

Hutson, S. 2006 Children Not at Chunchcmil: A Relational Approach to Young Subjects. In *The Social Experience of Childhood in Ancient Mesoamerica*, edited by. T. Ardren and S. Hutson, pp. 103–132. University Press of Colorado, Boulder.

Janik, L. 2000 The Construction of the Individual among North European Fisher-Gatherer-Hunters in the Early and Mid-Holocene. In *Children and Material Culture*, edited by J. Sofaer Derevenski, pp. 117–130. Routledge, New York.

Joyce, R. 2000 Girling the Girl and Boying the Boy: The Production of Adulthood in Ancient Mesoamerica. *World Archaeology* 31(30):473–483.

Joyce, R. 2006 Where We All Began: Archaeologies of Childhood in the Mesoamerican Past. In *The Social Experience of Childhood in Ancient Mesoamerica*, edited by T. Ardren and S. Hutson, pp. 283–302. University Press of Colorado, Boulder.

Kamp, K. 2001a Where Have All the Children Gone?: The Archaeology of Childhood. *Journal of Archaeological Method and Theory* 8(1):1–34.

Kamp, K. 2001b Prehistoric Children Working and Playing: A Southwestern Case Study in Learning Ceramics. *Journal of Anthropological Research* 57:427–450.

Kamp, K. 2002 Working for a Living: Children in the Prehistoric Southwestern Pueblos. In *Children in the Prehistoric Puebloan Southwest*, edited by K. Kamp, pp. 71–89. University of Utah Press, Salt Lake City.

Kamp, K., N. Timmerman, G. Lind, J. Graybill, and I. Natowsky 1999 Discovering Childhood: Using Fingerprints to Find Children in the Archaeological Record. *American Antiquity* 64(2):309–315.

Keith, K. 2006 Childcare, Learning, and the Distribution of Knowledge in Foraging Societies. In *Children in Action: Perspectives on the Archaeology of Childhood*, edited by J. E. Baxter, pp. 27–40. Archaeological Papers of the American Anthropological Association Volume 15. University of California Press, Berkeley.

King, S. 2006 The Marking of Age in Ancient Coastal Oaxaca. In *The Social Experience of Childhood in Ancient Mesoamerica*, edited by T. Ardren and S. Hutson, pp. 169–202. University Press of Colorado, Boulder.

Lamb, M. E., and B. Hewlett (editors) 2005 *Hunter-Gatherer Childhoods: Evolutionary, Developmental, and Cultural Perspectives.* Aldine Transaction Publishers, Somerset, New Jersey.

Lave, J., and E. Wenger 1991 *Situated Learning: Legitimate Peripheral Participation.* Cambridge University Press, Cambridge.

Lillehammer, G. 1989 A Child Is Born: The Child's World in an Archaeological Perspective. *Norwegian Archaeological Review* 22(2):89–105.

Lillehammer, G. 2000 The World of Children. In. *Children and Material Culture*, edited by J. Sofaer Derevenski, pp. 17–26. Routledge, New York.

Lopiparo, J. 2006 Crafting Children: Materiality, Social Memory, and the Reproduction of Terminal Classic House Societies in the Ulua Valley, Honduras. In *The Social Experience of Childhood in Ancient Mesoamerica*, edited by T. Ardren and S. Hutson, pp. 133–168. University of Colorado Press, Boulder.

Loren, D. D. 2007 In Contact: Bodies and Spaces in the 16th and 17th Century Eastern Woodlands. Alta Mira Press, Walnut Creek, California.

Loren, D. D., and M. Beaudry 2006 Becoming American: In Small Things Remembered. In *Historical Archaeology*, edited by M. Hall and S. Silliman, pp. 251–271. Blackwell, Oxford.

McCafferty, G., and S. McCafferty 2006 Boys and Girls Interrupted: Mortuary Evidence of Children from Postclassic Cholula, Puebla. In *The Social Experience of Childhood in Ancient Mesoamerica*, edited by T. Ardren and S. Hutson, pp. 25–52. University Press of Colorado, Boulder.

Meskell, L. 1994 Dying Young: The Experience of Death at Deir El Medina. *Archaeological Review from Cambridge* 13(2):35–46.

Meskell, L. 2004 *Object Worlds in Ancient Egypt: Material Biographies Past and Present.* Berg, Oxford.

Meskell, L. (editor) 2005 *Archaeologies of Materiality.* Blackwell, Oxford.

Miller, D. 2005 *Materiality.* Duke University Press, Durham.

Mizoguchi, K. 2000 The Child as a Node of Past, Present, and Future. In *Children and Material Culture*, edited by J. Sofaer Derevenski, pp. 141–150. Routledge, New York.

Park, R. 1998 Size Counts: The Miniature Archaeology of Childhood in Inuit Societies. *Antiquity* 72:269–281.

Perry, M. 2006 Redefining Childhood through Bioarchaeology: Towards an Archaeological and Biological Understanding of Children in Antiquity. In *Children in Action: Perspectives on the Archaeology of Childhood* edited by J. E. Baxter, pp. 89–114. Archaeological Papers of the American Anthropological Association Volume 15. University of California Press, Berkeley.

Rothschild, N. 2002 Introduction. In *Children in the Prehistoric Puebloan Southwest*, edited by K. Kamp, pp. 1–13. University of Utah Press, Salt Lake City.

Sanchez Romero, M. 2009 Childhood and the Construction of Gender Identities through Material Culture. *Childhood in the Past* 1(1):17–37.

Scott, Eleanor 1999 *The Archaeology of Infancy and Infant Death.* British Archaeological Reports Series S819. Archaeopress, Oxford.

Scott, Elizabeth 1994 *Those of Little Note: Gender, Race, and Class in Historical Archaeology.* University of Arizona Press, Tucson.

Shca, J. 2006 Child's Play: Reflections on the Invisibility of Children in the Paleolithic Record. *Evolutionary Anthropology* 15(6):212–216.

Sillar, B. 1994 Playing with God: Cultural Perceptions of Children, Play, and Miniatures in the Andes. *Archaeological Review from Cambridge: Perspectives on Children and Childhood* 13(2):47–63.

Smith, P. E. 2006 Children and Ceramic Innovation: A Study in the Archaeology of Children. In *Children in Action: Perspectives on the Archaeology of Childhood*, edited by J. E. Baxter, pp. 65–76. Archaeological Papers of the American Anthropological Association Volume 15, University of California Press, Berkeley.

Sofaer Derevenski, J. (editor) 1994a *Archaeological Review from Cambridge: Perspectives on Children and Childhood* 13(2).

Sofaer Derevenski, J. 1994b Where Are the Children?: Accessing Children in the Past. *Archaeological Review from Cambridge* 13(2):7–20.

Sofaer Derevenski, J. 1997 Engendering Children: Engendering Archaeology. In *Invisible People and Processes: Writing Gender and Childhood into European Archaeology*, edited by J. Moore and E. Scott, pp. 192–202. Leicester University Press, London.

Sofaer Derevenski, J. 2000 Material Culture Shock: Confronting Expectations in the Material Culture of Children. In *Children and Material Culture*, edited by, J. Sofaer Derevenski, pp. 3–16. Routledge, New York.

Spector, J. 1991 *What This Awl Means: Feminist Archaeology at a Wahpeton Dakota Village*. Minnesota Historical Society Press, Minneapolis.

Storey, R., and P. McAnany 2006 Children of K'axob: Premature Death in a Formative Maya Village. In *The Social Experience of Childhood in Ancient Mesoamerica*, edited by T. Ardren and S. Hutson, pp. 53–72. University Press of Colorado, Boulder.

White, C., and M. Beaudry 2009 Artifacts and Personal Identity. In *International Handbook of Historical Archaeology*, edited by T. Majewski and D. Gaimster, pp. 209–225. Springer, New York.

Wilkie, L. 2000 Not Merely Child's Play: Creating a Historical Archaeology of Children and Childhood. In *Children and Material Culture*, edited by J. Sofaer Derevenski, pp. 100–114. Routledge, New York.

Wood, E. 2009 Saving Childhood in Everyday Objects. *Childhood in the Past* 1(2):151–162.

CHAPTER TWO

Making Children Legitimate

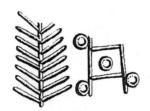

Negotiating the Place of Children and Childhoods in Archaeological Theory

Kathryn Kamp

Abstract   *Until the 1970s, with the rise of interest in individual artisans and the advent of gender archaeology, archaeologists tended not to attempt to identify the personal characteristics of the actors responsible for the archaeological remains they studied. However, they often implicitly assumed that adult males were the primary actors. Today, gender is seen as a legitimate, even necessary, focus of discussion, but adult is still the default and children are neglected. Nevertheless, given the high proportion of subadults in many of the societies studied by archaeologists and the proficiency of children at many tasks, it is really no more speculative to posit that children were responsible for many artifacts or artifact distributions than to say that adults were. For the archaeology of children to fully come of age as necessary and legitimate, those of us interested in the subject must demonstrate both the centrality of children to the functioning of society and a range of credible methods for studying children. "Finding" children requires the innovative use of method and theory as well as a reflective consideration of the aspects of children and childhoods being investigated. Archaeologists must consciously differentiate between several possible perspectives, including the possibly idealized views of the society being studied, a description of the "average" child's activities, and variability in the actual life experiences of individual children. A number of possible methodologies are evaluated and discussed in light of these issues.*

In a much-cited 1989 article, Lillehammer called for children to be seen and heard by archaeologists. Fifteen years later, Margarita Romero Sánchez (2004:278), speaking of the state of Spanish archaeology, still lamented, "Most archaeologists have felt that because they cannot identify age or gender in relation to activities in prehistoric societies, it is better to use the generic term 'man.' The use of this generic term 'man' has facilitated the idea that the 'others' are not important, or even present." She has joined a growing cadre of archaeologists (see Ardren 2006; Ardren and Hutson 2006; Baxter 2005c, 2006; Kamp 2001a, 2002; Neils and Oakley 2003; Sofaer Derevenski 2000a; and others) who are making personal characteristics such as age and gender one focus of inquiry, and, happily, this volume on prehistoric childhoods joins that effort.

In order to legitimate the inclusion of age categories so firmly that their consideration will become as normal a part of archaeological research as, for example, subsistence strategies, we need first to show that any description of a society that excludes children will not just be inadequate, but will be fundamentally flawed. Thus, as Baxter (2005a:1–2) states, "[T]he archaeology of childhood should not be considered an endeavor that is isolated or compartmentalized as a separate sphere of analysis but rather is a way to enrich and enhance our understanding of communities and cultures as a whole." Secondly, we need to demonstrate that it is possible, if not literally to "find" children, then at least to study them without any diminution of methodological rigor. Identities such as "baby," "toddler," "child," "adult," "girl," "boy," "woman," "man"—all social constructs— are always multifaceted, socially manipulated, and potentially interpreted from several perspectives. Thus, this methodological awareness must always explicitly consider which aspects of children and childhoods are being treated and which are, in fact, amenable to discussion with the particular evidence at hand.

THE INADEQUATE KNOWNS

Without even naming a time period or culture there are some things we can already say about the children and the childhoods of any time and place; nevertheless, all of these biological and cultural universals are very general. The cultural importance of the universals combined with their cross-cultural variability should convince us that the consideration of age variation is a critical topic for archaeological research and that we cannot rely on the simple use of cross-cultural regularities for our analysis, but must treat each culture as a unique case.

For example, we know that all human newborns require care and that it takes a period of some years for a child to grow to his or her full mental, social, and physical stature. We do not know, however, who the caregiver will be nor what types of activities will occupy the child as it grows. We do not even know at what point in the trajectory the individual will be viewed by its own culture as a mature adult. Furthermore, even this term is problematic, as adults themselves often progress through a series of stages.

We know that children comprise a substantial proportion of all societies, although computing the proportion of children in a particular past population is not a trivial task. Because young bones are more fragile, they may be systematically underrepresented in burial populations simply due to preservation. In addition, in some cultures children's remains are treated differently from adult remains, at least until certain ages or ceremonial stages are passed. Differential treatment may affect preservation or the location of final deposition (Kamp 1998). Since archaeologists do not usually sample all areas of a site equally, the proportions of a burial population recovered will depend heavily on where skeletal remains are deposited. In most cases, bodies buried near structures are most likely to be recovered and those deposited outside site boundaries, especially in scattered locations, are least likely. Nevertheless, demographic profiles from the present show that the proportion of children varies from 19 to 36 percent and is highest in populations with low life expectancies (Chamberlain 2000). Thus, for most of the past societies studied by archaeologists, children would have comprised a sizable part of the population.

We also know that during the period of maturation every child learns to speak a language and to function in a cultural setting. We know that from the instant of its birth, the child is enmeshed in a web of social interactions that includes individuals of all ages. We know that children can and do learn in a variety of ways, watching, trying, and simply experiencing the world around them with all of their available senses. We know that adults may teach children, but that perhaps even more often children learn by observation rather than structured lessons, and as much from other children as from adults. We know that child-rearing practices influence the distribution of knowledge across the social spectrum. For example, if children of both genders spend time with women, but girls are only rarely in the presence of adult males, men will understand the female world more than women will understand the male world (Keith 2005). Furthermore, we know that children, like adults, usually participate in all facets of the society. They are producers as well as consumers and participate in religious as well as secular spheres.

We know that adults have ideas about the meaning and place of children, that these conceptions vary with the age of the child, and that they structure many adult interactions with children. But we also know that the children themselves have varying degrees of latitude in structuring their own time and activities. The cultures of adults and children may overlap, but they are not identical. Similarly, children and the adults in their lives may sometimes believe their interests are in conflict, and children may use a variety of strategies to avoid adult control and to further their own goals. To use the current parlance: children have agency.

A cursory examination of most of the things we know about children and childhood reveals, not unexpectedly, that most of what we know is vague, at best. This follows directly from the most important thing we can affirm with confidence—that, like race and gender, children and childhood are culturally constructed. This means that, although we may realize that all societies perpetuate themselves by producing children, unless we examine the evidence from the particular case at hand, we don't know much about the costs and benefits of reproducing, the fertility rate, the economic roles of children, the ways adults do or do not try to control children's activities, the symbolic meanings of childhood, the subcultures that children devise for themselves and pass on to the next generation of youth, or any of the vast number of details that vary drastically from culture to culture. We do not even know the most basic and fundamental aspect of culture for a particular society—how the categories of childhood are defined. What *is* a child in our chosen time and place?

There is no natural childhood. From the moment an infant is born, and even before, there is little that we can confidently assume about the way the new person will be treated. The meaning of birth, the incidence of infanticide, birth ceremonies, the relative value and meaning of male versus female children, nursing practices, the identity of caregivers—none of these can just be assumed. Each will vary from culture to culture. This means that if, as interpreters of the past, we wish to include children and the nature of childhood in our discussions, it is vital that we refrain from making rash conclusions based on our own culturally conditioned stereotypes.

THE NEED FOR ARCHAEOLOGICAL STUDY OF CHILDREN AND CHILDHOODS

Perhaps the study of children and childhoods is not critical to an informed depiction of the past. Perhaps it is adults who are primarily responsible for the shape of social relations, the nature of cultural beliefs, and ultimately the majority of the material remains that archaeologists retrieve. If so, perhaps it is justifiable to simply ignore children's existence, pretending that the world is one of adults and adult concerns, and that variation due to age is simply too difficult to access. This argument sounds suspiciously parallel to those made before the advent of gender studies in archaeology; when men were considered the default, the existence of gender was either ignored altogether or Western gender patterns were assumed. Today, while not all studies explicitly consider gender, a considerable corpus of research does, and gradually gender is more central to all archaeological research.

Any thoughtful consideration of our, or any other society demonstrates that the inclusion of children in the story of the past is just as vital as the incorporation of women—that age can no more be ignored than gender. In all societies children comprise a substantial proportion of the population, they participate in all facets of the society to a greater or lesser degree, and their activities are not only necessary to the present, but help shape the face of the future. Given the high proportion of subadults in many of the societies studied by archaeologists and the proficiency of children at many tasks, it is really no more speculative to posit that children were responsible for many artifacts or artifact distributions than to say that adults were.

More importantly, in all societies there is enormous emotional and physical investment by adults in children. While the nuances of adult-child interactions vary considerably cross-culturally, in all societies children are vital for both the cultural success and physical continuity of the group as well as the personal success and happiness of many individuals. As such, many aspects of culture are intentionally shaped to facilitate child rearing and both groups and individuals often respond strongly to threats to their children. If children and their specific roles in the society being studied are not considered, population growth or the lack of it, economics, social relations, and even belief systems will be incompletely envisioned and may well even be misunderstood.

To ensure the continued development of the nascent study of children and childhoods of the past, I would like to argue here for three future developments in the field.

The first, continued research on the archaeological remains, I am confident will happen, and it is through this continued effort that additional methodologies as well as new insights into the past will be developed. The second relates specifically to the development of those methods and is the topic of the bulk of this chapter. Here I caution that, if we are to retain credibility while investigating children and childhoods, we must pay explicit attention to a discussion of which facets of children and childhood our data allow us to interpret. It is imperative that, for example, we not conflate a society's ideas about the nature of childhood with the actual realities of the life stage. Thus, that pictures of children may stereotypically show them only as happy and well tended, often playing, does not mean that actual children did not work, suffer abuse, or have severe medical problems. Thirdly, I would like to propose that archaeologists interested in children not disregard the importance of experimental and ethnoarchaeological research on children as important tools for developing both perspectives and methodologies.

The Need for Methodological Rigor

Let us consider in some detail the need for methodological rigor. There are at least six different types of intertwined potential foci for the study of past childhoods. (1) Every society has theories about children, childhood, and the stages of children's development. These notions, which I have termed the dominant discourse about childhood (Kamp 2005) after Bauman's (1996) definition, are primarily the creations of adults; although children themselves may adopt parts of the dominant discourse about them and reject other parts. (2) In each society there is some attempt by adults to influence the lives of children. These efforts may be large and very structured, as with formal school systems, or slight and very casual. (3) Children themselves have some agency, however, and they themselves not only react to the interventions of adults, but also create their own cultural forms and traditions. (4) These previously enumerated conditions plus cultural circumstances lead to what might be termed a "modal" childhood, some generalized idea of what childhood was like for the average child. This type of notion, while useful and probably unavoidable as an analytic and communicative device, needs to be approached with care, particularly in nonhomogeneous societies such as highly stratified societies or those with multiple types of residential or subsistence patterns, where it is undoubtedly more accurate to speak of multiple childhoods, even within a single culture. (5) The life history of a particular child, recognizing that no individual lives an "average" life and that variation in experience is important. (6) Finally, the perspective of children themselves must be acknowledged and separated from the adult perspective. As I discuss below, the types of evidence used to make arguments about each of these types of questions varies somewhat and, since different types of evidence yield alternative conclusions, it is important for the investigator to be clear about the focus of discussion.

I will briefly examine below a number of the types of evidence currently available and used by researchers to approach the topic of childhood, commenting on the way each relates to these six perspectives. It should however, be emphasized that the discussion will not claim to be a complete review of all the current approaches or literature, and is of necessity a simplification of the issues at hand because thankfully few researchers rely solely on a single type of evidence for their arguments.

TEXTS AND ART

Students of the past have often felt on the most secure ground when either written accounts or pictorial evidence are available. While neither should be discounted as valuable evidence, it is important to remember that both reflect the distinct perspectives of their producers, who are often writing or making art for a particular audience. Thus, both texts and art are frequently designed to promote particular perspectives, not to simply mirror the actual situation of either children or adults. As we all know, even a pre-Photoshop photograph represents a selective and biased view of reality. It seems most likely that, generally, both texts and pictures will present the dominant discourse about children and childhood, although ethnoarchaeological research is needed to systematically study this for modern and historic cases. Thus, patterns in these accounts will provide a cultural vision of the way children should act or be treated, more than a description of reality. The care with which these must be approached is illustrated by the disjunction between the textual and iconographic sources of information on Late Minoan women as caregivers (Olsen 1998). While Linear B tablets show a gender-segregated society, with children and even older boys grouped with women, artwork shows Late Minoan women mainly in nondomestic contexts.

In texts it is normally adults who are heard. As Golden (2003:54) comments of ancient Greece, "[T]heir [children's] voices are rarely audible. Baby talk in our sources represents what adults said to children and what they wanted to and expected to hear in return." Furthermore, it is likely that women, children, and especially daughters may be harder to access if men are the primary authors, sculptors, and painters and are not as interested in or knowledgeable about women's activities (Foley 2003). There are a few notable exceptions to this pattern, however—texts that are produced by children potentially allow us to view the world from their perspective. These include letters, diaries, and some artwork including graffiti (Baxter 2008; Hutson 2006). It must be remembered, however, that these childhood productions, like adult creations, have an intended audience—whether child or adult—and a desired message. Thus, the fourth-century letter from a Greek foundry apprentice who complains about his treatment, citing in particular excessive whipping, presumably is asking for some type of redress (Golden 2003).

The interpretation of children in artwork is made more difficult since it may be hard to differentiate children from adults (Beaumont 2003; Follensbee 2006; Rutter 2003), especially when artistic conventions dictate that subordinate status is indicated via miniaturization. Nevertheless, the use of texts and artistic renditions is particularly useful when it is a general cultural stereotype that is sought. Thus, it is possible to use texts and art to chart the ideal stages of childhood (Beaumont 2003; Joyce 2000; McCafferty and McCafferty 2006) or myths to describe the ideal Greek (Shapiro 2003) or Mayan

(Houston 2009) youth, but it should always be remembered that what is being recorded in art is often not lived experience, but dominant discourse.

THE SKELETAL REMAINS OF CHILDREN THEMSELVES

If texts and art provide a picture of the ideal childhood and its stages, the skeletal remains of the children themselves provide direct insight into portions of the lives of individual children as experienced by them and, when viewed in the aggregate, of patterns in children's lives. We can see evidence of nutrition and nutritional stress, illness, dental health, traumas such as broken bones, age at weaning, and even whether the child moved from one place to another during its maturation (Perry 2005; Sobolik 2002). Both physical examination and chemical analyses of bones and teeth provide indications of changes in health and diet as well as differences within populations and between the sexes (Wright and Schwarcz 1998). For example, DNA analysis provides a means for sexing skeletal remains, a notoriously difficult problem for individuals who died before reaching puberty. DNA analysis of the skeletal remains of children sacrificed to the Mesoamerican god Tlaloc, a god of rain, water, and fertility, but also associated with specific diseases, shows a predominance of males who were often in poor health (Berrelleza and Balderas 2006). This and other skeletal remains used as offerings to the gods reveal a portion of the story of children's religious and symbolic importance.

BURIAL TREATMENTS AND GRAVE FURNISHINGS

A death ceremonial expresses social relations between the dead and the living, and the treatment and deposition of the deceased's body is a statement of past, present, and future identity, often reflecting not only on the individual but also on the individual's group. As mentioned previously, because of differential preservation, children's remains are probably underrepresented in most mortuary data (Story and McAnany 2006). Further complicating the picture, adults and children may be buried in different contexts (King 2006; Nagar and Eshed 2001; Story and McAnany 2006). Differences in burial location may suggest that adults and children or children of different ages have different social or symbolic meanings and may be one indication of the stages in life that the dominant discourse prescribed for children. Often children are buried in domestic contexts, and burial near the household instead of in a more public place may suggest differences in the degree and type of intimacy (Joyce and Hendon 2000). Children are not always preferentially associated with the household, however. For example, in coastal Oaxaca, adults, but not children, are buried in houses (King 2006). King (2006) suggests this may indicate that children were not yet tied to specific houses because of bilateral kinship systems.

Adult and child burials may be very similar (McCafferty and McCafferty 2006; Story and McAnany 2006) or children may be interred with different types of offerings than adults (Story and McAnany 2006), suggesting that they may be viewed as qualitatively different. When older children are treated more similarly to adults than younger children, this may be an indication of their gradual transformation into adults. A similar situation sometimes occurs with respect to gender, with young children lacking gendered grave goods, which are present in adults' burials and with older children.

Many archaeologists have cautioned about the complexities of interpreting burial assemblages, given cultural variation in the types of meanings and ceremonials associated with death. Nevertheless, burials provide a window, not necessarily into the activities an individual did in life, what he or she owned, or even a personal, individual significance, but into the types of ritual deemed appropriate for that individual, given all the circumstances surrounding their life and death. In other words, like artwork and texts, burials include an element of the performative and are meant to communicate information potentially to both the living and the dead.

FINGER, FOOT, AND HAND PRINTS

In addition to their skeletons, individuals have left traces of their activities in the form of hand or foot prints. Experiments showing the relationship between characteristics of these hand and foot prints and the age of their producers have allowed researchers to identify some of them as the products of children (Kamp et al. 1999; Sharpe and van Gelder 2006). Sometimes the hand and foot prints represent purposeful acts; sometimes they were left by accident. These two types of actions—the purposeful and accidental—have different interpretations, given our earlier six categories of perspectives. The accidental prints left on ceramic figurines (Kamp 2001b), or linear B tablets (Sjöquist and Åström 1991) show that children were engaged in manufacturing. Other prints and hand marks were purposely made as artistic, symbolic, or communicative acts. Some of these may have been solely the result of children's actions, but others, such as the finger marks on the ceiling of the French Upper Paleolithic cave of Rouffignac (Sharpe and van Gelder 2006), undoubtedly required the assistance of an adult and must thus be discussed in terms of adult-child interactions. Guthrie (2005) has posited a considerable presence of children in Upper Paleolithic caves, based heavily on evidence of hand and foot prints.

ARTIFACTS

Some artifacts were made by children and others were merely used by them. Here the relationship of both child and adult to the artifact is critical to its interpretation. Are we looking at an attempt by adults to express their ideas of the nature of the child or to control the child's behavior? Or, in fact, are we viewing an element of a child's own agency or a children's culture? Artifacts designed by adults for children fall into a number of categories and in addition adults may encourage children to use objects originally constructed for adults or children may appropriate these objects, using them either for their original purposes or designing new uses.

Social identities are encoded in a variety of different types of artifacts, and material culture functions as an active medium of communication. Clothing and other types of adornment, including bodily modifications, transmit information about gender, social status, and age. Thus, apparel made by adults for use by children provides not only protection from the elements, but an expression of cultural, personal, and group identity. Only under very favorable circumstances of preservation, such as in wet or dry depositional contexts, has ancient clothing of fabric or leather survived. When jewelry is made of stone, shell, or bone, all less perishable, it survives with greater frequency. Even here, however, ornaments of fiber, feathers, and other perishable materials are underrepresented archaeologically. Pictorial and sculptural representations of clothing augment archaeologically preserved specimens. Age, gender, socioeconomic status, and membership in religious and social groups as well as other types of identity can all be indicated by clothing.

Clothing and hairstyles, as well as jewelry and bodily marking, are often indicators of age status as well as gender and other types of personal status. Children below a certain stage may wear no clothing or gender-neutral clothing. Trachman and Valdez Jr. (2006) argue that *Spondyllus* shell pendants sometimes found near the pelvis of formative Maya subadults may be the gender markers referred to by Diego de Landa. He reported that boys wore a small white bead in their hair and girls had a cord low-slung over their hips on which was fastened a shell. These shells were removed sometime between the ages of three and twelve in what Landa analogizes to a baptismal ceremony. Only after the completion of this ritual could children marry.

Whatever the clothing signifies, it is a general rule that clothes follow specific cultural rules, usually set by adults, at least for younger children. The clothing worn in artistic productions may well be different than the everyday clothing worn by the individuals or types being depicted. Similarly, that found in burials is in a special context, selected to communicate particular messages, and cannot be simply interpreted as everyday apparel.

Child-rearing devices are another type of artifact found on archeological sites, sometimes in burials, but more often in trash deposits. These include tools such as cradle boards, walkers, or cradles designed to hold children, infant and child feeders, and a variety of rattles and toys. While objects for the very young clearly reflect a dominant discourse about child rearing, toys are a more ambiguous category.

Miniature artifacts are often identified as toys, an inherently problematic characterization, since miniatures may have functioned instead as offerings or components of shaman's gear (Park 2005). Miniatures are sometimes included in graves or used as offerings in order to spare the cost of the full-sized object. Context may provide a clue to use. At Cholula, for example, the discovery of figurines in contexts such as children's graves and porch areas where children may well have played supports the hypothesis that some of them may have functioned as toys (McCafferty and McCafferty 2006). Other figurines, however, especially those with clear female characteristics, were deposited in wells, suggesting their use as offerings and part of a fertility complex. Furthermore, as Sofaer Derevenski (2000b) reminds us, children are surrounded by and constantly interacting with a range of everyday objects, and it is a fallacy to assume a simplistic association between children and miniaturization.

Even if objects designed for children's use are securely identified, their meaning still is in question. Are they to be viewed as mere amusements, designed to make the child happy, as educational vehicles for learning adult skills and/or values, as implements sized for use by a child but meant to facilitate useful work, or even as status objects fashioned to demonstrate adult affluence through conspicuous consumption? If adults are manufacturing playthings for children, it is clear that they are in some way attempting to structure the child's time and the question becomes, To what purpose? Through the material world adults, in part, fashion the child's reality and attempt to structure their cultural choices. Children may, of course, not always utilize these objects as envisioned by adults.

Some miniatures and toys are fashioned by children, however. I have, for example, argued on the basis of fingerprint evidence that children fashioned some of the small clay figurines found in Sinagua sites in the American Southwest. The play that children design for themselves provides one window into the child's world. Park (2005) notes that ethnographic Inuit children liked to play house and make miniature houses. These were of pebbles in summer, but complete ice houses in winter, furnished with minia-ture versions of adult tools. Patterns similar to the summer playhouses have been found archaeologically. Many times, however, we probably miss the toys that children made for themselves. Ethnographic examples suggest that many of the toys children make themselves are either of unaltered or minimally altered natural materials or of objects discarded by adults. We need more ethnoarchaeological studies to alert us to the patterns that might indicate a discarded or natural object being used as a plaything.

Some of the objects produced by children may have been playthings, but others were not. We know from ethnographic examples that children are often productive members of the workforce and, as such, it is not unlikely that some objects of children's manu-facture would have been for adult use. The products of children have sometimes been identified using fingerprints, as discussed above, but more often on the basis of qualities that suggest they are the results of efforts by novices (Bagwell 2002; Crown 1999, 2002; Grimm 2000; Högberg 2008; Menom and Varma 2011). While it is true that initially all children who learn craft production techniques must start out as learners, the assumption that all novice artisans are, in fact, children needs to be carefully assessed (Finlay 1997).

SPACE USE

Some of the earliest considerations of children saw their behaviors as merely disrupting the more interesting and interpretable artifact distributions left by adults (Hammond and Hammond 1981). We now know that children's activities are no more random than those of adults, and their effect on the landscape may be studied in similar ways. An important part of child socialization is teaching the appropriate places for particular types of activities (Baxter 2005b). Depending upon the cultural circumstances, children may be allowed great mobility or little. The adult rules often vary with the age and gender of the child. Since it may be in the child's interest to be near adults, but sheltered from their gaze to retain more autonomy, children may frequent locations on the fringes of sites or domestic areas. Children may find secret, special places that they frequent and that come to hold great significance for them, remembered even as adults (Sobel 1990).

Similarly the construction of structures such as forts may provide a children's environment free from adult interference (Sobel 1993). Such areas have been identified archaeologically (Baxter 2005b; Wilkie 2000), but probably often occur in areas of sites that are less investigated by archaeologists, and they simply may not be recognized as the result of children's activities. Thus, Hutson (2006) proposes that small shell fragments left in a number of abandoned rooms after the last sweeping, but while the walls would have been standing, may be the result of children's play activities.

The Role for Experiments, Ethnography, and Ethnoarchaeology

Scholars studying children tend to rely heavily on ethnographic analogies to bolster their interpretations of the roles children played in the past. Thus, when I argued that Sinagua children were probably an active part of the work force (Kamp 2002b), I used general cross-cultural patterns in the types of activities performed by children as well as information about what descendant Puebloan groups were known to have done during historic time periods to create a list of likely economic contributions for children. I then examined the tasks that the archaeological evidence revealed were, in fact, done at the Sinagua pueblo being studied. For ceramic manufacture, I was able to make an argument based on archaeological evidence in the form of fingerprints. Because some ethnographic studies had actually paid attention to both the roles of children in ceramic manufacture and the characteristics of the material assemblages associated with children (Donley-Reid 1990), and because ethnoarchaeological studies on ceramicists (Kramer 1997; Krause 1985) had paid some minimal attention to the roles of children, I was able to fortify the case for children's involvement in ceramics with reference to expected patterns in material culture. Ethnoarchaeologist William Longacre (1981) reports that among the Kalinga one of the most common causes of ceramic breakage is accidents by children who are in the process of fetching water, and Dennis (1940:83) records Hopi children collecting water using small vessels. Using these pieces of information, I plan to investigate the proposed children's participation in water acquisition with a study of the size of broken water jugs found near Sinagua reservoirs. For most of the tasks I proposed for children, the archaeological correlates are not obvious to me at this point, perhaps partially because of a paucity of ethnoarchaeological studies of the patterned relationships of children to the material world.

The pitfalls of relying too much on ethnographic analogy have been discussed frequently, so I will not belabor the point here. Suffice it to say that we need better methods for investigating a past informed by age. While there have been some ethnoarchaeological and experimental studies of children (for example, Bird and Bird 2000; Buchli and Lucas 2000; Ferguson 2008; Greenfield 2000), to date far too little ethnoarchaeology has been conducted specifically on the interrelationship between children and material culture.

By virtue of their smaller size children may relate to the environment differently from adults. Heft (1999) has argued the usefulness of using the concept of "affordances" for analyzing children's activities and their perception of their surroundings. This approach, originally developed by Gibson (1986) foregrounds the functional significance of the environment rather than its forms, in other words, it analyzes a landscape in terms of the opportunities it affords. Thus, rather than describing a landscape as including grass, trees, and rocks, it would be discussed in terms of the sit-able, climb-able, edible, hide-able, and throw-able, to list just a few possible affordances. One of the important characteristics of affordances is that they must always be viewed in terms of a particular individual and that person's mental and physical characteristics. A tree that is climb-able for one individual may not be accessible to someone of a different stature or climbing ability, or the second individual may simply have no interest in tree climbing.

CONCLUSION

The future of childhood studies is secure, but it is imperative that those of us interested in past children and childhoods prevent them from being isolated, a sideline of passing interest but not core to an understanding of societal dynamics and change. We certainly need to keep researching children for their inherent value, but we also have to consciously consider how children in a particular case study affected the trajectory of social and cultural development. In addition, and to have our efforts taken seriously, we need to be vigilant about the maintenance of rigor in our research and increase our knowledge of the systematic relationships between children and their material environments through experiments and ethnoarchaeological studies.

REFERENCES CITED

Ardren, T. 2006 Setting the Table: Why Children and Childhood Are Important in an Understanding of Ancient Mesoamerica. In *The Social Experience of Childhood in Ancient Mesoamerica*, edited by T. Ardren and S. R. Hutson, pp. 3–22. University of Colorado Press, Boulder.

Ardren, T., and S. R. Hutson 2006 *The Social Experience of Childhood in Ancient Mesoamerica*. University of Colorado Press, Boulder.

Bagwell, E. A. 2002 Ceramic Form and Skill: Attempting to Identify Child Producers at Pecos, New Mexico. In *Children in the Prehistoric Puebloan Southwest*, edited by K. A. Kamp, pp. 90–107. University of Utah Press, Salt Lake City.

Baumann, G. 1996 *Contesting Culture*. Cambridge University Press, London.

Baxter, J. E. 2005a Introduction: The Archaeology of Childhood in Context. In *Children in Action: Perspectives on the Archaeology of Childhood, Papers of the American Anthropological Association* 15, edited by J. E. Baxter, pp. 1–9. American Anthropological Association, Washington, D.C.

Baxter, J. E. 2005b Making Space for Children in Archaeological Interpretations. In *Children in Action: Perspectives on the Archaeology of Childhood, Papers of the American Anthropological Association* 15, edited by J. E. Baxter, pp 78–111. American Anthropological Association, Washington, D.C.

Baxter, J. E. 2005c *The Archaeology of Childhood: Children, Gender, and Material Culture*. Altimira, Walnut Creek, California.

Baxter, J. E. (editor) 2006 *Children in Action: Perspectives on the Archaeology of Childhood*. Archaeological Papers of the American Anthropological Association, Volume 15.

Baxter, J. E. 2008 Mimicry, Mimesis and Material Culture: Liminal Expressions of Identity and the Archaeological Record. Paper Presented at the Sixth World Archaeological Congress, Dublin, Ireland.

Berrelleza, J. A. R., and X. C. Balderas 2006 The Role of Children in the Ritual Practices of the Great Temple of Tenochtitlan and the Great Temple of Tlatelolco. In *The Social Experience of Childhood in Ancient Mesoamerica*, edited by T. Ardren and S. R. Hutson, pp. 233–248. University of Colorado Press, Boulder.

Beaumont, L. A. 2003 The Changing Face of Childhood. In *Coming of Age in Ancient Greece: Images from the Classical Past*, edited by J. Neils and J. H. Oakley, pp. 59–83. Yale University Press, New Haven.

Bird, D. W., and R. Bliege Bird 2000 The Ethnoarchaeology of Juvenile Foragers: Shellfishing Strategies among Meriam Children. *Journal of Anthropological Archaeology* 19:461–476.

Buchli, V., and G. Lucas 2000 Children, Gender, and the Material Culture of Domestic Abandonment in the Late Twentieth Century. In *Children and Material Culture*, edited by J. Sofaer Derevenski, pp. 131–138. Routledge, New York.

Chamberlain, A. 2000 Minor Concerns: A Demographic Perspective on Children in Past Societies. In *Children and Material Culture*, edited by J. Sofaer Derevenski, pp. 206–212. Routledge, New York.

Crown, P. L. 1999 Socialization in American Southwest Pottery Decoration. In *Pottery and People: A Dynamic Interaction*, edited by J. M. Skibo and G. M. Feinman, pp. 25–43. University of Utah Press, Salt Lake City.

Crown, P. L. 2002 Learning and Teaching in the Prehispanic American Southwest. In *Children in the Prehistoric Puebloan Southwest*, edited by K. A. Kamp, pp. 108–124. University of Utah Press, Salt Lake City.

Dennis, W. 1940 *The Hopi Child*. D. Appleton-Century, New York.

Donley-Reid, L. W. 1990 The Power of Swahili Porcelain, Beads, and Pottery. In *Powers of Observation: Alternative Views in Archaeology*, edited by S. M. Nelson and A. B. Kehoe, pp. 47–59. Archaeological Papers of the American Anthropological Association, No. 2. Washington, D.C.

Ferguson, J. R. 2008 The When, Where, and How of Novices in Craft Production. *Journal of Archaeological Method and Theory* 15:51–67.

Finlay, N. 1997 Kid Knapping: The Missing Children in Lithic Analysis. In *Invisible People and Processes: Writing Gender and Childhood into European Archaeology*, edited by J. Moore and E. Scott, pp. 203–212. Leicester University Press, London.

Foley, H. 2003 Mothers and Daughters. In *Coming of Age in Ancient Greece: Images from the Classical Past*, edited by J. Neils and J. H. Oakley, pp. 113–137. Yale University Press, New Haven.

Follensbee, B. 2006 The Child and the Childlike in Olmec Art and Archaeology. In *The Social Experience of Childhood in Ancient Mesoamerica*, edited by T. Ardren and S. R. Hutson, pp. 249–280. University of Colorado Press, Boulder.

Gibson, J. J. 1986 *The Ecological Approach to Visual Perception*. Lawrence Erlbaum Associates, Hillsdale, New Jersey.

Golden, M. 2003 Childhood in Ancient Greece. In *Coming of Age in Ancient Greece: Images from the Classical Past*, edited by J. Neils and J. H. Oakley, pp. 13–29. Yale University Press, New Haven.

Greenfield, P. 2000 Children, Material Culture, and Weaving: Historical Change and Developmental Change. In *Children and Material Culture*, edited by J. Sofaer Derevenski, pp. 72–89. Routledge, New York.

Grimm, L. 2000 Apprentice Flintknapping: Relating Material Culture and Social Practice in the Upper Paleolithic. In *Children and Material Culture*, edited by J. Sofaer Derevenski, pp. 53–71. Routledge, New York.

Guthrie, R. D. 2005 *The Nature of Paleolithic Art*. University of Chicago Press, Chicago.

Hammond, G., and N. Hammond 1981 Child's Play: A Distorting Factor in Archaeological Distribution. *American Antiquity* 46(3):634–636.

Heft, Harry 1999 Affordances of Children's Environments: A Functional approach to Environmental Description. In *Directions in Person-Environment Research and Practice*, edited by J. L. Nasar and W. R. E. Preiser. Ashgate, Aldershot, England.

Högberg, A. 2008 Playing with Flint: Tracing a Child's Imitation of Adult Work in a Lithic Assemblage. *Journal of Archaeological Method and Theory* 15(1):112–131.

Houston, S. 2009 A Splendid Predicament: Young Men in Classic Maya Society. *Cambridge Archaeological Journal* 19(2):149–178.

Hutson, S. R. 2006 Children Not at Chunchucmil: A Relational Approach to Young Subjects. In *The Social Experience of Childhood in Ancient Mesoamerica*, edited by T. Ardren and S. R. Hutson, pp. 103–131. University of Colorado Press, Boulder.

Joyce, R. A. 2000 Girling the Girl and Boying the Boy: The Production of Adulthood in Ancient Mesoamerica. *World Archaeology* 31(3):473–483.

Joyce, R. A. and J. Hendon 2000 Heterarchy, History, and Material Reality: "Communities" in Late Classic Honduras. In *The Archaeologiy of Communities*, edited by M. A. Canuto and J. Yaeger, pp. 143–169. Routledge, New York.

Kamp, K. A. 1998 Social Hierarchy and Burial Treatments: A Comparative Assessment. *Cross-Cultural Research* 32(1):79–115.

Kamp, K. A. 2001a Prehistoric Children Working and Playing: A Southwestern Case Study in Learning Ceramics. *Journal of Anthropological Research* 57:427–450.

Kamp, K. A. 2001b Where Have All the Children Gone?: The Archaeology of Childhood. *Journal of Archaeological Method and Theory* 8 (1):1–34.

Kamp, K.A. (editor) 2002a *Children in the Prehistoric Puebloan Southwest*. University of Utah Press, Salt Lake City.

Kamp, K. A. 2002b Working for a Living: Childhood in the Prehistoric Southwestern Pueblos. In *Children in the Prehistoric Puebloan Southwest*, edited by K.A. Kamp, pp. 71–89. University of Utah Press, Salt Lake City.

Kamp, K. A. 2005 Dominant Discourses; Lived Experiences: Studying the Archaeology of Children and Childhood. In *Children in Action: Perspectives on the Archaeology of Childhood, Papers of the American Anthropological Association* 15, edited by J. E. Baxter, pp. 115–122. American Anthropological Association, Washington, D.C.

Kamp, K. A., N. Timmerman, G. Lind, J. Graybill, and I. Natowsky 1999 Discovering Childhood: Using Fingerprints to Find Children in the Archaeological Record. *American Antiquity* 64(2):309–315.

Keith, K. 2005 Childhood Learning and the Distribution of Knowledge in Foraging Societies. In *Children in Action: Perspectives on the Archaeology of Childhood, Papers of the American Anthropological Association* 15, edited by J. E. Baxter, pp. 27–40. American Anthropological Association, Washington, D.C.

King, S. M. 2006 The Marking of Age in Ancient Coastal Oaxaca. In *The Social Experience of Childhood in Ancient Mesoamerica*, edited by T. Ardren and S. R. Hutson, pp. 169–200. University of Colorado Press, Boulder.

Kramer, C. 1997 *Pottery in Rajasthan: Ethnoarchaeology in Two Indian Cities.* Smithsonian Institution Press, Washington, D.C.

Krause, R. A. 1985 *The Clay Sleeps: An Ethnoarchaeological Study of Three African Potters.* The University of Alabama Press, Tuscaloosa.

Lillehammer, G. 1989 A Child Is Born. The Child's World in an Archaeological Perspective. *Norwegian Archaeological Review* 22(2):89–105.

Longacre, W. 1981 Kalinga Pottery: An Ethnoarchaeological Study. In *Pattern of the Past*, edited by I. Hodder, G. Isaac, and N. Hammond, pp. 49–66. Cambridge University Press, Cambridge.

McCafferty, G. G., and S. D. McCafferty 2006 Boys and Girls Interrupted: Mortuary Evidence of Children from Postclassic Cholula Puebla. In *The Social Experience of Childhood in Ancient Mesoamerica*, edited by T. Ardren and S. R. Hutson, pp. 25–52. University of Colorado Press, Boulder.

Menon, J., and S. Varma 2011 Children Playing and Learning: Crafting Ceramics in Ancient Indor Khera. *Asian Perspectives* 49 (1):85–109.

Nagar, Y., and V. Eshed 2001 Where Are the Children? Age-dependent Burial Practices in Pequ'in. *Israel Exploration Journal* 51(1):27–35.

Neils, J., and J. H. Oakley (editors) 2003 *Coming of Age in Ancient Greece: Images of Childhood from the Classical Past.* Yale University Press, New Haven.

Oakley, J. H. 2003 Death and the Child. In *Coming of Age in Ancient Greece: Images from the Classical Past*, edited by J. Neils and J. H. Oakley, pp. 163–194. Yale University Press, New Haven.

Olsen, B. A. 1998 Women, Children, and the Family in the Late Aegean Bronze Age: Differences in Minoan and Mycenaean Constructions of Gender. *World Archaeology* 29(3):380–392.

Park, R. W. 2005 Growing Up North: Exploring the Archaeology of Childhood in the Thule and Dorset Cultures of Arctic Canada. In *Children in Action: Perspectives on the Archaeology of Childhood, Papers of the American Anthropological Association* 15, edited by J. E. Baxter, pp. 53–64. American Anthropological Association, Washington, D.C.

Perry, M. A. 2005 Redefining Childhood through Bioarchaeology: Toward an Archaeological and Biological Understanding of Children in Antiquity. In *Children in Action: Perspectives on the Archaeology of Childhood, Papers of the American Anthropological Association* 15, edited by J. E. Baxter, pp 89–111. American Anthropological Association, Washington, D.C.

Romero Sánchez, M. 2004 Children in the Southeast of the Iberian Peninsula during the Bronze Age. *Ethnographisch-Archäologische Zeitschrift* 45:377–387. ·

Rutter, J. 2003 Children in Aegean Prehistory. In *Coming of Age in Ancient Greece: Images from the Classical Past*, edited by J. Neils and J. H. Oakley, pp. 31–57. Yale University Press, New Haven.

Shapiro, H. A. 2003 Fathers and Sons, Men and Boys. In *Coming of Age in Ancient Greece: Images from the Classical Past*, edited by J. Neils and J. H. Oakley, pp. 85–111. Yale University Press, New Haven.

Sharpe K., and L. van Gelder 2006 The Study of Finger Flutings *Cambridge Archaeological Journal* 16(3):281–295.

Sjöquist, K.-E., and P. Åström 1991 *Knossos: Keepers and Kneaders.* SIMA PocketBook 82, Göteberg.

Sobel, D. 1990 A Place in the World: Adults' Memories of Childhood's Special Places. *Children's Environments Quarterly* 7(4):5–12.

Sobel, D. 1993 *Children's Special Places: Exploring the Role of Forts, Dens, and Bush Houses in Middle Childhood.* Zephyr, Tucson.

Sobolik, K. 2002 Children's Health in the Prehistoric Southwest. In *Children in the Prehistoric Puebloan Southwest*, edited by K. A. Kamp, pp. 125–151. University of Utah Press, Salt Lake City.

Sofaer Derevenski, J. 2000a *Children and Material Culture*. Routledge, New York.

Sofaer Derevenski, J. 2000b Material Culture Shock: Confronting Expectation in the Material Culture of Children. In *Children and Material Culture*, edited by J. Sofaer Derevenski, pp. 3–16. Routledge, New York.

Story, R., and P. A. McAnany 2006 Children of K'axob: Premature Death in a Formative Maya Village. In *The Social Experience of Childhood in Ancient Mesoamerica*, edited by T. Ardren and S. R. Hutson, pp. 53–72. University of Colorado Press, Boulder.

Trachman, R. M. and F. Valdez Jr. 2006 Identifying Childhood among the Ancient Maya. In *The Social Experience of Childhood in Ancient Mesoamerica*, edited by T. Ardren and S. R. Hutson, pp. 73–100. University of Colorado Press, Boulder.

Wilkie, L. 2000 Not Merely Child's Play: Creating a Historical Archaeology of Children and Childhood. In *Children and Material Culture*, edited by J. Sofaer Derevenski, pp. 206–212. Routledge, New York.

Wright, L. E., and H. P. Schwarcz 1998 Stable Carbon and Oxygen Isotopes in Human Tooth Enamel: Identifying Breastfeeding and Weaning in Prehistory. *American Journal of Physical Anthropology* 106:1–18.

CHAPTER THREE

Method and Theory for an Archaeology of Age

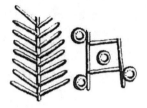

Scott R. Hutson

Abstract   *The question of whether children are visible or invisible follows previous questions about whether women, kinship systems, or even sexuality are archaeologically visible. Indeed, visibility is the central metaphor for considering the archaeological record. However, the notion of visibility often brings with it an undesired ontological position in which the agent that sees is an active subject and that which is seen becomes a passive object. "Seeing" children therefore runs the risk of rendering children as static objects. In this chapter, I approach young people in the ancient past from a relational perspective that blends objectivity and subjectivity. This approach also requires consideration of the other age groups with whom children act. More broadly, an archaeology of childhood should be an archaeology of age. The question of the visibility of children also introduces methodological questions about the kinds of evidence that permit discussion of children in the past. I argue that archaeologists studying children and actors of other ages can use both smoking guns and less direct forms of evidence. The chapter focuses on figurines but also makes suggestions for useful approaches to architecture. Approaches to figurines should embrace not just what figurines represent, but how they were used and who made them. With regard to architecture, children incorporate built environments into their sense of self by dwelling in them and creating their place in the world through them. Thus, people shape buildings but buildings also shape people. In this process of mutual construction, childhood is critical. Lived space shapes children's sensibilities and, roughly following these sensibilities, children will later grow up to produce and reproduce these spaces and the social conventions surrounding them. To undertake an analysis of this in the past, we do not need to "see" direct signatures of children in the past. I highlight this point with data from the Classic period Maya area and Çatalhöyük.*

INTRODUCTION

The subtitle of the IEMA Visiting Scholars Conference posed the question of whether children are visible or invisible in the archaeological record. With the encouragement of the IEMA editorial board, I have abandoned an Old World case study and addressed this question more broadly. In this chapter, I discuss two issues raised by the conference subtitle. The first issue regards a polarity—children as active subjects or passive objects—brought about by tropes of vision and visibility. The second issue regards the kinds of evidence that can be used to speak about ancient children in the context of archaeology's empirical legacy. I will discuss these issues with reference primarily to figurines but will also make tentative suggestions about approaches to the built environment. I begin by elaborating on the interrelated issues of vision and evidence. Such an elaboration requires contextualizing the archaeology of childhood within archaeologies of identity and the kinds of social relations at their core.

IDENTITY, RELATIONALITY, AND VISION

The archaeology of childhood is an archaeology of identity. As such, it resembles archaeologies of gender, ethnicity, sexuality, etc. An interest in relations unites these archaeologies and gives them their vitality. Identity is a process. More specifically, it is the process of identification, of establishing (and challenging) relations of similarity and difference that affect who we understand ourselves to be, who others understand us to be, and how these understandings condition our possibilities for action in the world (Jenkins 2004). Archaeologists have come to understand that relations of similarity and difference arise from interactions between people (as well as with the material world). Therefore, archaeologies of identity cannot be archaeologies of specific groups of people, but of relations between groups and how the actors in these groups relate to material culture. This is because the identity of any specific group depends on its relationships to other groups and to the material milieu. For example, the archaeology of gender cannot merely be an archaeology of women (Conkey and Gero 1991). Rather, it must be an archaeology of the processes by which people of multiple genders come to understand each other and relate to each other based on the association of patterns of action with sexed bodies (Butler 1993). Likewise, the archaeology of childhood cannot be an archaeology of children. Rather, it must be an archaeology of the processes by which people relate to each other based on expectations of performance and competency associated with age. In other words, archaeologists interested in children must consider themselves as engaging not in an archaeology of children, but an archaeology of age (Gilchrist 2000). They must attend to how age-based identities come into being as a result of the interactions and relationships between people at different stages of the life cycle. Therefore, the success of an archaeology of children must be measured on the basis of how quickly it relinquishes a focus on children alone and embraces the analysis of multiple age groups. In other words, following the logic proposed for the study of women in archaeology (Tringham 1991:115), we cannot merely add children and stir. Rather, we must step back and reconsider the relations between actors of all ages and consider how these relations configure age categories such as childhood.

Recognizing that the study of children is a study of identity highlights the notion that the study of children should be inherently relational. A relational perspective maintains that people derive their sense of identity from the objects, activities, and social relations in which they are entangled (Gell 1998; Heidegger 1996 [1927]; Strathern 1988). This entanglement furnishes people with the projects, purposes, and dispositions that guide them and allow them to cope with the world. A relational view conceives of the self not as individualized, sealed off, and independent, but rather as a node in an open network connecting other people, places, and things (Latour 1993; Law and Callon 1992). Relations in these networks not only help solidify what are at root unstable identities, they also affect the patterns of action associated with any particular group. With regard to age, Giddens states that the socialization of children "is not simply that of the child, but of the parents and others with whom the child is in contact, and whose conduct is influenced by the child just as the latter's is by theirs" (Giddens 1979:139). Relational approaches in archaeology that have made the boldest efforts to avoid subject/object dichotomies would add that material things (Olsen 2003; Webmoor and Witmore 2008) and landscapes (Tilley 1994) also shape and are shaped by this experience of socialization.

Since an archaeology of age is a relational archaeology, we must be very careful about the kinds of relationships toward which our language predisposes us. In the modern world, vision reigns over the other senses and visual metaphors permeate our language (Jay 1993). Do such metaphors aid or inhibit our investigation? In particular, does the language of visibility embed assumptions about how we go about studying children? Does it embed assumptions about what kinds of beings children are? In archaeology, Lazzari (2003) has noted that the concept of visibility harbors a pair of deeply rooted ways of thinking. First, vision presumes a dichotomy between the seeing subject and the seen object. The eye sees everything but itself, thus creating a sharp distinction between objects in sight and the viewer, who is not in the picture. Such vision—objectifying, totalizing, disembodying—affords the viewer a neutral, detached, distanced perspective that forfeits the possibility of situated, experiential understandings of the world (Haraway 1988). Second, vision embeds power relations into this dichotomy between subject and object. De Certeau (1984) commented on the mastery afforded by views from above and Said (1979) elaborated how the colonial gaze helped justify colonial subordination. Archaeologists are more likely to be familiar with Foucault's (1977[1975]) discussion of how space can be organized (in prisons, schools, hospitals, etc.) to permit the kind of visual surveillance and examinations necessary for discipline and punishment. Therefore, to make children visible risks objectifying them as the passive objects of a powerful gaze. Yes, we want to be able to "see" evidence of children, but if we agree with Giddens's statement that children influence the lives of people of other ages (see also Baxter 2005:32–34; Kamp 2001a:26–27), we also want to conceive of children in ways that render them active subjects in their own right.

Thus, our first impulse is to resist the way in which the language of vision positions children and to switch them from objects to subjects. This would seem to address the problem of power relations. However, in switching children from objects to subjects, our intervention leaves intact the dichotomy between subject and object. Rather than questioning the dichotomy, we have simply shifted children from one pole to the other. Getting out of this trap requires recognizing the paradox of subjectivity. On the one hand, humans are subjects: active beings that have the agency to transform society, the physical world, and their positions within these realms. On the other hand, humans cannot become acting subjects without being subjected to a constellation of social norms, mannerisms, and expectations. Subjection is the precondition for subjecthood. In other words, humans are always both subject and object. I will address this paradox more concretely in the discussion of the relationship between children and architecture.

EVIDENCE

The question of the visibility of children also directs attention to the method and theory of the archaeology of age. Can we talk about children if we cannot "see" them? Highly visible data pertaining to children in archaeology include toys, things made by children, burials of children, and representations of children. These data are often called "smoking guns" (Conkey and Gero 1991:17), "direct" data (Lucy 2005:46), or "index artifacts" (Prine 2000:201). It is said that these kinds of data can be isolated as pertinent to ancient experiences or understandings of children. For example, in the burial of a seven-year-old, no one doubts that other people, often adults, prepared the burial, but we also do not doubt that the human remains and what they may illustrate about diet, for example, speak loudly about the life experience of that child. Likewise, although an adult may have produced a figurine that depicts a woman cradling a child, aspects of the appearance of the child certainly express attitudes toward children. Nevertheless, pitfalls present themselves even to researchers that do have "smoking guns," such as dozens of stone tools knapped by children. These cases, in which children can be isolated from other actors, tempt us to focus only on children—to isolate them—without considering children's relations to society as a whole, thus abandoning the possibilities of a relational approach.

The study of children faces a more pressing challenge, however, when smoking guns are not available. If, for example, a large corpus of figurines lacks examples that clearly depict children, should we abandon any attempt to consider age-based identity? I argue that it would be shortsighted to postpone an analysis of age until smoking guns become available (Hutson 2006; Lucy 2005). Such a postponement recalls the problem identified a quarter-century ago by feminist archaeologists: we cannot afford to ignore a whole class of people while waiting for direct evidence of their actions (Conkey and Spector 1984; Kamp 2001a; Scott 1997:5). Continuing the parallel with studies of gender bears important realizations for a study of age. Wylie (1991:32–24) argued that the complaint that archaeological data are too limited to address gender (or age) does not justify postponing the study of gender (or age). This is because archaeologists do not necessarily wait on the data, as if data were active and the interpreters of that data were passive. Data become evidence of sociocultural phenomena only when archaeologists take the initiative of building a body of linking principles. Thus, rather than contenting themselves with sitting back and waiting for smoking guns, archaeologists can in fact confront the issue head on by engaging in actualistic studies that make relevant the data already at hand. I will return to an example of actualistic studies in the section below on figurines.

Stated differently, useful data are always at hand, even if they do not come in the form of smoking guns. In the same way that all archaeological records contain evidence of women (what ancient societies lacked females?), all archaeological records contain evidence of children (what ancient societies lacked children?). Given that half of the living individuals in many prehistoric populations were under the age of 20 and perhaps a third under the age of 10, young people certainly contributed to the archaeological record (Chamberlain 1997:249; Grimm 2000:53; Sofaer Derevenski 1997). They ate from and broke some of the pots archaeologists recover, they wore down the buildings and floors archaeologists unearth, and they contributed their labor to the households archaeologists reconstruct. Much like engendering the past (Conkey and Gero 1991:17) or sexualizing the past (Voss and Schmidt 2000:6–7), writing children into the past must begin even in the absence of smoking guns, direct evidence, or index artifacts. To postpone a critical inquiry into childhood silently reproduces current understandings of childhood and diverts us from asking productive and transformative questions about differences between people in the past (Conkey and Gero 1991:12).

Regardless of the methodological insights gained from other archaeologies of identity, encouraging archaeologists to look beyond index artifacts and smoking guns will be a challenge given archaeology's historical legacy of empirical, object-focused approaches. In the United States, archaeology developed in the context of museums whose major imperative was, for varied reasons, to acquire objects (Hinsley 1992). The obsession with empirical objects continued into the cultural historical era of the twentieth century, when archaeologists prioritized the expansion of their data sets, as opposed to addressing broader questions about ancient life (Taylor 1948). Though processual archaeologists attempted to replace empiricism with what they thought was hypothetico-deductivism (Salmon 1976), the kind of hypothesis testing favored by, for example, Binford (1983) was in many ways hostile to archaeologies of identity (Wylie 1991). I consider only the hostility engendered by a relational approach. First, archaeologies of identity are interested not in objects but in relations between people. Objects can be made to speak relatively unambiguously about some aspects of prehistory (Hawkes 1954), such as climate and subsistence (the macrosystemic variables Binford favored). However, the link between objects and social relations is ambiguous, more amenable to hermeneutic forms of inquiry than to hypothesis testing (Hodder and Hutson 2003).

What are the possibilities and prospects for coping with such ambiguity? Can we disambiguate the archaeological signatures of one age group from another? In other words, what are the prospects for attributing material culture to children as opposed to adults? In the sections below, I present examples of research that offer successful responses to these questions. Some of the strongest research has come from the study of lithics (Finlay 1997; Grimm 2000; Högberg 2008; Pigeot 1990). In the interest of brevity, I limit my examples to clay figurines and architecture. The examples nevertheless show a breadth of interpretive challenges: whereas the architecture example works without the help of smoking guns, archaeologists working with figurines have performed the actualistic studies that find them. As I will show, this has required a move toward indexicality. Below, I discuss this movement as a shift away from what figurines represent or the meanings they symbolize and toward the conditions of their production and aspects of their use.

FIGURINES

Figurines are often defined as durable, three-dimensional, miniature representations of humans, animals, or other phenomena (Bailey 1996). Nevertheless, we must think twice about the project of isolating figurines from other images and defining them in the abstract, because ancient understandings of figurines may have been inseparable from other images that were neither durable, nor three-dimensional, nor miniature in scale, nor representational (Joyce 2002; Meskell et al. 2008:141; Rollefson 2008:388). Figu-rines are notoriously difficult to interpret. Bailey (2005:84–85) puts it well when he states that "it is most probable that any one figurine was understood, used if you wish, in different ways by different people, or by the same person in different contexts and different places, or in the company of different people, or at different phases of different spectator's lives." In other words, we can never be certain about what figurines meant (see also Lesure 2002).

In 2002, Richard Lesure proposed a "rudimentary synthesis" of the different ways archaeologists approach ancient figurines. Lesure's synthesis focused explicitly on what figurines mean, and, in particular, the gender of figurines from early villages. Other authors examining figurines from early villages, such as Rosemary Joyce (2007), consider not just *what* they mean, but *how* they mean. However, neither Lesure nor Joyce implies an either/or dichotomy between what an object means and how it is meaningful. Some archaeologists, such as cognitive processualists, endorse this dichotomy and claim that we can understand how symbols were used without any reference to what they meant (Renfrew 1994:6). I would reject such a dichotomy. Despite well-intentioned attempts, it is impossible to avoid imputing meaning to the archaeological record (Hodder and Hutson 2003). Even the process of describing and categorizing material from the past loads this material with assumptions about its meaning (Hodder 1999:53; Spector 1993; see also Foucault 1990[1966]:xv). For example, ideas about the meaning of death inevitably and often unconsciously smuggle their way into explanations of the function of burials. To take a separate example from figurine studies, some publications of Neolithic figurines explicitly attempt to avoid the attribution of meaning by restricting themselves to extraordinarily detailed measurements (e.g., Vajsov 1992). Bailey (2005:13–14) argues that these studies fetishize figurines: though the authors may say nothing about the meaning of figurines, the disproportionate attention they give to figurines speaks loudly about their assessment of them as meaningful in the past.

Looking at what figurines mean requires attention to who made them, who used them, and how they were used. This Peircean take on meaning is broader than the tradi-tional Saussurean paradigm because it recognizes that the relations between figurine (the signifier) and meaning (the signified) are not always arbitrary (Preucel and Bauer 2001).

Rather than meaning always being arbitrary, meaning may stem from iconicity—what figurines resemble—and indexicality—the materials out of which they are made, the contexts in which they were found, or their presence among or physical contact with other things, such as figurine makers and users. This approach is not new. Indeed, many studies (discussed below) have looked at, for example, indexical aspects of figurines—who made figurines and how they were used—before the contributions of Peircian semiotics were explicitly promoted in archaeology.

CHILDREN AS FIGURINE MAKERS

Some of the best work on who made figurines has followed Wylie's recommendation to take the initiative of using actualistic studies to build principles that link behavioral dynamics with archaeological residues. For example, Kamp et al. (1999) have used fingerprint analyses to determine the age of people who shaped ancient clay artifacts such as figurines and pots. In particular, they synthesized contemporary data on ridge breadth measurements of the fingerprints of men, women, boys, and girls of multiple different ages and ethnicities and found that certain ranges of fingerprint breadths correspond almost exclusively to the fingers of children. They applied this method to Sinagua animal figurines from the 11th to 13th centuries A.D. in central Arizona (anthropomorphic figurines are rare among the Sinagua; Kamp and Whittaker 1999:79). Kamp et al. (1999) found that the average age of figurine producers was between 11 and 13 years, with some figurines made by children no more than five years old. Unpublished research by Warren Barbour on fingerprints from figurines at the central Mexican site of Teotihuacan in the first half of the first Millennium also addresses the question of children producing figurines (Barbour, personal communication 2010). These studies help our understanding of the past because they enable us to specify the ages of figurine makers. If we know that children produced figurines, this aids our interpretation of children's lives and experiences.

Knowing with certainty what was made by children also allows us to generalize characteristics of children's production. Such characteristics serve as tools for bridging arguments: identifying these same characteristics in objects without fingerprints may help us identify who produced such objects. Research by Crown (1999, 2001) and Bagwell (2002) has shown that children's incompletely developed motor skills result in noticeable ceramic production characteristics. For ceramic figurines, Kamp et al. (1999) also noted that ancient figurines made by children often have lumpy surfaces, little detail, and poor attachments between appendages and torsos (Kamp 2001b; Kamp et al. 1999). Other characteristics of figurines made by children include asymmetrical forms, coarse surface finishes, and uneven thicknesses of the figurine. In a study published in 1975, Brown asked children of different ages to create human figures with clay. Though Brown's study was primarily geared toward measuring stages of cognitive development, it adds additional expectations for what figurines produced by children might look like. By age six, most children in the study could make human figures, and these figures typically consist of a single chunk of clay shaped into a continuous head/torso—a stalk—lacking much detail. In my presentation for the IEMA conference, I used the above aspects of figurines known to have been produced by children to argue that figurines with similarly youthful production characteristics in Central Mexico during the Postclassic period and Anatolia in the Pre-Pottery Neolithic were also produced by children.

It is important to note that adults who are also shaping clay for the first time may produce figurines with some of the same characteristics. Furthermore, in the U.S. Southwest, Puebloan adults with advanced skills sometimes purposefully produce poorly made ceramics for ritual deposits (Bartlett 1934; Crown 2001:454). Therefore, figurines exhibiting beginner's characteristics are not an infallible signature of children's production. This makes independent lines of evidence such as fingerprinting increasingly important.

The possibility that children made figurines is intriguing because if we can identify children's production, there is a possibility for identifying how children's innovations contributed to society at large. In the conclusion to her pathbreaking article "Where Have the Children Gone?" Kathryn Kamp (2001a:26–27) states: "We need to allow children the possibility of agency. . . . Children learn from adults and act as the recipients of culture, but children also learn from other children, innovate, and pass their innovations on to other children and perhaps adults as well" (see also Sillar 1994). Wallaert-Pêtre's (2001) ethnoarchaeology of potting communities in Cameroon suggests that the degree to which children as producers of material culture have the leeway to innovate depends on whether a particular craft is considered "open" or "closed." In closed situations, conformity is a very important ideal, experimentation is discouraged, and outside ideas are not welcome. In contrast, learners in open situations use trial and error, have little fear of exploring foreign styles, and enjoy the challenge of new tasks. Patricia Crown's (2001) investigation of pottery made by children in the American Southwest suggests that Hohokam and Mimbres pottery making align closely with the distinction between closed and open learning situations. Among the Mimbres, who emphasized creativity, children had a freer hand in painting pots. As a result, Mimbres potters produced an explosion of innovative compositions and their ceramic sequence was characterized by rapid changes in technology and designs (see DeBoer's [1990] study of Shipibo-Conibo potters for an account of how specific innovations relate to interpersonal dynamics among potters' teachers and families). The point here is that archaeologists have shown that children's learning processes can lead to innovations that carry over into adult domains (Crown 2001; Smith 2005).

Even when children's production does not lead to innovation, their participation in the creation of material culture gives them an active role in the process of socialization (Baxter 2005:24–27). Children do not receive knowledge from adults passively like a bank receiving a deposit, but rather, in crafting anthropomorphic figures with their own hands, they come to learn socially constructed understandings of the human body and reproduce these understandings in durable media (Joyce 2002). A series of studies from Mesoamerica has shown that the human body can be depicted in myriad ways, which means that how a society chooses to depict the human body represents a very narrow vision among a universe of possibilities, therefore establishing a selective ideal of what is proper (Bachand et al. 2003; Joyce 1998). Kuijt and Chesson's (2005, 2007) studies of figurines in the Levant recognize this point, which can be expanded, I believe, when considering children as figurine makers. When children produce human figurines, they are re-producing a very particular theory of the body. Thus, children become instrumental in the process of reproducing not just the material heritage of a society but also the ideals and norms that perpetuate social structure (Lopiparo 2006).

FIGURINES AS TOYS

Long ago, Peter Ucko (1968; see also Voigt 2000), working with a collection of figurines from Predynastic Egypt and Neolithic Crete, outlined a framework of expectations entailed by the hypothesis that figurines were used as toys. Here, I limit my attention to a few areas where the framework could be expanded or reworked. In terms of context, Ucko argued that we would not expect figurines to appear in ritual contexts if they were used as toys. Furthermore, if children held them dear, figurines should be found in burials of children. In Mesoamerica, McCafferty and McCafferty (2006) note that figurines from the site of Cholula satisfy both of these expectations. Figurines were most often found in nonceremonial porch contexts where children likely played. In the rare instances when they are found in burials, they accompany children, though two were found with adult females. Given recent consideration of the blurred line between ritual and other daily practices (Brück 1999; Hutson and Stanton 2007; McAnany 2010), and between child's play and the sacred (Hutson 2011; Sillar 1994), Ucko's notion of a purely ritual space devoid of toys or other profane materials should be considered critically.

In terms of wear patterns, figurines used as toys should have substantial wear from being handled actively. Such handling should result in breaks at points of structural weakness. Though figurines used in rituals may also have substantial wear, Voigt (2000; cf. Meskell et al. 2008) argues that such figurines may have a different breakage pattern than figurines used as toys. Specifically, using data on figurines from Çatalhöyük, she argues that figurines with intentional damage at places of structural strength may have been made for the sole purpose of ritual termination. Wilkie (2000) provides a case study from historic period California in which children appear to have intentionally destroyed ceramic dolls at points of structural strength. In Wilkie's interpretation, however, the behavior that caused the damage was more ritualistic than mere child's play. Meskell et al. (2008) also build an argument for the religiosity of pre-pottery figurines at Çatalhöyük by attending to wear patterns and the context of discard. The advantage of the Meskell et al. study is that it recognizes that the overwhelming majority of Çatalhöyük figurines have very little in common with the rarest and most famous figurines such as the seated woman with felines. Furthermore, it recognizes that the large body of simplistic figurines is quite different from later Pottery Neolithic figurines and that we must be extremely cautious in applying interpretations abstracted from the Pottery Neolithic. Finally, Ucko suggested that figurines used as toys would be small. This is unremarkable given that it is difficult for small children to play with unwieldy objects. Yet we can go beyond the question of why toys are small and ask a more stimulating question: What effects do small objects have on the people handling them? Stated differently, What kinds of experience does a reduction in scale make possible (e.g., Bailey 2005)?

These kinds of questions again favor a shift from asking what figurines mean to asking how they are meaningful. Though tantalizing, such questions are admittedly difficult to address with archaeological data.

FIGURINES AS VEHICLES OF MAGIC

Childbirth is not only a defining event in the life cycle of both the child and the parent, it is also a critical juncture in which people of multiple generations mutually implicate each other in the process of maintaining the viability of the population as a whole (e.g., Cyphers-Guillen 1993). A second usage of figurines that relates to an archaeology of age occurs when adults use them as vehicles of magic to protect the health of children and to improve the odds of healthy childbirth (Rollefson 2008:408; Voigt 2000:269). Such discussions align well with the project suggested in my introduction: pursuing childhood by looking at linkages across age groups and between people and things. Rollefson has made a case for the use of figurines as vehicles of magic in the Southern Levant during the Middle Pre-Pottery Neolithic B (MPPNB). More specifically, the notion that Levantine figurines have to do with fertility and childbirth comes from what Rollefson (2008:408) cites as the abundance of pregnant figurines from the Southern Levant in the MPPNB. Rollefson (2008) argues that a concern for successful pregnancy makes sense because the expanded demand for labor in the Neolithic would have caused families to desire more children. Demographic data suggest that women were indeed having more children in the PPNB (Guerrero et al. 2008). However, the fertility argument does not seem to hold for some sites with large figurine collections, such as Ain Ghazal (McAdam 1997:139) and Çatalhöyük (Meskell et al. 2008:148), where the vast majority of anthropomorphic figurines are not pregnant.

Rollefson's argument is one of many that use the conditions of life in the Pre-Pottery Neolithic to explain the uses of figurines. In this case, the shift to agriculture creates a demand for labor that selects for giving birth to more children. A shortcoming of such an explanation is that the time scale of the shift to agriculture is very different from the time scale of figurine production (Lesure 2002:592). In other words, the shift to a diet based on domesticates took place gradually, over the course of hundreds or even thousands of years. Figurines, on the other hand, were probably produced in a matter of days. For figurine production to be seen as a response to the shift to agriculture, people must have palpably experienced this shift in particular moments. However, since this shift took place gradually, we cannot be certain that people ever consciously noticed it.

Whether or not growing demands for agricultural labor spurred the desire to have children, childbirth amounts to nothing less than the physical regeneration of society; one would expect people to bracket it with an array of powerful rites and material culture calibrated to stack the odds in favor of safe, successful pregnancies. The higher mortality rates of ancient societies made childbirth even more risky and successful pregnancies a matter of magic. With help from ethnohistory and archaeological context, Brumfiel and Overholtzer build a strong case that figurines served as the vehicles of such magic. In Central Mexico during the Postclassic period shortly before the Spanish conquest, hollow figurines with rattles depict what Brumfiel and Overholtzer (2009:312–315; Overholtzer 2005) believe to be the three stages of women's reproduction: not pregnant, pregnant, and holding a child. These figurines are found in habitation rooms and sweat baths at the site of Cihuatecpan. Aztec informants told the sixteenth-century Spanish Friar Bernardino de Sahagun (1950–1982) that "sweat baths were places where women received regular treatments before and after childbirth to ensure reproductive success" (Brumfiel and Overholtzer 2009:313). Furthermore, the hollowness of these figurines may be directly implicated in the rituals as decoys onto which bad luck could be diverted. Since unhealthy babies were, according to Sahagún, dry like a hollow gourd or pottery rattle and since women took precautions to avoid this, the hollow rattle figurines may have been used to attract dryness and channel it away from the womb. Other Aztec ethnohistoric sources also remark on the use of figurines in fertility ceremonies as well as curing ceremonies; Friar Diego Durán noted that children wore idols around the neck as protection from illness (Smith 2002:106). In colonial Mexico, *idol* referred to anthropomorphic figures, that is, figurines.

YOUTHFUL ENCHANTMENT

I have discussed three associations between children and figurines. First, there is the possibility that children made some figurines. Second, children may have played with some of the figurines as toys. Third, figurines may have been used as vehicles of magic for the benefit of children's health. The first two associations are indexical in the sense that they imply actual physical contact between figurines and children. Is it possible that these two indexical associations between children and figurines gave figurines some of the potency that allowed them to be used as protective magic? Sillar (1994) suggests precisely this possibility in his case from Andean South America: the importance of figurines as offerings comes from the fact that children played with them. In other words, the indexical associations that figurines acquire serve as a "first step" (Joyce 2007:101) for understanding their symbolic meanings, such as their role in ensuring good health. This gains plausibility for the Andes, as well as among the Aztecs, because childhood in these societies was a time of purity that aided communication with the gods (Cobo 1990; Román Berrellaza and Chávez Balderas 2006; Sillar 1994). Indeed, at many different times and places, such as early modern Europe, the perceived inexperience and innocence of children were thought to give them privileged links to the sacred (Hamann 2006:211). For the Aztecs, child sacrifice gave force to requests for rain (Durán 1951). In this context it is not even necessary that any specific child had an indexical association with a particular figurine used as an offering as long as the figurine was made to look "childish." Here I have in mind the ethnographic example of Puebloan adults intentionally producing small, poorly made pottery vessels—the kinds of miniatures often made by children (Bagwell 2002:95; Bartlett 1934; Crown 2001:454)—as offerings. Investigating the associations—symbolic, indexical, iconic—between children and figurines in a variety of contexts—Central Mexico, the Andes, the Levant—contributes an anthropological perspective to our understanding of the past. Finding common patterns and deviations from patterns enriches our sense of humanity in its multiple guises.

ARCHITECTURE

In the introduction, I suggested that an archaeology of childhood shares an important feature with archaeologies of identity: the need to examine not just a single group of people (in this case children), but to examine relations between multiple groups and between people and material culture. Looking at architecture is important because it highlights relations between people and material culture and gives material culture an active role in this relationship. Buildings physically forge a dialogue with people as people pass through them. People must move in certain ways and assume certain postures within and around buildings simply to avoid collisions. In repeating these motions day after day, humans become subject to buildings, come into rhythm with their walls, walkways, steps, and other features. Buildings therefore actively inculcate ways of carrying oneself. Though children are born into built environments that they themselves did not build, they incorporate these environments into their subjecthood by dwelling in them and creating their place in the world through them. In this way, buildings shape subjects. British prehistorians have made a similar point with respect to the ways in which Neolithic monuments mold ancient subjects by positioning and orienting people's bodies (Barrett 1994; Thomas 1993; Tilley 1994). More recently, and in a slightly different vein, Gosden (2005:202) has stated that "environments into which children were born and socialized internalize a set of spatial and social rules whose power lay in the fact that they were obeyed unconsciously rather than being formally taught."

The way in which buildings shape subjects can be seen most clearly when people reproduce these buildings later in life. The architecture shapes the child's sensibilities and, roughly following these sensibilities, the full-grown person will later shape new architecture based on these sensibilities. The child is the parent of the adult: "Adult's perceptual categories are from time to time infused with emotions that surge out of early experiences" (Tuan 1977:20; see also Ingold 2000:186). This principle can be seen in the dominant residences of two contiguous houselots—'Aak and Muuch—from the ancient Maya site of Chunchucmil, Yucatan, Mexico. Analyses presented elsewhere (Hutson 2010) suggest that the 'Aak houselot was built first and people from the 'Aak houselot splintered off and built the neighboring Muuch houselot.

The main residences at the two houselots (structures S2E2-13 in Muuch and S2E2-22 in 'Aak) have nearly identical construction techniques, floor plans, and dimensions. However, other fully excavated residences at Chunchucmil differ drastically from structures S2E2-13 and S2E2-22 (see Hutson 2010, Figure 4.5). The fact that the similarities between these two buildings are not shared in other buildings suggests that there was no widely held template, either habitual and unspoken or explicit and geomantic, of the proper floor plan at the site. The explanation that best accounts for the similarities between the two buildings is that members of the 'Aak houselot fissioned and founded the Muuch houselot (for more on household fissioning in the Maya area, see Haviland 1988:121; Manzanilla and Barba 1990:44; Tourtellot 1983). In other words, Structures S2E2-13 and S2E2-22 are similar because the people who built S2E2-13 in the Muuch houselot originally lived in or around S2E2-22 in the 'Aak houselot. Congruent to the notion of buildings as structuring structures (Bourdieu 1977; Donley-Reid 1990), the founders of the Muuch group grew up dwelling in S2E2-22 and when it came time to build S2E2-13, they followed the dispositions durably imposed in them from first relating to S2E2-22. In constructing S2E2-13, they produced a design whose fidelity to S2E2-22 stands as a materialization of this relation between people and house. Tilley (2004:118) puts it well: "Moving into and around and encountering architectural spaces clearly has direct physical effects on the body and creates a set of expectations with regard to future encounters." The design of S2E2-13 reproduces not only the sedimented spatial experiences of the builders' childhoods as spent in structure S2E2-22, but also that of the elders and the ancestors. To quote Joyce (Meskell and Joyce 2003:51): "Participation in the bodily experience of ancestors was an effect produced in the bodies of young people by their experience of the same architectural settings used by their predecessors." Such a study helps our understanding of the past because we have narrowed the list of explanations for similarities and differences across time, space, and form. In other words, we can state that similarities in building form are due not to a timeless, site-wide template, but to the specific experiences of particular people across the life cycle.

Another example of the way in which buildings inculcate ways of carrying oneself comes from excavations at Çatalhöyük. Hodder and Cessford (2004:18) argue that architecture helps embed social rules and dispositions as people go about their daily tasks: "As a child grows up within routinized domestic space, it learns that particular practices, movements, ways of holding oneself, deferential gestures, and so on are positively valued while others are not." Within houses at Çatalhöyük, floors were a mosaic of different heights, different matting, different degrees of cleanliness, and different kinds of plaster. Such floors, as well as mantles and walls, divided domestic space into many different areas, and particular areas—hearth areas versus areas with subfloor burials—had particular symbolic associations. Children "would have learned the social world at least partly in terms of this material-social-spatial map" (Hodder 2006:187). Learning such rules of order—what things could be done in what spaces—created discipline in the absence of centralized leadership.

Winston Churchill (cited in Hall 1966:106) declared that buildings shape their builders as much as the builders shape buildings (see also Tilley 2004:138). The case studies discussed above accord with this sentiment. Objects act upon humans who then reproduce more objects in a similar style (Gosden 2005). In this sense, the building is caught up in the process of subjectification insofar as the relations that constitute subjects cannot exist without being materialized in space. Yet if people are inextricably bound to each other, new buildings would be exact replicas of old buildings. We would not be able to explain why building conventions change over time. We can escape this bind by fleshing out the paradox of subjectivity mentioned in the first section of the chapter. Children are subjected to the sense of order that buildings cultivate, but this subjectification also makes them acting subjects: culturally intelligible people whose actions are taken seriously by others. Though predispositions, norms, rules, senses of space shape action, they do not determine outcomes entirely: not all actions blindly replicate conventions. Some actions tinker with norms, citing them differently. And when a culturally intelligible actor does things slightly differently, others may follow. This perspective (Sewell 1992) allows for change over time and provides a mechanism by which actors strongly embedded within systems of rules and regulations can nevertheless work to change them. Indeed, in both the Chunchucmil and Çatalhöyük cases, later structures are not identical replicas of earlier structures, despite all their similarities.

Conclusion

One of the most exciting breakthroughs in locating the actions of ancient children has been work that establishes children as makers of material culture. In the case of ceramic figurines, studies of fingerprint breadth measurements provide an excellent example of archaeologists engaging in the kind of middle range work that produces uncontestable signatures of children in the past. Yet I have argued in this chapter that the absence of uncontestable signatures does not prevent us from coming to know about childhood in the past. Specifically, examples of stone tools, pots, figurines, and art that appear to be made by novices are strong candidates for classification as the work of children. These cases can be strengthened by additional observations. For example, in the case of pottery, the small size of some novice vessels suggests that they were made by younger people, a claim strengthened by ethnographic observations of children working on smaller scales. An alternative approach to being able to talk about childhood in the past considers the relationships between children and other actors. This kind of approach, which can be termed relational, aligns the study of childhood with other studies of identity in the past, such as the study of gender.

Many relational approaches emphasize the key roles played by material culture. In this chapter I considered the relationship between people and built space. We know that both adults and children populated ancient buildings. Though we may not always be able to detect how people of different ages used the same space, the case studies from Chunchucmil (Mexico) and Çatalhöyük (Turkey) suggest that the organization of space inculcates a "way of being," starting from a person's earliest years. Whether we refer to this way of being as a sociospatial map, a *habitus*, or a set of proxemic expectations, the important point is that people reproduced similar spatial arrangements once they grew old enough to rebuild their world. Childhood experiences are fossilized in these built worlds, providing a route to considering processes of acculturation even in the absence of smoking guns of childhood, such as representations of children or bodily remains of children.

Recognizing that newer buildings are not exact replicas of older buildings emphasizes the point that children are both subjects and objects. They are shaped by the worlds they inhabit but in being shaped, they become proper, intelligible subjects authorized to shape the world, if but a little. The trope of visibility presumes a viewing subject and a viewed object. Understanding the paradox that humans are both active and passive, subject and object, eases some of the dichotomizing tension embedded in tropes of visibility. Considering children as potters or molders of figurines can make this logic more concrete. As discussed above, in cultures where innovation is frowned upon and there are few opportunities for innovation, children and adults nevertheless reproduce their social and material worlds. Thus, agents are active and powerful in the very moment that they are constrained by the weight of tradition. On the other hand, in contexts where innovation is encouraged, tradition still constrains or guides the children's and adults' creativity. The conditions for the possibility of innovation involve the prior existence of rich representational traditions that afford a wealth of models that serve as jumping-off points for new models. In other words, creativity is nurtured by situations where there is already much to copy (Wilson and Wilson 1977). The case of child sacrifice provides the most startling illustration of the paradox of how children can be both powerful and powerless, subject and object. Both the Aztecs and Incas viewed childhood as a time of purity. Children's perceived inexperience and innocence made them ritually potent, bringing them closer to the gods. This potency made them appropriate as sacrificial offerings. Thus, the perceived power of children made some into mortal victims.

ACKNOWLEDGMENTS

I thank Ian Kuijt and Frank Hole for commenting on this manuscript. I also thank the College of Arts and Sciences at the University of Kentucky for granting me the teaching leave that made possible the completion of this manuscript. Finally, I thank Güner Coşkunsu for inviting me to participate in the IEMA Visiting Scholar Conference, for bringing together a terrific set of speakers, and for skillfully editing the essays.

REFERENCES CITED

Bachand, H., R. A. Joyce, and J. A. Hendon 2003 Bodies Moving in Space: Ancient Mesoamerican Human Sculpture and Embodiment. *Cambridge Archaeological Journal* 13(2):238–247.

Bagwell, E. 2002 Ceramic Form and Skill: Attempting to Identify Child Producers at Pecos Pueblo, New Mexico. In *Children in the Prehistoric Puebloan Southwest*, edited by K. A. Kamp, pp. 90–107. The University of Utah Press, Salt Lake City.

Bailey, D. W. 1996 Interpretation of Figurines: The Emergence of Illusion and New Ways of Seeing. *Cambridge Archaeological Journal* 6(2):291–295.

Bailey, D. W. 2005 *Prehistoric Figurines: Representation and Corporeality in the Neolithic.* Routledge, London.

Barrett, J. C. 1994 *Fragments from Antiquity: An Archaeology of Social Life in Britain, 2900–1200 B.C.* Blackwell, Oxford.

Bartlett, K. 1934 *The Material Culture of Pueblo II in the San Francisco Mountains, Arizona.* Museum of Northern Arizona Bulletin 7. Northern Arizona Society of Science and Art, Flagstaff.

Baxter, J. E. 2005 *The Archaeology of Childhood: Children, Gender and Material Culture.* Altamira, Walnut Creek, California.

Binford, L. R. 1983 *In Pursuit of the Past.* Academic Press, London.

Bourdieu, P. 1977 *Outline of a Theory of Practice.* Cambridge University Press, Cambridge.

Brown, E. V. 1975 Developmental Characteristics of Clay Figures Made by Children from Age Three through Eleven. *Studies in Art Education* 16(3):45–53.

Brück, J. 1999 Ritual and Rationality: Some Problems of Interpretation in European Prehistory. *European Journal of Archaeology* 2(3):313–344.

Brumfiel, E. M., and L. Overholtzer 2009 Alien Bodies, Everyday People, and Hollow Spaces: Embodiment, Figurines, and Social Discourse in Postclassic Mexico. In *Mesoamerican Figurines: Small-Scale Indices of Large-Scale Social Phenomena*, edited by C. T. Halperin, K. A. Faust, R. Taube, and A. Giguet, pp. 297–323. University Press of Florida, Gainesville.

Butler, J. 1993 *Bodies that Matter: On the Discursive Limits of Sex*. Routledge, New York.

Chamberlain, A. T. 1997 Commentary: Missing Stages of Life—Towards the Perception of Children in Archaeology. In *Invisible People and Processes: Writing Gender and Childhood into European Archaeology*, edited by J. Moore and E. Scott, pp. 248–250. Leicester University Press, London.

Cobo, B. 1990 [1653] *Inca Religion and Customs*. Translated by R. Hamilton. University of Texas Press, Austin.

Conkey, M. W., and J. Gero 1991 Tensions, Pluralities, and Engendering Archaeology: An Introduction to Women in Prehistory. In *Engendering Archaeology: Women and Prehistory*, edited by M. W. Conkey and J. Gero, pp. 3–30. Blackwell, Oxford.

Conkey, M. W., and J. Spector 1984 Archaeology and the Study of Gender. In *Advances in Archaeological Method and Theory*, edited by M. B. Schiffer, pp. 1–38. Academic Press, New York.

Crown, P. L. 1999 Socialization in American Southwest Pottery Decoration. In *Pottery and People: A Dynamic Interaction*, edited by J. M. Skibo and G. M. Feinman, pp. 25–43. University of Utah Press, Salt Lake City.

Crown, P. L. 2001 Learning to Make Pottery in the Prehispanic American Southwest *Journal of Anthropological Research* 57(4):451–469.

Cyphers-Guillen, A. 1993 Women, Ritual, and Social Dynamics at Ancient Chalcatzingo. *Latin American Antiquity* 4(3):209–224.

De Certeau, M. 1984 *The Practice of Everyday Life*. Translated by S. Rendall. University of California Press, Berkeley.

DeBoer, W. R. 1990 Interaction, Imitation, and Communication as Expressed through Style: The Ucayali Experience. In *The Uses of Style in Archaeology*, edited by C. Hastorf and M. W. Conkey, pp. 82–104. Cambridge University Press, Cambridge.

Donley-Reid, L. W. 1990 A Structuring Structure: The Swahili House. In *Domestic Architecture and the Use of Space*, edited by S. Kent, pp. 114–126. Cambridge University Press, Cambridge.

Durán, Fray D. 1951 *Historia de las Indias de Nueva España y Islas de Tierra Firme*, Volumes 1 and 2. Editora Nacional, Mexico City.

Finlay, N. 1997 Kid Knapping: The Missing Children in Lithic Analysis. In *Invisible People and Processes: Writing Gender and Childhood into European Archaeology*, edited by J. Moore and E. Scott, pp. 203–212. Leicester University Press, London.

Foucault, M. 1977 [1975] *Discipline and Punish: The Birth of the Prison*. Translated by A. Sheridan. Vintage, New York.

Foucault, M. 1990 [1966] *The Order of Things*. Translated by A. Sheridan. Vintage, New York.

Gell, A. 1998 *Art and Agency*. Clarendon, Oxford.

Giddens, A. 1979 *Central Problems in Social Theory*. University of California, Berkeley.

Gilchrist, R. 2000 Archaeological Biographies: Realizing Human Life-cycles, –courses, and –histories. *World Archaeology* 31(3):325–328.

Gosden, C. 2005 What Do Objects Want? *Journal of Archaeological Method and Theory* 12(3):193–211.

Grimm, L. 2000 Apprentice Flintknapping: Relating Material Culture and Social Practice in the Upper Paleolithic. In *Children and Material Culture*, edited by J. Sofaer Derevenski, pp. 53–71. Routledge, London.

Guerrero, E., S. Naji, and J.-P. Bocquet-Appel 2008 The Signal of the Neolithic Demographic Transition in the Levant. In *The Neolithic Demographic Transition and its Consequences*, edited by J.-P. Bocquet-Appel and O. Bar-Yosef, pp. 57–80. Springer, New York.

Hall, E. T. 1966 *The Hidden Dimension*. Doubleday, New York.

Hamann, B. E. 2006 Child Martyrs and Murderous Children: Age and Agency in 16th Century Transatlantic Conflicts. In *The Social Experience of Childhood in Ancient Mesoamerica*, edited by T. Ardren and S. R. Hutson, pp. 205–233. University Press of Colorado, Boulder.

Haraway, D. 1988 Situated Knowledges: The Science Question in Feminism and the Privilege of Partial Perspective. *Feminist Studies* 14(3):575–599.

Haviland, W. 1988 Musical Hammocks at Tikal: Problems with Reconstructing Household Composition. In *Household and Community in the Mesoamerican Past*, edited by R. Wilk and W. Ashmore, pp. 121–134. University of New Mexico Press, Albuquerque.

Hawkes, C. 1954 Archaeological Theory: Some Suggestions from the Old World. *American Anthropologist* 56:155–168.

Heidegger, M. 1996 [1927] *Being and Time*. Translated by J. Stambaugh. State University of New York Press, Albany.

Hinsley, C. M. 1992 The Museum Origins of Harvard Anthropology. In *Science at Harvard University: Historical Perspectives*, edited by C. A. Elliott and M. W. Rossiter, pp. 121–145. Lehigh University Press, Bethlehem, Pennsylvania.

Hodder, I. 1999 *The Archaeological Process*. Blackwell, Oxford.

Hodder, I. 2006 *The Leopard's Tale: Revealing the Mysteries of Çatalhöyük*. Thames and Hudson, London.

Hodder, I., and C. Cessford 2004 Daily Practice and Social Memory at Çatalhöyük. *American Antiquity* 69(1):17–40.

Hodder, I. and S. R. Hutson 2003 *Reading the Past*. 3rd edition. Cambridge University Press, Cambridge.

Högberg, A. 2008 Playing with Flint: Tracing a Child's Imitation of Adult Work in a Lithic Assemblage. *Journal of Archaeological Method and Theory* 15:112–131.

Hutson, S. R. 2006 Children not at Chunchucmil: A Relational Approach to Young Subjects. In *The Social Experience of Childhood in Ancient Mesoamerica*, edited by T. Ardren and S. R. Hutson, pp. 103–132. University Press of Colorado, Boulder.

Hutson, S. R. 2010 *Dwelling, Identity and the Maya: Relational Archaeology at Chunchucmil*. Altamira, Lanham, Maryland.

Hutson, S. R. 2011 The Art of Becoming: The Graffiti of Tikal, Guatemala. *Latin American Antiquity* 22: 403–426.

Hutson, S. R., and T. W. Stanton 2007 Cultural Logic and Practical Reason: the Structure of Discard in Ancient Maya Houselots. *Cambridge Archaeological Journal* 17(1):123–144.

Ingold, T. 2000 *The Perception of the Environment: Essays on Livelihood, Dwelling, and Skill*. Routledge, London.

Jay, M. 1993 *Downcast Eye: The Denigration of Vision in Twentieth-Century French Thought*. University of California Press, Berkeley.

Jenkins, R. 2004 *Social Identity*. 2nd edition. Routledge, London.

Joyce, R. A. 1998 Performing the Body in Prehispanic Central America. *Res: Journal of Anthropology and Aesthetics* 33:147–165.

Joyce, R. A. 2002 Comment on Lesure. *Current Anthropology* 43(4):602–603.

Joyce, R. A. 2007 Figurines, Meaning, and Meaning-making in Early Mesoamerica. In *Image and Imagination: A Global Prehistory of Figurative Representation*, edited by C. Renfrew and I. Morley, pp. 101–110. McDonald Institute for Archaeological Research, Cambridge.

Kamp, K. A. 2001a Where Have all the Children Gone?: The Archaeology of Childhood. *Journal of Archaeological Method and Theory* 8(1):1–34.

Kamp, K.A. 2001b Prehistoric Children Working and Playing: A Southwestern Case Study in Learning Ceramics. *Journal of Anthropological Research* 57(4):427–450.

Kamp, K. A., N. Timmerman, G. Lind, J. Graybill, and I. Natowsky 1999 Discovering Childhood: Using Fingerprints to Find Children in the Archaeological Record. *American Antiquity* 64:309–315.

Kamp, K. A. and J. Whittaker 1999 *Surviving Adversity: The Sinagua of Lizard Man Village.* University of Utah Anthropological Papers 121, Salt Lake City.

Kuijt, I., and M. S. Chesson 2005 Lumps of Clay and Pieces of Stone: Ambiguity, Bodies, and Identity as Portrayed in Neolithic Figurines. In *Archaeologies of the Middle East: Critical Perspectives*, edited by S. Pollock and R. Bernbeck, pp. 152–183. Blackwell, Malden, Massachusetts.

Kuijt, I., and M. S. Chesson 2007 Imagery and Social Relationships: Shifting Identity and Ambiguity in the Neolithic. In *Image and Imagination: A Global Prehistory of Figurative Representation*, edited by C. Renfrew and I. Morley, pp. 211–226. McDonald Institute for Archaeological Research, Cambridge.

Latour, B. 1993 *We Have Never Been Modern.* Harvester-Wheatsheaf, New York.

Law, J., and M. Callon 1992 The Life and Death of an Aircraft: A Network Analysis of Technical Change. In *Shaping Technology/Building Society*, edited by W. E. Bijker and J. Law, pp. 21–52. MIT Press, Cambridge.

Lazzari, M. 2003 Archaeological Visions: Gender, Landscape and Optic Knowledge. *Journal of Social Archaeology* 3(2):194–222.

Lesure, R. 2002 The Goddess Diffracted: Thinking about the Figurines of Early Villages. *Current Anthropology* 43(4):587–610.

Lucy, S. 2005 The Archaeology of Age. In *The Archaeology of Identity: Approaches to Gender, Age, Status, Ethnicity, and Religion*, by M. Díaz-Andreu, S. Lucy, S. Babić, and D. N. Edwards, pp. 43–66. Routledge, New York.

Lopiparo, J. 2006 Crafting Children: Materiality, Social Memory, and the Reproduction of Terminal Classic House Societies in the Ulua Valley, Honduras. In *The Social Experience of Childhood in Mesoamerica*, edited by T. Ardren and S.R. Hutson, pp. 133–170. University Press of Colorado, Boulder.

Manzanilla, L., and L. Barba 1990 The Study of Activities in Classic Households: Two Case Studies from Coba and Teotihuacan. *Ancient Mesoamerica* 1:41–49.

McAdam, E. 1997 The Figurines from the 1982–5 Seasons of Excavations at Ain Ghazal. *Levant* 29:115–145.

McAnany, P. 2010 *Ancestral Maya Economies in Archaeological Perspective.* Cambridge University Press, Cambridge.

McCafferty, G., and S. D. McCafferty 2006 Boys and Girls Interrupted: Mortuary Evidence of Children from Postclassic Cholula, Puebla. In *The Social Experience of Childhood in Ancient Mesoamerica*, edited by T. Ardren and S. R. Hutson, pp. 25–53. University Press of Colorado, Boulder.

Meskell, L., and R. A. Joyce 2003 *Embodied Lives.* Routledge, London.

Meskell, L., C. Nakamura, R. King, and S. Farid 2008 Figured Lifeworlds and Depositional Practices at Çatalhöyük. *Cambridge Archaeological Journal* 18(2):139–161.

Olsen, B. 2003 Material Culture after Text: Re-Membering Things. *Norwegian Archaeological Review* 36(2):87–104.

Overholtzer, L. M. 2005 *The Kneeling Mexica Women: Evidence for Male Domination or Gender Complementarity?* Unpublished Senior Honors Thesis, Department of Anthropology, University of California at Berkeley.

Pigeot, N. 1990 Technical and Social Actors. Flint Knapping Specialists and Apprentices at Magdalenian Etiolles. *Archaeological Review from Cambridge* 9(1):126–141.

Preucel, R. W., and A. A. Bauer 2001 Archaeological Pragmatics. *Norwegian Archaeological Review* 34(2):85–96.

Prine, E. 2000 Searching for Third Genders: Towards a Prehistory of Domestic Space in Middle Missouri Villages. In *Archaeologies of Sexuality*, edited by R. A. Schmidt and B. L. Voss, pp. 197–219. Routledge, London.

Renfrew, C. 1994 Towards a Cognitive Archaeology. In *The Ancient Mind: Elements of a Cognitive Archaeology*, edited by C. Renfrew, pp. 3–12. Cambridge University Press, Cambridge.

Rollefson, G. O. 2008 Charming Lives: Human and Animal Figurines in the Late Epipaleolithic and Early Neolithic Periods in the Greater Levant and Eastern Anatolia. In *The Neolithic Demographic Transition and its Consequences*, edited by J.-P. Bocquet-Appel and O. Bar-Yosef, pp. 287–313. Springer, Netherlands.

Román Berrellaza, J. A., and X. Chávez Balderas 2006 The Role of Children in the Ritual Practices of the Great Temple of Tenochtitlan and the Great Temple of Tlatelolco. In *The Social Experience of Childhood in Ancient Mesoamerica*, edited by T. Ardren and S. R. Hutson, pp. 235–250. University Press of Colorado, Boulder.

Sahagún, B. de 1950–1982 *The Florentine Codex.* Translated by Arthur J. O. Anderson and C. E. Dibble. Monographs of the School of American Research, Santa Fe, and University of New Mexico Press, Albuquerque.

Said, E. 1979 *Orientalism.* Vintage, New York.

Salmon, M. 1976 Deductive Versus Inductive Archaeology. *American Antiquity* 41:376–381.

Scott, E. 1997 Introduction: On the Incompleteness of Archaeological Narratives. In *Invisible People and Processes: Writing Gender and Childhood into European Archaeology*, edited by J. Moore and E. Scott, pp. 1–14. Leicester University Press, London.

Sewell, W. H., Jr. 1992 A Theory of Structure: Duality, Agency and Transformation. *American Journal of Sociology* 98(1):1–29.

Sillar, B. 1994 Playing with God: Cultural Perceptions of Children, Play, and Miniatures in the Andes. *Archaeological Review from Cambridge* 13(2):47–63.

Smith, M. E. 2002 Domestic Ritual at Aztec Provincial Sites in Morelos. In *Domestic Ritual in Ancient Mesoamerica*, edited by P. Plunket, pp. 93–114. Cotsen Institute of Archaeology, Los Angeles.

Smith, P. E. 2005 Children and Ceramic Innovation: A Study in the Archaeology of Children. In *Children in Action: Perspectives on the Archaeology of Childhood*, edited by J. E. Baxter, pp. 65–76. Anthropological Papers of the American Anthropological Association, Number 15. American Anthropological Association, Washington, D.C.

Sofaer Derevenski, J. 1997 Engendering Children, Engendering Archaeology. In *Invisible People and Processes: Writing Gender and Childhood into European Archaeology*, edited by J. Moore and E. Scott, pp. 192–202. Leicester University Press, London.

Spector, J. 1993 *What This Awl Means.* Minnesota Historical Society Press, St. Paul.

Strathern, M. 1988 *The Gender of the Gift: Problems with Women and Problems with Society in Melanesia*. University of California Press, Berkeley.

Taylor, W. 1948 *A Study of Archaeology*. Southern Illinois University Press, Carbondale.

Thomas, J. 1993 The Hermeneutics of Megalithic Space. In *Interpretative Archaeology*, edited by C. Tilley, pp. 73–98. Berg, Oxford.

Tilley, C. 1994 *A Phenomenology of Landscape: Places, Paths, and Monuments*. Berg, Providence, Rhode Island.

Tilley, C. 2004 *The Materiality of Stone: Explorations in Landscape Phenomenology*. Berg, Oxford.

Tourtellot, G. 1983 An Assessment of Classic Maya Household Composition. In *Prehispanic Settlement Patterns: Essays in Honor of Gordon R. Willey*, edited by E. Vogt and R. Leventhal, pp. 35–54. Peabody Museum of Archaeology and Ethnology, Harvard University, Cambridge.

Tringham, R. 1991 Households with Faces: The Challenge of Gender in Prehistoric Architectural Remains. In *Engendering Prehistory*, edited by J. M. Gero and M. W. Conkey, pp. 93–131. Blackwell, Oxford.

Tuan, Y.-F. 1977 *Space and Place: The Perspective of Experience*. University of Minnesota Press, Minneapolis.

Ucko, P.J. 1968 *Anthropomorphic Figurines of Predynastic Egypt and Neolithic Crete with Comparative Material from the Prehistoric Near East and Mainland Crete*. A. Szmidla, London.

Vajsov, I. 1992 Antropomorphnata Plastika na Kulturata Hamandzhiya. *Dobrudzha* 9:35–71.

Voigt, M. M. 2000 Çatal Höyük in Context: Ritual at Early Neolithic Sites in Central and Eastern Turkey. In *Life in Neolithic Farming Communities: Social Organization, Identity, and Differentiation*, edited by I. Kuijt, pp. 253–294. Kluwer Academic/Plenum, New York.

Voss, B. L., and R. A. Schmidt 2000 Archaeologies of Sexuality: An Introduction. In *Archaeologies of Sexuality*, edited by R. A. Schmidt and B. L. Voss, pp. 1–34. Routledge, London.

Wallaert-Pêtre, H. 2001 Learning How to Make the Right Pots: Apprenticeship Strategies and Material Culture, a Case Study in Handmade Pottery from Cameroon. *Journal of Anthropological Research* 57(4):471–493.

Webmoor, T., and C. L. Witmore 2008 Things Are Us. *Norwegian Archaeological Review* 41(1):53–66.

Wilkie, L. 2000 Not Merely Child's Play: Creating a Historical Archaeology of Children and Childhood. In *Children and Material Culture*, edited by J. Sofaer Derevenski, pp. 100–114. Routledge, London.

Wilson, B., and M. Wilson 1977 An Iconoclastic View of the Imagery Sources in the Drawings of Young People. *Art Education* 30:5–11.

Wylie, A. 1991 Gender Theory and the Archaeological Record: Why Is There No Archaeology of Gender? In *Engendering Archaeology*, edited by M. W. Conkey and J. M. Gero, pp. 31–54. Blackwell, Oxford.

CHAPTER FOUR

Bodies and Encounters

Seeing Invisible Children in Archaeology

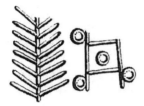

Joanna Sofaer

Abstract *The study of children in archaeology has frequently been framed in terms of their visibility or rather, in many cases, their invisibility. This chapter examines why the in/visibility of children remains such a persistent theme by scrutinizing some of the theoretical and methodological underpinnings of existing approaches to the study of children in archaeology. In particular, it explores the ways that investigating children in the past has become dependent upon the presence of child bodies in archaeological contexts. I argue that the archaeological need to have a visible body in order to "do" the archaeology of children creates significant and unnecessary restrictions to inquiry. As a response, I examine other possibilities for accessing children in the past by reconsidering the role of the child body and the perceived need for its visibility in archaeological contexts.*

THE VISIBILITY AND INVISIBILITY OF CHILDREN IN ARCHAEOLOGY

The study of children in archaeology has frequently been framed in terms of the visibility or rather, in many cases, the invisibility of children in the past. Despite a recent surge in scholarship, more than twelve years since the first publications on children in archaeology, it seems to have been difficult for the discipline to move beyond this question of in/visibility. Although the contextually dependent natures of "children" and "childhood" now form key foci of investigation, and there has been welcome expansion of the range of periods and places in which children have been examined, much of this work constitutes case studies rather than a radical reappraisal of the ways that past children might be encountered. In this chapter, I want to explore why the in/visibility of children remains such a persistent theme by scrutinizing some of the theoretical and methodological underpinnings of existing approaches to the study of children in archaeology. My particular focus is the child body, since the absence or presence of child bodies frequently forms the basis for archaeological assessments of in/visibility. I want to argue that the archaeological need to have a visible body in order to "do" the archaeology of children creates significant and unnecessary restrictions to enquiry. In response to the limitations of current approaches, I want to examine what other possibilities there might be for accessing children in the past by reconsidering what we mean by the child body and the perceived need for its visibility in archaeological contexts.

SETTING THE IN/VISIBILITY AGENDA

Concern with the in/visibility of children in the archaeological record was first voiced in the late 1980s and 1990s when children were identified as a distinct social category worthy of study in archaeology (Crawford 1991; Lillehammer 1989; Moore and Scott 1997; Roveland 1997; Sofaer Derevenski 1994a). This work followed the precedent set by early Gender Archaeology, which commented upon women as a hitherto archaeologically marginalized social group in order to generate more rounded interpretations of the past (e.g., Classen 1992; Gero and Conkey 1991). Since children must have been part of ancient societies, it was argued that archaeological interpretations also needed to "put them back into the past" in order to create more authentic versions of human history. Capturing the mood, publications were given titles such as "Where Are the Children?" (Sofaer Derevenski 1994b), "Invisible People and Processes" (Moore and Scott 1997), or "Where Have All the Children Gone" (Kamp 2001a).

    To fulfill this brief, much of the early research on children concentrated on identifying the kinds of archaeological materials in which children could be recognized. This also made the point that the omission of children from archaeological interpretation was more a question of investigator bias than of the potential of archaeological contexts for social interpretations. "Seeing" children sometimes involved the identification of specific forms of child-associated material culture, most readily described as toys or childcare paraphernalia (see Egan 1998; Kamp 2001a; Wileman 2005), and miniatures (e.g., Park 1998), but also including material interventions by children (e.g., Hammond and Hammond 1981; Kamp 2001b; Wilkie 2000). More frequently, however, researchers turned to settings in which children themselves were physically present, such as mortuary contexts (e.g., Lucy 2005; Meskell 1994; Rega 1997; Scott 1991) or iconographic representations and figurines (e.g., Janssen and Janssen 1990; Joyce 2000); whereas a specific material culture of children often proved difficult to definitively identify, the body was perceived as offering incontrovertible and ready opportunities to document children in the past.

    More often than not, the identification of children has required investigators to identify child bodies. Scholars have investigated specific locations where children's bodies were found through mortuary studies (e.g., Borić and Stefanović 2004; Mays 1993; McKerr et al. 2009; Scott 1993; Smith and Kahila 1992), asked how children were depicted (e.g., Beaumont 2000; Golden 1990; Janssen and Janssen 1990), described what children's bodies looked like in terms of their skeletal remains (e.g., Bogin 1999; Humphrey 2000; Lewis 2007; Lorentz 2008; Scheuer and Black 2000), or recorded imprints of child bodies as footprints, finger impressions, or paintings (e.g., Guthrie 2005; Kamp et al. 1999; Roveland 2000). This focus on the body has been extended in the theoretical development of life course perspectives and discussions of child identity. Here, associations between objects and bodies of different ages and sex have been used to characterize children in relation to others, rather than taking them to be a predefined or self-evident category (e.g., Gowland 2006; Joyce 2000; Sánchez-Romero 2008; Sofaer Derevenski 2000a).

An often tacit concern with the body has therefore come to dominate the archaeological study of children. Indeed, within the discipline the body has become almost a sine qua non for childhood studies. Nonetheless, a methodologically driven focus on the body also creates problems for archaeology. In particular, a focus on the body means that children become inaccessible in situations where there are no child bodies. This means that, for example, there are almost no studies of children in domestic contexts, the exceptions being historical settings with documentary evidence (e.g., Baxter 2005; Wilkie 2003). Yet these are contexts that one might expect children to have inhabited. Archaeological attitudes to the child body thus beg a series of questions: What do we stand to gain from a study of children if it is only to show what we already know: that children existed in the past? Is it possible to archaeologically access children in contexts where there are no child bodies? Furthermore, as it stands, the notion of in/visibility implies that children are passive—that they need to be "made visible"—but could it be possible to investigate child action? In order to answer these questions it is useful to take a step back to more closely examine the role of the child body in archaeology.

THE BODY IN THE ARCHAEOLOGY OF CHILDREN

The body is critical to understanding children as a category since it is body difference that makes a child a child as opposed to any other age-related category. In particular, intense and rapid whole body changes that occur during the early years of life are seen as characteristic of children (Prout 2000). Changes to the physical body, such as the development of secondary sex characteristics, are frequently understood in terms of a shift in social identity away from child to adult as the body is given symbolic and moral value (James 1993; Prendergast 2000). Understandings of the child body are therefore both material and social (Prout 2000). For archaeologists working with the physical remains of children the notion of body change is particularly powerful because of the sheer number of changes and their clarity in the human skeleton (Sofaer 2006).

Yet, as many researchers have pointed out it, it is not enough simply to identify immature bodies as children since cultural categorizations of children are variable. Who is a child in one society, is not in another (Welinder 1998). In taking this approach, archaeologists have been heavily influenced by anthropological and sociological insights pointing to variability in social perceptions and definitions of children and childhood (see Bluebond-Langer and Korbin 2007; Montgomery 2009). Many archaeological studies have therefore attempted to identify children by locating culturally specific boundaries of childhood through associations between material culture and age categories (e.g., Crawford 1991; Gowland 2001, 2006; Lucy 2005). On their own, however, statements regarding the culturally variable nature of the child category and the claim for children as illuminating cultural difference tend to be trite if they are not accompanied by a more penetrating analysis (Montgomery 2009:12).

Furthermore, the way that the child body is methodologically placed in such analyses means that archaeologists have found it difficult to move toward an understanding of archaeological children that links the materiality of the body and the social in a satisfying way (Sofaer 2006). In other words, standard archaeological method makes associations between bodies of designated chronological ages and forms of material culture, where age is determined through a combination of osteological and dental estimates. This kind of approach treats the child body as universal, inasmuch as stereotypes of the physiologically "normal" child are used as templates for how children are expected to look at certain ages (Steedman 1995). Thus, while the method of artifact association allows for the investigation of the range of expression in what past people may have made of the body, there is little room for understanding variability and cultural contingency of the body itself, since the body is taken for granted (Sofaer 2006). Children thus continue to be interpreted within a naturalistic frame. In such analyses, material culture acts as symbolic capital that confers identity upon the user or owner (Budden and Sofaer 2009). This places children as passive recipients of identity overlaid on the body, which acts as a kind of substrate. This in turn means that the kinds of questions that can be asked of child bodies are somewhat reduced.

Although an understanding of categories is important, since people operate in the world by recognizing these (Sørensen 2000), the method of artifact association, as it is frequently deployed, clearly has drawbacks in relation to the study of children. In order to move beyond these, it may be useful to rethink the relationship between the child body and material culture and to consider what kinds of new questions or insights this might provoke.

MATERIAL CULTURE, THE BODY, AND AN ARCHAEOLOGY OF ONTOGENY

The first step in such a reconsideration is to address the preconception that in order to "see" children in the archaeological record it is necessary to identify a child-specific material culture either by direct association with child bodies or independently of these. Children, as other social categories, live in a world of objects. From the moment they are born, they are surrounded by the material culture of their society. In order to examine the relationship between children and material culture it is not therefore necessary to a priori posit or determine a suite of distinctive child objects (Wood 2009), even though these may exist in some settings in the form of toys, child care paraphernalia, or other kinds of objects. Having accepted this point, the issue then becomes how to understand and analyze the relationship between children and material culture if objects are not exclusive to a particular social category, while acknowledging that objects may simultaneously have different meanings to different people (cf. Baxter 2005).

One way forward is to consider the effects of material culture on the people who live with it. It has long been understood that environmental conditions impact on human growth and nutrition (see Bogin 2001; Coleman 1995). Similarly, a range of studies have argued that the emotional and psychological development of children is affected in various ways by the social, emotional, and cultural contexts of their care (see Bretherton 1997; Butterworth and Harris 1994; Valsiner and Rosa 2007). Given that material culture also forms part of the environment in its broadest sense, it may be useful to think about material culture in relation to human development.

Material culture has a profound impact on human development through the process of ontogeny (Sofaer 2011; Toren 1999). Following Toren (1999, 2001, 2007) human ontogeny can be understood as a process of self-creation or autopoesis of the "whole person." It is an embodied and ongoing process grounded in active engagement with one's surroundings in which cognitive development is a material phenomenon; learning how to behave in an appropriate manner involves changes to both mind and body as physical and inseparable entities (Ingold 2001; Sofaer 2006; Toren 1999). In this phe-nomenologically inspired perspective there is no need to posit a dialectical relationship between mind and body, biology and culture, or individual and society (Toren 2003). People are historical accumulations of experience whose contingency is linked to their relations to other people and to objects. In other words, people literally make themselves through learning in a social setting. They literally embody their histories and the histories of their relations with others and the material world (Toren 1999:2). Bodies will therefore develop differently under different material conditions.

This emphasis on the body differentiates the notion of ontogeny from the more frequently used concept of socialization (Sofaer 2011). It also foregrounds the ways that people are active in their own development through learning that they need to "belong" in a given social context, rather than implying a top-down view of culture imposed on passive individuals (Toren 2007). In terms of ontogeny, intersubjectivity is vital to human development since a person's moment-to-moment encounters with the material world are always and inevitably mediated by relations with others. It is the differences and similarities in encounters with others and the material world that result both in unique experiential histories for each person, as well as shared experiences at a given historical moment (Toren 2003).

In this view people are not biological containers to be simply filled up with culture (Ingold 1998) but actively engage with the world in and through their bodies. Body actions and expressions therefore become key to understanding and investigating the contextually specific material circumstances of human development. For example, in her ethnographic study of child cognition and the learning of hierarchy in Fiji, Toren (1999) describes how the deportment and spatial disposition of the child body manifests the phenomenology of learning in Fijian longhouses. The embodiment of behavior is key to the process by which behaviors are understood over time and to the reproduction of ritual and ritualized behavior (Toren 1999). This does not mean, however, that children necessarily act like mini-adults. Indeed, in Toren's example children have to accommodate adult concerns by sitting, crawling, walking, clapping, or taking food in the prescribed manner. Here the body is critical to simultaneously learning and expressing behavior appropriate to one's particular age and position in the social hierarchy.

Embodied engagement with the material world thus involves learning gestures, or "techniques of the body" (Mauss 1935), appropriate to one's society and place within it. These techniques are learned body actions, which are not just expressive of social values imposed on the body but are acquired skills that develop in specific settings in particular ways depending on the surrounding environment in its broadest sense, including caregivers, objects, and the physical landscape (Ingold 1998). Techniques of the body are thus fundamental to the social and cultural context of daily life and it is not possible to separate learning to do things from learning to do things in the approved manner of one's society (Ingold 1998:26). Importantly for archaeology, techniques may be closely related to the form of material culture enabling a working back from object forms to the body actions, or rather range of potential body actions or postures, involved in their use. Thus, Leroi-Gourhan (1971 [1943]) famously presented different ways that individual objects belonging to a single class of artifact were used in culturally specific ways linked to their form. For example, contrasting basket forms could be carried with a tumpline, on the head, on the back, or in the hand. Likewise, objects with blades were classified into those involving different kinds of gestures including those that require the blade to be pushed, lanced with the point down, or pushed with a striker (Leroi-Gourhan 1971 [1943]). This, then, is not just about what something is used for—the much vaunted relationship between form and function that underpins a great deal of archaeological interpretation—but is also about *how* it is used. It therefore offers insights into the nature of gestures that need to be learned.

Ethnoarchaeological studies in the French tradition have employed this approach to analyze in detail the gestures and skills required to learn crafts such as bead making or pottery manufacture (Roux 2000; Roux and Corbetta 1990). Ergonomic analyses have also been deployed to investigate the complexity of muscle actions involved in apparently simple tasks such as sitting or brushing teeth (Arcadio et al.1973). More recently, some Scandinavian archaeologists have begun to document studies of movement in relation to the use of material culture. Using filming techniques to record and visualize the breakdown of body movements into individual actions, and inspired by notations used in dance choreography to write down this movement choreography, they have moved from experimental work to the actions involved in making past objects (Bender Jørgensen 2006). Høgseth (2007), for example, has used this approach to study the actions involved in Medieval carpentry. He recorded axe and saw marks on timbers in buildings and through experimental work identified body actions that would be required to make those marks. Within Anglo-American archaeology however, despite some exceptions, investigations of body gestures have received relatively little attention (Ingold 2001; Sofaer 2006).

Body gestures need to be learned, but this process—through material encounters and intersubjectivity—is not confined to children. It takes place throughout the life course as people move through categories of age as well as of gender and status, and accumulate material and intersubjective experiences. There is, therefore, no fundamental ontological difference per se between children and other age categories (Sofaer Derevenski 2000b; Sofaer 2011). Instead, the difference between children and other social categories is one of degree; younger individuals are particularly plastic and, having less of a reservoir of experience, are exposed to a greater number of new experiences and therefore subject to more rapid development. Furthermore, while body difference defines children, this is also the case for other age categories such as the elderly (Appleby 2010); bodies are defined not only in their own terms but in relation to others.

The implications of the ontological similarity between children and other categories for archaeological method are profound since it means that the study of human ontogeny does not require us to predefine what a child *is* before we can explore human development. Nor does it deny the existence of culturally contingent social categories. Instead, it creates a new set of challenges about the nature of human experience in terms of the ways that meanings and interactions may alter as people's understandings change and accumulate with age. This perspective invites us to think about material culture in relation to the processes that underpin the creation of social categories, rather than the description of those categories alone. It offers analytical possibilities for exploring common developmental experiences in particular times and places in terms of what people needed to learn in order to "belong" to a particular society, as well as more detailed investigations of the ontogeny of people belonging to particular social groups/categories (Sofaer 2011). In other words, what the often used term *cultural difference* means in practice; the things that we all learn in our society that allow us to "fit in," but that also provide for culture shock when we go somewhere very different.

Tracing Ontogeny in the Archaeological Record

Given my arguments above, exploring human ontogeny in the archaeological record requires tracing learned embodied interaction with material culture. Of course, not all interactions with material culture will be archaeologically accessible, but it is possible to suggest two general levels on which such interactions may be explored archaeologically. These can be briefly summarized as learning to *make* objects and learning to *use* objects. The distinction between making and using is to some extent artificial but provides clarity in the provision of examples and involves different pathways in order to investigate them. The first involves following the process of learning to make objects by identifying patterns of error (inappropriate body actions) fossilized in archaeological material. The second examines the ways that "finished" material culture creates body gestures (appropriate body actions), which have to be learned in order to use finished objects.

Ontogeny 1: Learning to Make Things

In recent years there has been increasing focus on identifying apprenticeship in the material record in ethnographic contexts and in the past (e.g., Crown 1999; Ferguson 2008;

Wendrich 2012). While apprentices need not necessarily be children (Ferguson 2008), since the learning of craft skills may require considerable training and practice, many ethnographic studies suggest that the learning of traditional craft skills (whether formally or informally) can begin early in life (Greenfield 2000; Grimm 2000). Furthermore, the development of craft skills is a very physical process that requires the craftsperson to engage bodily with his or her material and tools (Budden and Sofaer 2009). The production of different kinds of objects requires different suites of body actions from the maker, who has to engage with varying technical requirements and tools. It therefore constitutes the development of embodied knowledge (Sofaer and Budden 2012).

Research has examined apprenticeship in a range of materials including flint knapping (Grimm 2000; Pigeot 1990), pottery manufacture (Budden 2008; Crown 1999; Sofaer and Budden 2012), bead making (Roux 2000), and weaving (Greenfield 2000). Much of this work has typically focused on identifying the presence of novices by identifying technical errors in working toward an "ideal" object type at different stages of the manufacturing process or *chaîne opératoire*. For example, at the French Upper Palaeolithic site of Solvieux, a novice knapper was identified through his/her relative lack of control over basic technical principals (Grimm 2000). These technical errors in core reduction reflect body gestures that were inappropriate to the task.

Yet at Solvieux, the apprentice knapper was not alone. S/he appears to have been guided by a master (Grimm 2000). While research on apprenticeship in the archaeological record has typically been expressed in terms of identifying novices at work through the identification of technical error it can also be understood in ontogenetic terms. The development of craft skills is a product of the relationship between the learner and others in society, whether by observation and imitation, informal instruction or formal guidance (Baxter 2005; Crown 2001, 2002; David 1990; Michelaki 2008; Sofaer and Budden 2012). Learning to make things is an intersubjective process in which learners join a community of practice (Lave and Wenger 1991). It implies a learning process in which less experienced makers of objects learn how to craft things from more experienced makers. In other words, the errors visible in archaeological material do not just represent the development of technical skill but represent the process of ontogeny itself; the "becoming" of a knapper, a potter, a weaver, or a smith.

Within communities of practice, learning takes place through different kinds of "participation frameworks" in which apprentices learn through participating in the practices of experts (Lave and Wenger 1991). Such frameworks offer a range of different social and pedagogical models for the nature of the master-apprentice relationship. It can involve scaffolded (highly structured) or unscaffolded (relatively independent trial and error) learning (Gosselain 1992, 1998; Greenfield 2000; Greenfield, Maynard, and Childs 2000; Wallaert-Pêtre 2001). In scaffolded learning, learners are guided by teachers who provide practical help and verbal direction in accordance with the developmental level of the learner (Greenfield 2000). Advice is freely available and learners observe and follow models presented by more skilled practitioners. In strongly scaffolded situations, teachers intervene before learners have the opportunity to make errors, and learners have little chance to make mistakes, innovate, or experiment. Thus, the transmission of traditional ways of doing things is ensured (Greenfield 2000). By contrast, in unscaffolded learning, learners are offered very little guidance. This leads to a much higher rate of error but also encourages innovation and experimentation (Greenfield 2000; Greenfield, Maynard, and Childs 2000). By examining the patterns of error in objects it is possible to explore the nature of relationships at play between individual learners and more experienced craftspeople, and thus further explore the process of ontogeny.

In a recent study of ceramics from the Middle Bronze Age site of Százhalombatta in Hungary, Budden (2008) found a relatively high frequency of technical errors in simple vessel types such as cups, while complex fine wares with well-prepared clays showed very few such errors. She argued that this showed the presence of apprentice potters practicing and making mistakes on simpler forms, while more proficient potters produced more complicated vessels using better quality resources where there may have been a lower tolerance for error (Budden 2008; Budden and Sofaer 2009). She also identified a number of "mixed message" pots that can be interpreted as the product of more than one hand, with people of different skills and experience collaborating together (Budden 2007; Sofaer and Budden 2012), this feature has also been noted in other rather different ceramic assemblages (cf. Crown 2007). These vessels indicate that more experienced help was available to guide learner potters, either by being assisted through the input of more experienced helpers, or where learners were encouraged to add to their skills by working on pots made by more experienced potters.

The evidence from Százhalombatta therefore points to a range of competencies—a situation that might be expected when beginners or apprentice potters who have not yet acquired a full range of skills work alongside more experienced ones—although the existence of errors in less technically complex vessel forms suggests that potters were allowed to make their own mistakes (Sofaer and Budden 2012). Furthermore, synchronic and diachronic variation in vessel form suggest that innovation was possible, albeit within strict rules surrounding the "correct" culturally acceptable way to make a pot (Budden and Sofaer 2009). Learning at Százhalombatta may therefore have been lightly or moderately scaffolded; novice potters frequently worked on their own but acted within a wider environment where they were able to draw on the help and support of others (Sofaer and Budden 2012).

ONTOGENY 2: LEARNING TO USE THINGS

Just as learning to make things is an ontogenetic process, so too is learning to use objects in a culturally appropriate manner. The body is a prerequisite for the interaction between people and objects and it is through this interaction that bodies themselves develop. For example, learning to write involves not only a knowledge of letters and numbers but a learned bodily understanding of how to grip a pencil, press down on the page with just the right amount of weight, and how to move it in the correct way to draw the desired figure. Learning to write is therefore a collaboration between the body and the object that takes place in a social setting, through which the body develops as it becomes more practiced. Malafouris (2008:115) broadens this argument by suggesting that material culture has the ability to change and shape bodies by transforming and extending the boundaries of "body schema"; the neuronal map associated with body positions that he places at the center of his understanding of embodied cognition.

Since the material world is critical to human development, an understanding of the ways that bodies and objects work together can be used to explore human ontogeny. This may be particularly useful in exploring ontogenetic changes over time, since the acquisition of particular socially appropriate body movements in relation to new or different objects will result in contrasts in learning experiences. I have recently argued that changes in pottery forms and their distribution within houses at the Bronze Age tell at Százhalombatta had an impact on human ontogeny through altering social dynamics and body gestures in relation to changes in movement through domestic space (Sofaer 2011). So-called typological changes thus, in fact, represent ontogenetic changes. To further illustrate what I mean, it is useful to give an additional example.

Bronze weaponry is a well-documented feature of the European Bronze Age. It is found in hoards, as single finds, and in graves. The sequence of development of European Bronze Age weaponry is well documented. In general, there is a move from small daggers to dirks and rapiers by the Middle Bronze Age, and to swords in the later Middle Bronze Age. This reflects changes in styles of combat. While daggers may have been "last chance" close-quarters weapons or used as pocket knives, rapiers are long thin thrusting weapons, which required greater precision than daggers and which would have required a degree of training in their use (Osgood et al. 2000). The swords take a range of forms with the general development of a leaf-shaped blade suited to a slashing or cut-and-thrust type of action (Harding 1999; Osgood 2000 et al.). Although not all swords were used in combat (some being symbolic objects), many display evidence of blade damage as a result of combat and subsequent resharpening (Bridgford 1997; Kristiansen 1984, 2002).

Each of these different types of weapons requires different skills, fighting techniques, and learned body movements. In particular, the development of the sword changed body action substantially. As Malafouris (2008:118) puts it in his discussion of Mycenaean swords as body parts, the sword "draws out of the . . . body a novel predisposition for action not previously available." The development of defensive equipment, including shields, helmets, corselets, and greaves, which are known particularly from the Late Bronze Age, also speaks to distinct fighting styles in which the body moved in particular ways. To be a warrior it was not enough simply to hold a weapon. To be involved in combat—even if ritual or symbolic—meant that the warrior knew how to *use* a weapon and this must have been a learned skill. Training for combat involves learning how to hold, swing, and sheath a weapon, simultaneously developing endurance, musculature, and neuronal and motor pathways. For these skills to be effectively developed, and in order to capitalize on the plasticity and strength of youth, training may begin at a young age. Spartan boys famously began their military training at the age of seven years (Cartledge 2003). Similarly, the path to becoming a Medieval knight also began at about age seven or eight, when boys left the care of women to become pages or to be placed into the care of male tutors, with training as squires starting between ages 10 and 14 (Orme 1984). Ethnographic examples from the Americas and Papua New Guinea reveal boys "playing" war from an early age

(Vandkilde 2007). Becoming a warrior is therefore about developing the body knowledge that underpins being part of that category; it is gaining identity through doing. As such, the development of knowledge and age are inextricably linked together.

In mortuary contexts, European Bronze Age weaponry is almost exclusively associated with males (Vandkilde 2007; Wilson 2007). This association between people and objects has led to widespread interpretations of an elite male warrior aristocracy (Kristinansen 1999; Treherne 1995; Vandkilde 2003, 2007). Discussions have also considered different institutional forms of warriorhood and the social structuring of martial identities, with particular focus on contextual differences in the ages of people buried with weapons (Vandkilde 2007; Wilson 2007). Irrespective of the age of person with whom weapons were deposited, what is important for an understanding of ontogeny is that being a warrior is an intersubjective experience on at least two levels. First, as Vandkilde (2007:80) points out, being a warrior is, like any other social identity, "individually felt and collectively shared." Second, combat and learning to fight necessarily involves at least one, if not many, other people to fight against (cf. Vandkilde 2007).

Shifts in weapon types and combat techniques that we see in the archaeological record thus reveal diachronic shifts in human experience that are the consequence of material changes. Different ways of fighting will, in turn, lead to different ontogenies, resulting in physically different kinds of human bodies. Yet the relationship between objects and human ontogeny is not one way. Just as ontogeny is the product of intersubjectivity and experiences of the material world, so it is that experiences can also lead to changes in material culture (Sofaer 2011). Intriguingly, some Bronze Age rapiers appear to have been used in an unsuitable (and perhaps more natural) slashing movement, shown by tears found on the rivet holes of the handles of such weapons and some iconographic depictions (Harding 1999; Osgood et al. 2000). The experience and consequences of using rapiers in this way may have led to the typological changes seen in the archaeological record and the development of the sword. New and different weapon types may therefore have been the product of previous accumulated understandings. As Toren (2007: 23) puts it, "Children are born into a world in the making that was already rendered meaningful in all its material aspects, and with time they [make] these meanings anew." This reconfiguration happens through interactions with others and the constant negotiation and assimilation of understandings. Such a process provides for a relationship between changes in social organization and material change where one need not precede the other. It may be this never-ending body-centered learning—rather than abstract processes of "typological development," "evolution," or "innovation"—that underpins material change (Sofaer 2011).

CONCLUSION

Rather than helping archaeologists to "do" an archaeology of children, a frequent focus on the in/visibility of children in the archaeological record has inadvertently created methodological barriers to understanding children in the past. The requirement for a child body in order to evidence children in the past has not only made it impossible to "see" them in contexts where bodies are not physically present, but has also detracted from understanding *why* the study of children is a worthwhile endeavor.

In this chapter, I have argued that rethinking the methodological issues posed by child bodies offers the possibility to access children in contexts where physical bodies are not present. I have suggested that this may be done by widening archaeological understandings of the relationship between bodies and objects. In addition to the ways that material culture acts as a signifier of identity, it is useful to understand *how bodies interact with the material world* in order to ask questions about human development. Since different forms of material culture have the potential to produce qualitatively different kinds of bodies (Sofaer 2006, 2011; see also Malafouris 2008), understanding the ways that people learn to make and use the material world allows us to ask one of the fundamental questions of human life: "How do people become who they are?" (Toren 1999). Seen through this lens, a focus on children is important because it highlights human ontogeny. For although ontogeny is a lifelong process, the plasticity and rapidity of human development in the early years are particularly critical. Ontogeny is the counterpart to the construction of social categories (Sofaer 2011).

An archaeology of ontogeny is challenging. It asks us to consider the body in ways that focus on the implications of bodily difference in relation to the material world, rather than the presence or absence of objects linked to the physical body per se. It provokes ambitious questions about the material and social conditions under which human development takes place. Furthermore, the reflexive and intersubjective nature of human development also hints at a means by which active human experience can lead to alteration of the material world. Yet, these same challenges also mean that encountering the "invisible" body is also full of archaeological possibilities.

REFERENCES CITED

Appleby, J. 2010 Why We Need an Archaeology of Old Age, and a Suggested Approach. *Norwegian Archaeological Review* 43(2):145–168.

Arcadio, F., A. Moulay, and P. Chauvinc 1973 *Gestes de la Vie Qotidienne*. Masson et Cie, Editeurs, Lyon.

Baxter, J. E. 2005 *The Archaeology of Childhood. Children, Gender and Material Culture*. AltaMira Press, Walnut Creek, California.

Beaumont, L. 2000 The Social Status and Artistic Representation of "Adolescence" in Fifth Century Athens. In *Children and Material Culture*, edited by J. Sofaer Derevenski, pp. 39–50. Routledge, London.

Bender Jørgensen, L. 2006 *Embodying Belief: Practice as a Form of Knowledge*. Paper presented at the 12th Annual European Archaeological Association Meeting, Cracow.

Bluebond-Langner, M., and J. Korbin 2007 Challenges and Opportunities in the Anthropology of Childhoods: An Introduction to "Children, Childhoods, and Childhood Studies." *American Anthropologist* 109:241–246.

Bogin, B. 1999 *Patterns of Human Growth*. Cambridge University Press, Cambridge.

Bogin, B. 2001 *The Growth of Humanity*. Wiley-Liss, New York.

Borić, D., and S. Stefanović 2004 Birth and Death: Infant Burials from Vlasac and Lepenski Vir. *Antiquity* 78:526–546.

Bretherton, I. 1997 Bowlby's Legacy to Developmental Psychology. *Child Psychiatry and Human Development* 28(1):33–43.

Bridgford, S. 1997 Mightier than the Pen? An Edgewise Look at Irish Bronze Age Swords. In *Material Harm: Archaeological Studies of War and Violence*, edited by J. Carman, pp. 95–115. Cruithne Press, Glasgow.

Budden, S. 2007 Renewal and Reinvention: The Role of Learning Strategies in the Early to Late Middle Bronze Age of the Carpathian Basin. Unpublished PhD Dissertation, University of Southampton.

Budden, S. 2008 Skill Amongst the Sherds: Understanding the Role of Skill in the Early to Late Middle Bronze Age in Hungary. In *Breaking the Mould: Challenging the Past through Pottery*, Proceedings of the 3rd International Conference on Prehistoric Ceramics. University of Manchester, 6–8 October 2006, edited by I. Berg, pp. 1–17. BAR International Series 1861, Oxford.

Budden, S., and J. Sofaer 2009 Non-Discursive Knowledge and the Construction of Identity. Potters, Potting, and Performance at the Bronze Age Tell of Százhalombatta, Hungary. *Cambridge Archaeological Journal* 19(2):203–220.

Butterworth, G., and M. Harris 1994 *Principles of Developmental Psychology: An Introduction*. Psychology Press, Hove.

Cartledge, P. 2003 *The Spartans: The World of the Warrior-Heroes of Ancient Greece*. The Overlook Press, Woodstock.

Classen, C. 1992 *Exploring Gender through Archaeology*. Prehistory Press, Madison.

Coleman, D. 1995 Human Migration: Effects on People, Effects on Populations. In *Human Variability and Plasticity*, edited by C. G. Nicholas Mascie-Taylor and B. Bogin, pp. 115–145. Cambridge University Press, Cambridge.

Crawford, S. 1991 When Do Anglo-Saxon Saxon Children Count? *Journal of Theoretical Archaeology* 2:17–24.

Crown, P. 1999 Socialization in American Southwest Pottery Decoration. In *Pottery and People: A Dynamic Interaction*, edited by J. Skibo and G. Feinman, pp. 25–43. University of Utah Press, Salt Lake City.

Crown, P. 2001 Learning to Make Pottery in the Prehispanic American Southwest. *Journal of Anthropological Research* 57:451–469.

Crown, P. 2002 Learning and Teaching in the Pre-Hispanic American Southwest. In *Children in the Puebloan Southwest*, edited by K. Kamp, pp. 108–124. University of Utah Press, Salt Lake City.

Crown, P. 2007 Life Histories of Pots and Potters: Situating the Individual in Archaeology. *American Antiquity* 72:677–690.

David, N. 1990 *Vessels of The Spirit: Pots and People in North Cameroon* (Video). University of Calgary.

Egan, G. 1998 Miniature Toys of Medieval Childhood. *British Archaeology* 35:10–11.

Ferguson, J. 2008 The When, Where and How of Novices in Craft Production. *Journal of Archaeological Method and Theory* 15:51–67.

Gero, J., and M. Conkey 1991 *Engendering Archaeology*. Blackwell, Oxford.

Golden, Mark 1990 *Children and Childhood in Classical Athens*. Johns Hopkins University Press, Baltimore.

Gosselain, O. 1992 Technology and Style: Potters and Pottery among the Bafia of Cameroon. *Man* 27:559–586.

Gosselain, O. 1998 Social and Technical Identity in a Clay Crystal Ball. In *The Archaeology of Social Boundaries*, edited by M. Stark, pp. 78–106. Smithsonian Institution Press, Washington, D.C.

Gowland, R. 2001 Playing Dead: Implications of Mortuary Evidence for the Social Construction of Childhood in Roman Britain. In *Tenth Annual Theoretical Roman Archaeology Conference*, edited by G. Davies, A. Gardner, and K. Lockyear, pp. 152–168. Oxbow, Oxford.

Gowland, R. 2006 Ageing the Past: Examining Age Identity from Funerary Evidence. In *Social Bioarchaeology of Funerary Remains*, edited by R. Gowland and C. Knüsel, pp. 143–154. Oxbow, Oxford.

Greenfield, P. 2000 Children, Material Culture, and Weaving: Historical Change and Developmental Change. In *Children and Material Culture*, edited by J. Sofaer Derevenski, pp. 72–86. Routledge, London.

Greenfield, P., A. Maynard, and C. Childs 2000 History, Culture, Learning, and Development. *Cross Cultural Research* 34(4):351–374.

Grimm, L. 2000 Apprentice Flintknapping: Relating Material Culture and Social Practice in the Upper Palaeolithic. In *Children and Material Culture*, edited by J. Sofaer Derevenski, pp. 53–71. Routledge, London.

Guthrie, R. D. 2005 *The Nature of Palaeolithic Art*. University of Chicago Press, Chicago.

Hammond, G., and N. Hammond 1981 Child's Play: A Distorting Factor in Archaeological Distribution. *American Antiquity* 46:634–636.

Harding, A. 1999 Warfare: A Defining Characteristic of Bronze Age Europe? In *Ancient Warfare*, edited by J. Carman and A. Harding, pp. 157–173. Sutton, Stroud.

Humphrey, L. 2000 Growth Studies of Past Populations: An Overview and an Example. In *Human Osteology in Archaeology and Forensic Science*, edited by M. Cox and S. Mays, pp. 23–38. Greenwich Medical Media, London.

Høgseth, H. 2007 The Craftsman's Toolbox. An Investigation of Embodied Knowledge as Reflected in Archaeological Timbers Dated to the 11th Century AD. Unpublished PhD Dissertation, Norwegian University of Science and Technology, Trondheim.

Ingold, T. 1998 From Complimentary to Obviation: on Dissolving the Boundaries Between Social and Biological Anthropology, Archaeology, and Psychology. *Zeitschrift für Ethnologie* 123:21–52.

Ingold, T. 2001 Beyond Art and Technology: the Anthropology of Skill. In *Anthropological Perspectives on Technology*, edited by M. Schiffer pp. 17–31. University of New Mexico Press, Albuquerque.

James, A. 1993 *Childhood Identities: Self and Social Relationships in the Experience of the Child*. Edinburgh University Press, Edinburgh.

Janssen, R., and J. Janssen 1990 *Growing Up in Ancient Egypt*. The Rubicon Press, London.

Joyce, R. 2000 Girling the Girl and Boying the Boy: The Production of Adulthood in Ancient Mesoamerica. *World Archaeology* 31(3):473–483.

Kamp, K. 2001a Where Have all the Children Gone? The Archaeology of Childhood. *Journal of Archaeological Method and Theory* 8(1):1–29.

Kamp, K. 2001b Prehistoric Children Working and Playing: A Southwestern Case Study in Learning Ceramics. *Journal of Anthropological Research* 57:427–450.

Kamp, K., N. Timmerman, G. Lind, J. Graybill, and I. Natowsky 1999 Discovering Childhood: Using Fingerprints to Find Children in the Archaeological Record. *American Antiquity* 64(2):309–315.

Kristiansen, K. 1984 Krieger und Hauptlinge in der Bronzezeit Dänemarks. Ein Beitrag zur Geschichte des bronzezeitlichen Schwertes. *Jahrbuch des Römisch-Germanisches Zentralmuseums* 31:187–208. Mainz.

Kristiansen, K. 1999 The Emergence of Warrior Aristocracies in Later European Prehistory and Their Long-Term History. In *Ancient Warfare*, edited by J. Carman and A. Harding, pp. 175–189. Sutton, Stroud.

Kristiansen, K. 2002 The Tale of the Sword—Swords and Swordfighters in Bronze Age Europe. *Oxford Journal of Archaeology* 21(4):319–332.

Lave, J., and E. Wenger 1991 *Situated Learning: Legitimate Peripheral Participation*. Cambridge University Press, New York.

Leroi-Gourhan, A. 1971 [1943]. *L'Homme et la Matière*. Editions Albin Michel, Paris.

Lewis, M. 2007 *The Bioarchaeology of Children: Perspectives from Biological and Forensic Anthropology*. Cambridge University Press, Cambridge.

Lillehammer, G. 1989 A Child Is Born: The Child's World in an Archaeological Perspective. *Norwegian Archaeological Review* 22(2):89–105.

Lorentz, K. 2008 From Bodies to Bones and Back: Theory and Human Bioarchaeology. In *Between Biology and Culture*, edited by H. Schutkowski, pp. 273–303. Cambridge University Press, Cambridge.

Lucy, S. 2005 The Archaeology of Age. In *The Archaeology of Identity: Approaches To Gender, Age, Status, Ethnicity, and Religion*, edited by M. Diaz-Andreu, S. Lucy, S. Babić, and D. Edwards, pp. 43–66. Routledge, London.

Malafouris, L. 2008 Is it "Me" or is it "Mine"? The Mycenaean Sword as a Body-Part. In *Past Bodies. Body-Centred Research in Archaeology*, edited by D. Borić and J. Robb, pp. 115–123. Oxbow Books, Oxford.

Mauss, M. 1935 Les Techniques du Corps. *Journal de Psychologie* 32:271–293.

Mays, S. 1993 Infanticide in Roman Britain. *Antiquity* 67:883–888.

McKerr, L., E. Murphy, and C. Donnelly 2009 I Am Not Dead, but Do Sleep Here: The Representation of Children in Early Modern Burial Grounds in the North of Ireland. *Childhood in the Past* 2(1):109–131.

Meskell, Lynn 1994 Dying Young: The Experience of Death at Deir el Medina. *Archaeological Review from Cambridge* 13(2):35–45.

Michelaki, K. 2008. Making Pots and Potters in the Bronze Age Maros Villages of Kiszombor-Új-Élet and Kláraflava-Hajdova. *Cambridge Archaeological Journal* 18(3):327–352.

Montgomery, H. 2009. *An Introduction to Childhood: Anthropological Perspectives on Children's Lives*. Wiley-Blackwell, Oxford.

Moore, J., and E. Scott (editors) 1997 *Invisible People and Processes. Writing Gender and Childhood into European Archaeology*. Leicester University Press, London.

Orme, N. 1984 *From Childhood to Chivalry: the Education of the English Kings and Aristocracy 1066–1530*. Methuen, London.

Osgood, R., S. Monks, and J. Toms 2000 *Bronze Age Warfare*. Sutton Publishing, Stroud.

Park, R. 1998 Size Counts: The Miniature Archaeology of Childhood in Inuit Societies. *Antiquity* 72:269–281.

Pigeot, N. 1990 Technical and Social Actors: Flintknapping Specialists at Magdalenian Etoilles. *Archaeological Review from Cambridge* 9(1):126–141.

Prendergast, S. 2000 "To Become Dizzy in Our Turning": Girls, Body-Maps and Gender as Childhood Ends. In *The Body, Childhood, and Society*, edited by A. Prout, pp. 101–24. Macmillan, Basingstoke.

Prout, A. 2000 Childhood Bodies: Construction, Agency, and Hybridity. In *The Body, Childhood, and Society*, edited by A. Prout, pp. 1–18. Macmillan, Basingstoke.

Rega, E. 1997 Age, Gender, and Biological Reality in the Early Bronze Age Cemetery at Mokrin. In *Invisible People and Processes*, edited by J. Moore and E. Scott, pp. 229–247. Leicester University Press, London.

Roux, V. (editor) 2000 *Cornaline de l'Inde: Des Pratiques Techniques de Cambay aux Techno-systèmes de l'Indus*. Editions de la Maison des Sciences de L'homme, Paris.

Roux, V., and D. Corbetta 1990 *Le Tour du Potier: Spécialisation Artisanale et Compétences Techniques*. CNRS, Paris.

Roveland, B. 1997 Archaeology of Children. *Anthropology Newsletter* 38(4):14.

Roveland, B. 2000 Footprints in the Clay: Upper Palaeolithic Children in Ritual and Secular Contexts. In *Children and Material Culture*, edited by J. Sofaer Derevenski, pp. 29–38. Routledge, London.

Sánchez-Romero, M. 2008 Childhood and the Construction of Gender Identities through Material Culture. *Childhood in the Past* 1:17–37.

Scheuer, L., and S. Black 2000 *Developmental Juvenile Osteology*. Academic Press, San Diego, California.

Scott, E. 1991 Animal and Infant Burials in Romano-British Villas: A Revitalization Movement. In *Sacred and Profane: Proceedings of a Conference on Archaeology, Religion, and Ritual, Oxford, 1989*, edited by P. Garwood, D. Jennings, R. Skeates, and J. Toms, pp. 115–121. Oxford Committee for Archaeology, Institute of Archaeology, Oxford.

Scott, E. 1993. Images and Contexts of Infants and Infant Burials: Some Thoughts on Cross-Cultural Evidence. *Archaeological Review from Cambridge* 11:77–92.

Smith, P., and G. Kahila 1992 Identification of Infanticide in Archaeological Sites: a Case Study from the Late Roman-Early Byzantine Periods at Ashkelon, Israel. *Journal of Archaeological Science* 19:667–75.

Sofaer Derevenski, J. (editor) 1994a Perspectives on Children and Childhood. *Archaeological Review from Cambridge* 13(2).

Sofaer Derevenski, J. 1994b Where Are the Children? Accessing Children in the Past. *Archaeological Review from Cambridge* 13(2):7–20.

Sofaer Derevenski, J. 2000a Rings of Life: The Role of Early Metalwork in Mediating the Gendered Life Course. *World Archaeology* 31(3):389–406.

Sofaer Derevenski, J. 2000b Material Culture Shock. Confronting Expectations in the Material Culture of Children. In *Children and Material Culture*, edited by J. Sofaer Derevenski, pp. 3–16. Routledge, London.

Sofaer, J. 2006 *The Body as Material Culture. A Theoretical Osteoarchaeology*. Cambridge University Press, Cambridge.

Sofaer, J. 2011 Human Ontogeny and Material Change at the Bronze Age Tell of Százhalombatta, Hungary. *Cambridge Archaeological Journal* 21(2):217–27.

Sofaer, J., and S. Budden 2012 Many Hands Make Light Work: Embodied Knowledge at the Bronze Age Tell at Százhalombatta, Hungary. In *Embodied Knowledge*, edited by M. L. S. Sørensen, L. Bender Jørgensen, and K. Rebay-Salisbury, pp. 117–27. Oxbow Press, Oxford.

Steedman, C. 1995 *Strange Dislocations: Childhood and the Idea of Human Interiority 1780–1930*. Harvard University Press, Cambridge.

Sørensen, M. L. S. 2000 *Gender Archaeology*. Polity Press, Cambridge.

Toren, C. 1999 *Mind, Materiality and History: Essays in Fijian Ethnography*. Routledge, London.

Toren, C. 2001 The Child in Mind. In *The Debated Mind. Evolutionary Psychology versus Ethnography*, edited by H. Whitehouse, pp. 155–179. Berg, Oxford.

Toren, C. 2003 Becoming a Christian in Fiji: An Ethnographic Study of Ontogeny. *Journal of the Royal Anthropological Institute* 9(4):709–727.

Toren, C. 2007 Sunday Lunch in Fiji: Continuity and Transformation in Ideas of the Household. *American Anthropologist* 109(2):285–295.

Treherne, P. 1995 The Warrior's Beauty: The Masculine Body and Self-Identity in Bronze Age Europe. *Journal of European Archaeology* 3(1):105–144.

Valsiner, J., and A. Rosa (editors) 2007 *The Cambridge Handbook of Sociocultural Psychology*. Cambridge University Press, Cambridge.

Vandkilde, H. 2003 Commemorative Tales: Archaeological Responses to Modern Myth, Politics, and War. *World Archaeology* 35(1):126–144.

Vandkilde, H. 2007 *Culture and Change in Central European Prehistory*. Aarhus University Press, Aarhus.

Wallaert-Pêtre, H. 2001. Learning How to Make the Right Pots: Apprenticeship Strategies and Material Culture, a Case Study in Handmade Pottery from Cameroon. *Journal of Anthropological Research* 57:471–492.

Welinder, Stig 1998 The Cultural Construction of Childhood in Scandinavia, 3500 BC–1350 AD. *Current Swedish Archaeology* 6:185–204.

Wendrich, W. (editor) 2012 *Archaeology and Apprenticeship: Acquiring Body Knowledge in the Ancient World*. University of Arizona Press, Tucson.

Wileman, J. 2005 *Hide and Seek. The Archaeology of Childhood*. Tempus, Stroud.

Wilkie, L. 2000 Not Merely Child's Play: Creating a Historical Archaeology of Children and Childhood. In *Children and Material Culture*, edited by J. Sofaer Derevenski, pp. 100–113. Routledge, London.

Wilkie, L. 2003 *The Archaeology of Mothering: An African-American Midwife's Tale*. Routledge, New York.

Wilson, J. 2007 *The Social Role of the Elderly in the Early Bronze Age of Central Europe*. Unpublished PhD Dissertation, University of Cambridge, Cambridge.

Wood, E. 2009 Saving Childhood in Everyday Objects. *Childhood in the Past* 2(1):151–162.

CHAPTER FIVE

Modern Biases, Hunter-Gatherers' Children

On the Visibility of Children in Other Cultures

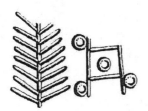

Nurit Bird-David

Abstract   *In this chapter, I consider a fundamental problem weighing on the growing comparative research of children, in response to the growing call to redress their previous invisibility. I explore implicit biases inherent in using the English language concept "children" in cross-cultural research. This English language word has its cultural, historical, and ontological antecedents. I examine some of these biases, pitted against the ethnography of contemporary hunter-gatherers. I focus on the lived realities of children in these societies, and on the symbolic meanings of the indigenous concepts of them. Their cases, I argue, suggest that in some social contexts (not necessarily restricted to hunter-gatherers) children and parents are better studied and made visible as* inseparable *subjects and constructs. "Children" are better explored* relationally, *rather than as a separate class and population.*

The end of the twentieth century saw a surge of concern about the absence of children in archeological and anthropological studies, leading to increasing efforts to redress the problem and make children visible. The resulting comparative research has become highly visible through mushrooming conferences and workshops, many publications and special issues in leading journals. But does this visible research effectively make visible the children's own lived realities in the diverse societies across the time and space in which it is pursued? I maintain that it is instructive to ask this question at this moment in the expansion of this valuable research enterprise.

The problems involved in the universal extension of analytical concepts that come from the scholars' own lived worlds are well known. Consider, for example, the distorting effect of using the orthodox concept of "economy" in the study of very small-scale hunter-gatherer societies. Coming from large-scale modern lived worlds, this concept instills its institutional and domain-segregated biases into hunter-gatherers' ethnographies. Their foraging pursuits are subsequently studied, for instance, as "economic" and "subsistence" activities, skewing the manifold experiences they constitute for those who pursue them, and their bearings on these people's senses of themselves and their worlds. Yet, much as the use of such analytical concepts is problematic—so, no less, is their avoidance. Their use cannot be completely avoided. The best we can do, then, is to use these concepts with cultivated awareness and attentiveness to the biases and distortions they sneak into the analysis. Reflecting on the cultural antecedents of our key analytical categories that are used in writing ethnographies in our language about the life worlds of other peoples can significantly contribute to better understanding their worlds (see Bird-David 2008). The fact that an ethnographic analysis is written in English should not be left transparent when a word such as (the English) "children" carries a complex collection of historical and cultural antecedents.

In this chapter, I give attention to the concept of "children" pitted against hunter-gatherers' lived realities, especially hunter-gatherers of the kind I know from my own ethnographic fieldwork among a South Indian group known locally as Nayaka (among other ethnic names). I conducted fieldwork among one local Nayaka group during 1978–79, and revisited them in 1989, 2001, and 2012. I use the generalizing term *hunter-gatherers* as a useful label, without belittling the diversity and the complex changes undergone by the communities that are typed in this way. "Hunter-gatherers" is an analytical prism through which we look comparatively at these diverse indigenous peoples, and regard them as "cases" in our own discussions. While using the term, I give analytical primacy not to their mode of subsistence and their techniques as done in some scholarly traditions, but to their ways of seeing their world, their modes of sociality, and their epistemologies and ontologies.

The present chapter draws on two earlier publications, and pursues their concerns further. In the first one, I examined why the children of hunter-gatherers had been invisible, and why it is important to study them from a cultural perspective. In the second, I examined through the prism of child feeding, how—far from being passive and dependent as the terms *feeding children* and *nurturing children* imply—hunter-gatherer children are active agents who contribute to food sharing. In the last-mentioned publication I pursued what I called "bi-focal ethnography," which is the strategy I further pursue here as I discuss below several antecedents of the (English) concept of "children" that I suggest can lead astray child-focused hunter-gatherer ethnographers. I pay attention to whether infants count as children; whether children are passive and dependent on adults; whether children should be approached as a separate class and population; and whether "parents and children" symbolizes descent and substitute generations. These are conventional modern antecedents of the concept of children, which I argue constrain understanding both hunter-gatherers' children, and hunter-gatherers' meanings of children. Some of these modern biases have been extensively pointed out, especially regarding children as passive and dependent. I argue that looking at them as a class of active agents still bears modern biases. They should be looked at in a relational context, examining children's relations with adults, just as gender studies, on which their study is sometimes modeled, is about women in the context of women-men relations.

Do Infants Count as Children?

One aspect of the concept of "children" that concerns me as a student of hunter-gatherers who is writing in English, is the blurred distinction between children and infants. Furthermore, it is how often infants are considered as the prototype children. An English dictionary defines "infant" as "a child during the earliest period of its life, esp. before he or she can walk," and in Law as "a person who is not of full age, esp. one who has not reached the age of 18 years; a minor."[1] The use of the word is traced back to the fourteenth century, literally meaning "one unable to speak."[2] Parents normally experience the difference between caring for babies and older children, even in the basic routines of the parents' everyday life, such as how much the parents sleep, when they eat, and how easily they can leave the children at home and go out. Yet, from the state's point of view, the term *children* includes "infants." Or, the two are used synonymously, in various contexts, such as the parents' legal responsibility, some statistical surveys, welfare benefits, and so on and so forth. In these contexts, "children" refers to people right from their birth to attaining legal majority.

At the same time, the young child is implicitly regarded as the prototype "child" in many regards. Consider, for example, cultural and scientific discourses on "child development" and "child care" that are commonly taken to refer to young children. The surge of popular and scientific interest over the years in birth, nursing, nurturing, mother-baby bonding, infants' physical, cognitive, and emotional development, and such issues—indeed in "having babies"—places babies at the hub of the interest in children. Handbooks on childcare overwhelmingly focus on the early years, as do studies in the child development research tradition. For example, within the prolific field of child development, the feeding of children with solid food has been a relatively understudied area and still gets rare mention in recent anthologies. One can provocatively say that the child's calendar is like the famous Nuer cattle-clock; in the latter, the morning has far more temporal distinctions than the rest of the day because it is then that many tasks are carried out. In the former, at the early years of childhood far more developmental stages are distinguished than in the children's later years. There is a case for saying that perceiving the birth of a human being as the beginning of the transformation from nature to society underscores these emphases and interests. The dramatic events from this perspective take place in the first transformative years during which the newborn becomes a person. And, yet, the concept of "children" encompasses persons from birth to legal majority. Furthermore, young infants are commonly regarded as the prototype child. These antecedents of the concept of "children" can bias child-focused research in other societies and cultures, and numb ethnographic attentiveness to other diverse cultural sensibilities and perspectives.

Ethnographers of hunter-gatherer societies largely focused to date on babies and infants. While in hunter-gatherers' own cultural and ontological terms, a clear distinction is sometimes made between babies and older children: in some hunter-gatherer cases, infants are not yet regarded as children, and as persons in their own right. They are regarded, for example, as embryonic human beings, and as spirits who take a human form until, with the appearance of their first teeth, they become fully humans. When infants die, in some cases, they are not buried as other members of the community. Their bodies are discarded in a casual way, without wailing; the houses and camps in which they live are not abandoned. In some cases, their death is viewed as simply the failed birth of persons who will subsequently try getting born a second time. In yet some other cases, babies are not named until they are capable of walking by themselves and engaging in conversation with others, and it is only from then that they are regarded as children.

Going hand in hand with such concepts, young infants are rarely on their own and, at the same time, rarely the object of concern about how they are developing. It has been commonly observed among hunter-gatherers that babies are constantly held, touched, or kept near others. Quantitative observations carried out suggest that, in some cases, they are held 98 percent of the time when awake, and 94 percent of their sleep time. They are held by their mother or father, and otherwise by a host of allo-parents who live close to the parents in the little partitioned hunter-gatherers' hamlet, or "camp." The proximity of relatives, along with an absence of baby-care equipment and accessories, at once enable and perpetuate holding the baby almost all of the time.

This constant "being with" someone else, in turn, enables the babies' active involvement in their own nurturing, which means as well that they are not the constant focus of adults' gaze and attention. Quantitative studies in central Africa have recorded the extent to which hunter-gatherers' babies initiate their own nursing far more than agricultural neighbors' babies. Barry Hewlett reports, for example, that Aka infants took the breast 58 percent of the time while their Ngandu neighbors did so only two percent. Hirasawa reports that sedentarized hunter-gatherer Baka infants still initiated more than 70 percent of the nursing sessions. In the Nayaka case, where self-nursing similarly occurs extensively, this is possible as mothers carry the babies on their side when walking and on their lap when sitting, which allows the babies to reach by themselves, when they want, their mother's bare or loosely covered breast. Some studies showed that hunter-gatherers' infants also decide when to stop breastfeeding, without overt parental guidance or coercion, while among neighboring farmers, mothers overtly strive by various means to wean children from the breast.

Young toddlers' active involvement with their "caregivers"—note the inherent bias in this English concept that a priori frames children as recipients and objects of care—is apparent also in other ways. Toddlers in hunter-gatherer societies are reported in some cases to go for cuddles to their parents far more than the parents pick them up. Barry Hewlett reported, for example, that after Lamb's study of American parents' reasons for picking up their children, he tried the same study among the Aka, only to find out in a very short time that the results of such a study would be limited for them. The Aka, he found out, seldom picked up the infant voluntarily; the infant more often than not initiated and completed the action itself by climbing into the parent's lap, or it was transferred from someone else. In my own fieldwork, I did not see Nayaka adults coo to babies, or talk with babies who cannot yet talk back, in a sort of play-dialogue (responding to the infants' imagined questions or asking them questions the infants are imagined to reply; or playing interactively with the infants in any other nonverbal way aimed to trigger an interactive response). Just as the infants initiate their own feeding, weaning, and cuddling, so they initiate two-way dialogues and interaction with others when they are ready and able to do so.

From the perspective of child development research, such ethnographic observations are read as evidence that hunter-gatherer babies are strikingly autonomous agents from an early age. With a cultivated awareness of how antecedents of the English analytical term *children* directs investigation, these accounts simultaneously can be read as indicators that infants—unlike older children—are not yet approached as persons in their own right. This reading concurs with the above-mentioned hunter-gatherers' cultural views of infants as not yet persons but merely embryonic human beings and spirits.

Are Children Passive and Dependent on Adults?

Other aspects of "children" that concern me—as mentioned, as a student of hunter-gatherers who writes about them in English—are the related concepts of children's passivity, fragility, and dependence. These historical and cultural antecedents of "children" are among those most addressed in the new children's research paradigms, precluding a need to elaborately recycle them here. Margaret Mead's words from the early twentieth century can be cited for a sense of what scholars at that time tended to universalize and now question and redress. Mead posited—and assumed this to be universal—that parent-child relationships are fundamentally structured by the understanding that "to the adults, children everywhere represent something weak and helpless, in need of protection." Frequently acknowledging Aries's contribution, extensive research has argued since then for the recent European historical and cultural roots of seeing children as innocent and vulnerable, and of speaking about children in terms of "needs" (see Levine and New 2008). Studies of hunter-gatherers made their contribution to this growing research enterprise.

Hunter-gatherers' ethnographers who focused on children (here, referring to the age range of roughly four to 16) demonstrated the children's involvement in and contribution to the procuring of food, both for themselves and for their community. In many cases, children accompanied adults in foraging pursuits, and in some cases they played their part along with the adults. In Mbuti net hunting, for example, children held the nets with the women, while the men chased game into the nets. Among Nayaka, children participated in gathering sikai beans for sale (the beans are used in the local industry as a gentle detergent for cleaning jewels). While men climbed up the high trees on which the sikai creeper grew and shook the creepers' branches until the beans fell down, the women and children collected the beans from the ground. Hadza children as young as five years of age gathered fruit and hunted lizards efficiently on their own. Meriam children collected seashells on their own, providing nearly 50 percent of their own caloric intake by their own hunting and gathering. Ethnographers noted that children from a very early age carried and used adult-sized tools, including sharp knives that could injure them.

Children were also involved in some cases in the sharing of large game animals, which is a key event among many hunter-gatherers. Nayaka children, for example, assisted in the butchering and the division of the game: they gathered vessels or plantain leaves and brought them to where the meat was cut; they held a torch if the butchering took place at night; they held the animal's limbs to ease its cutting; they playfully monitored the equal distribution of meat chunks between families, and then carried the portions to the families. Children were taken into account in the division of the meat between families: a bigger share was given to families with more children.

In many cases, children took part in rituals alongside adults. Evocative films shot on the !Kung medicine dance and on Baka performances, for example, show young children clapping hands alongside adults, not to mention infants nestling on the adults' laps, in the darkness of the night. Richard Katz reported the striking case of a young !Kung boy (11 or 12 years old) who had experienced the altered state of consciousness (*kia*), though he did not perform as healer.

Lastly, ethnographers noted how little hierarchical one-way parental teaching and instruction is bestowed on hunter-gatherers' children, who are encouraged and allowed to develop their own knowledge from direct experience, trial and error, and from partic-ipation in most—if not all—adults' activities and affairs. The children not only accom-panied adults in most activities but they were not prohibited from using all their tools, including those which in the "dependent and weak" child paradigm would be considered highly dangerous and better kept outside the reach of children. Children were generally indulged by their parents, who rarely admonished them. If the parents lost control over a particularly mischievous child, they—not the children—were, in some cases, admonished by adult bystanders. Naveh evocatively describes the closest example of parental teaching that he saw among the Nayaka he studied: a father dismantles a trap which his son has not assembled very well. The son watches as the father does it again without any words of criticism or instruction. Naveh further describes children's games through which they learn to hunt: for example, two children playing a hunter and its prey, exercising different ways of trapping. The child playing the game not only mimicked the animal (walking on all fours, etc.), but he also voiced aloud the thoughts of the prey.

ARE CHILDREN A SEPARATE CLASS OR POPULATION?

The growing call over the last two decades to study the previously neglected population of children, in their own right, with their own cultures and worlds—indeed, even as a "minority group" and a "subaltern culture"—is entangled with yet another antecedent of "children" that concerns me in my capacity as a student of hunter-gatherers who writes their ethnography in English. In such uses, the term *children* receives what can be described as essentialist and separatist readings. An understanding of children is brought to the forefront in these readings, which depicts them as persons who are in a particu-lar age range: persons who are young, persons who are not adults, persons that, as one English dictionary defines them, are "between birth and full growth" or "between birth and puberty."[3] This implies to no small extent investigating them in essentialist terms as a distinguished kind of being, whose characteristic range of behaviors, capabilities, perspectives, and worlds—normalized and/or actual—are explored. And, in turn, this entails among others a sense of "children" as the plurality of such beings, each one as an individual of this kind, abstracted from the web of relations in which s/he lives, and considered as a member of this class with others of her/his kind. And this further encourages investigating their commonality as same-and-separate beings (or their diversity within this commonality), in an implicit binary opposite to adults as their "other."

Now, in large-scale and age-regulated nation-states, a child society or population is a visible concrete entity: suffice it to imagine the pupils of a small school (say, in England) with a child population easily outnumbering the entire population of a hunter-gatherer local group or band. These children spend a considerable part of their everyday life at school, and then also in various child extracurricular activities. In the domain-split large-scale world, there are many child-focused niches in the form of child-targeted productions, consumption, circulation, advertisements, theatre, books, and many more. In such a multidomain environment, it is perfectly acceptable to speak about the children's populations, worlds, and cultures.

But when it comes to hunter-gatherers, this view is highly problematic. A distinguishing characteristic of those hunter-gatherers, previously described as "band societies" for this reason, is their very small total populations and their very small local groups or bands. Estimates of their total population size may be questioned, given unreliable official censuses in the marginal areas in which many of these peoples live, let alone given that ethnic classifications were imposed on them from the outside. But the order of size is clear. The average size of populations profiled in *The Cambridge Encyclopedia of Hunters and Gatherers* is 6,197 (for the South Asian population, 2,535), while many well-known examples number fewer than one thousand persons each. The size of local groups, or bands, is more reliable. After all, ethnographers can reliably count even the fluid numbers of people who live together in a local group, where they themselves often live during their studies. In the landmark symposium, *Man the Hunter*, attention was drawn to what were then described as the "magic numbers" in hunter-gatherer studies. Most striking and enduring were the "magic numbers" of 25 to 50 persons as the most frequently reported size of local groups, or bands.[4] Now, if there are 25 to 50 persons (including men, women, and children) in a local group, there are between one to two dozen children, of all ages, at that, in such a group.[5]

For each age range that we may want to focus on, there are very few children. They live inseparably with all the others, adults and other children. It is vital to remember that prior to colonial and state interference, and in a modified way that continues today in many cases, hunter-gatherer hamlets or camps were very small. Men, women, and children lived very closely together. In some cases, the traditional camps were composed of only a few dwellings. The dwellings stood close to one another out of choice rather than from a lack of space, amid the natural surroundings (forest, tundra, desert, etc.). When weather permitted, a great deal of domestic life took place outside the dwellings in the open: for instance, cooking, eating, bathing infants, and bathing in the river. People rarely slept alone—which in some cases locally signaled social pathology. Children commonly slept with their parents, or their friends' parents. As mentioned above, they joined adults in subsistence pursuits and communal ceremonies.

It is true that children also played on their own, and in some cases even hunted and gathered on their own (see above). The separatist focus in child-focused hunter-gatherer ethnographies on what children do—rather than on whom and where they do it—makes it difficult to assess where such children-only economic activities and games fit within the general close living of adults and children in traditional hunter-gatherers' settlements. For the Nayaka local group I studied, I can say that children played on their own and went occasionally on child-only expeditions (such as fishing). But this took place in the vicinity of the hamlet, and only occasionally interrupted the everyday flow of communal life where children and adults were hardly separate as classes or categories. Of course, there can be expected variations among hunter-gatherers as to how much time their children would spend on their own, and how much with parents and older relatives. But generally, it is fair to say that looking at children as a separate class or population, with their own world, is farfetched in traditional hunter-gatherers communities, where, on the contrary, adult-child communities are the predominant frame of social life.

ARE "PARENTS-CHILDREN" A SYMBOL OF REPRODUCTION AND SUBSTITUTE GENERATIONS?

As a cultural anthropologist, I am particularly concerned with what "children" symbolically stands for—or, rather, as I argue, "children and parents." This is the last antecedent of "children" which I consider in this brief chapter. "Parents and children" is a conventional English phrase that suggests subsequent generations, generations that follow one another. The concept of "generation" is such that, as Ingold put it, "with each new generation, those preceding it regress ever further into the past." One generation goes and the other comes, each superseding the other. This image ignores the commonplace overlap between parents and children, who share lives for a significant period of their lifetimes. This symbolic sense of "parents and children" further frames each as a separate and autonomous class.

In his *Death is the Mother of Beauty*, the cognitive linguist and literary critic Mark Turner showed how the parent-child terms constitute basic conceptual metaphors that are deeply seated in "our" cognitive structures. Obviously, Turner refers to English language parent-child terms, and hence his "our" refers conservatively to English speakers' cognitive structures. His analysis usefully illustrates the point I make and is worthy of a detailed mention. Turner examines the abundant metaphorical uses of "parents-children" terms in the body of high canon poetry in English from Chaucer to Wallace Stevens. (In literary language, Turner maintains, writers constantly explore conceptual and linguistic structures, pushing them to see how they respond, and where they break. Therefore, the common processes of ordinary language are seen there in their highest relief and most compelling manifestation [198/:13]). Turner discovers thousands of parent-child metaphorical uses, far more than there are for any other kinship term, as for example, "necessity is the mother of invention," "a child of evil," "fear, father of cruelty," "trade is the mother of money." With Lakoff and Johnson, Turner assumes that English speakers can invent and understand infinite examples at the level of particular words, because all the examples derive from a few basic metaphors at the conceptual level. Using standard cognitive linguist procedures, Turner draws on what he construes as "our" (read conservatively: English speakers') knowledge of kinship in analyzing these basic metaphors. In what follows I skim only the thin surface of his complex analysis for my present purposes.

One basic conceptual metaphor—which is manifested, for example, in the literary metaphor "a child of evil" (meaning the child is evil)—foregrounds the idea that children inherit salient features of their parents. Similarities observed between parent and child, whether in physical form or character (e.g., both are tall, or both are grumpy) are commonly reasoned in terms of inheritance, which is conveyed in expressions such as "she is her mother's daughter," "like mother, like daughter" (Turner 1987:22). This idea is articulated with the conceptual metaphor that a quality, a trait—in our case, evil—can be personified as a person, including the parent from whom the child inherits this salient characteristic. Another basic conceptual metaphor—which is manifested, for example, in the proverb, "necessity is the mother of invention" (meaning invention springs from necessity, or invention is the result of necessity as its condition, or invention is the outcome of necessity as its cause or, to use another metaphor, necessity gives birth to invention)—exemplifies the idea that "children spring from their parents" (Turner 1987: 22). The parent is the known origin or cause of the child. Yet, a third basic conceptual metaphor—which is manifested in the linguistic concept of "mother-node" (Turner 1987:23), or to add my own examples, the computer's "motherboard" and mother company—shows the idea that a child, "certainly during gestation," is part of the mother (Turner 1987:23), which articulates with another basic conceptual metaphor, which is that "a whole is made of its parts" (Turner 1987:23).

As a word combination, the English terms *parents and children* connote, then, relations of origin, causality, transmission, similarity, functional hierarchy, and containment. They suggest sequential "parent" and "child," like cause and result, origin and offspring, past and present. What these concepts conceal is as intriguing as what they show: a parent-child coevalness. In connoting inheritance, reproduction of substance, cause and result, and whole-part inclusion, they conceal parents-children living together. For this reason, these English language terms are extremely tricky when it comes to hunter-gatherer cases.

These connotations conceal what for Nayaka—and I believe for other hunter-gatherers—is the salient feature of "parents and children," and what these relations symbolize for them. Rather than subsequent generations—one coming after the other, substituting for one another, carrying the same substance or property through time—parents and children here almost connote the opposite, to wit, close shared living together, mutual attentiveness and concern, belonging, and a sense of shared identity. The attention here focuses on the overlap between parents and children, who live together for a considerable part of their lives. Children share their lives with parents not only as young children who live in the parents' households but they continue to share a communal life with parents also when they grow up and set up their own families. Growing up is not identified in this case with a separation from the parents as an expression of individual autonomy and independence, as it is the connotation of yet another antecedent of the English sense of nurturing children. Rather than a separate class of a particular kind of beings, humans in a particular age range and/or particular development stages, "children" in hunter-gatherer cases foregrounds a sense of "children of" (Bird-David 2005a): children of parents, children who live with parents, children within a child/parent relation rather than just young persons in and for themselves. And precisely because hunter-gatherer children are active contributors to their communities, rather than passive dependents (as discussed above), "children of" connotes mutual care, sharing, and growing old together, rather than reproduction, descent, and substitute generations. The words *children of* connote reproducing relations of sharing and caring continuously in time, rather than transmission of material, biological or psychological property.

CONCLUSIONS

From the vantage point of their marginality, hunter-gatherers can contribute a cautionary note to the burgeoning studies of children in response to the growing call to redress their previous invisibility in anthropological and archeological studies. Their cultures should draw attention to the fact that this seductive call can trap anthropologists and archeologists within their own cultural and ontological terms and tensions as they use the English word *children* as a universal analytical category. Through the case of hunter-gatherers I hope to have shown in this chapter that in some social contexts (not restricted to "hunter-gatherers") the terms *children* and *parents* may be better studied and made visible as inseparable subjects and constructs. In some cultural contexts (not unique to "hunter-gatherers") "children" may be better explored relationally rather than as a separate class and population.

NOTES

1.   http://dictionary.reference.com/browse/infants, October 19, 2010.
2.   http://dictionary.reference.com/browse/infants, October 19, 2010.
3.   http://dictionary.reference.com/browse/children, February 5, 2010.
4.   These numbers were not questioned later, as were two other mentioned numbers: "500" as the size of the dialectical band, and "1000 or fewer" as the total population (Lee and DeVore 1968:245–247).
5.   Child-focused research involving hunter-gatherers—based on follow-up individual observations in more than one local group in order to reach sizeable samples—reach child populations in the order of about 50 children.

REFERENCES CITED

Agland, P. 1987 *Baka: The People of the Rainforest*. Great Britain: 104 min.
Aries, P. 1973 [1960] *Centuries of Childhood*. Penguin, Harmondsworth.

Bird-David, N. 1987 The Kurumbas of the Nilgiris: An Ethnographic Myth? *Modern Asian Studies* 21:173–189.

Bird-David, N. 1990 The Giving Environment: Another Perspective on the Economic System of Gatherer-Hunters. *Current Anthropology* 31(2):183–196.

Bird-David, N. 1992 Beyond the Original Affluent Society: A Culturalist Reformulation. *Current Anthropology* 33(1):25–47.

Bird-David, N. 1994 Sociality and Immediacy: Or Past and Present Conversations on Bands. *Man* 29(3):583–603.

Bird-David, N. 1999 Animism Revisited: Personhood, Environment and Relational Epistemology. *Current Anthropology* 40(Supplement):S67–91.

Bird-David, N. 2005 The Property of Relations: Modern Notions, Nayaka Contexts. In *Property and Equality. Vol 1 Ritualization, Sharing, Egalitarianisn*, edited by T. Widlock and W. G. Tadesse. Bergham, Oxford.

Bird-David, N. 2005a Studying Children in "Hunter-Gatherer" Societies: Reflections from a Nayaka Perspective. In *Hunter-Gatherer Childhoods: Evolutionary, Developmental, and Cultural Perspectives*, edited by B. S. Hewlett and E. L. Michael, pp. 92–105. Aldine, New Brunswick and London.

Bird-David, N. 2008 Feeding Nayaka Children and English Readers: A Bifocal Ethnography of Parental Feeding in "The Giving Environment." *Anthropological Quarterly* 81(3):523–550.

Bird-David, N. 2009 Indigenous Architecture and Relational Senses of Personhood: A Cultural Reading of Changing Dwelling Styles among Forest-Dwelling Foragers. *Design Principles & Practices: An International Journal* 3(5):203–210.

Bird, D. W., and R. Bliege Bird 2005 Mardu Children's Hunting Strategies in the Western Desert, Australia. In *Hunter-Gatherer Childhoods: Evolutionary, Developmental, and Cultural Perspectives*, edited by B. S. Hewlett and M. E. Lamb, pp. 129–146. Aldine, New Brunswick and London.

Dettwyler, K. A. 1989 Styles of Infant Feeding: Parental/Caretaker Control of Food Consumption in Young Children. *American Anthropologist* 91(3):696–703.

Endicott, K. M., and K. L. Endicott 2008 *The Headman was a Woman*. Wavekand, Long Grove, Illinois.

Fouts, H. N., and M. E. Lamb 2005 Weanling Emotional Patterns among the Bofi Foragers of Central Africa: The Role of Maternal Availability. In *Hunter-Gatherer Childhoods: Evolutionary, Developmental,and Cultural Perspectives*, edited by B. S. Hewlett and M. E. Lamb, pp. 309–322. Aldine, New Brunswick and London.

Gardner, P. M. 1966 Symmetric Respect and Memorate Knowledge: The Structure and Ecology of Individualistic Culture. *Journal of South Eastern Anthropology* 22:389–415.

Hart, J. A. 1978 From Subsistence to Market: A Case Study of the Mbuti Net Hunters. *Human Ecology* 6(3):325–353.

Hawkes, K., and N. Blurton-Jones 2005 Human Age Structures, Paleodemography and the Grandmother Hypothesis. In *Grandmotherhood: The Psychological, Social, and Reproductive Significance of the Second Half of Life*, edited by E. Voland, A. Chasiotis, and W. Schiefenhovel, pp. 118–176. Rutgers University Press, New Brunswick.

Hawkes, K., O'Connell, J. F., Blurton-Jones, N. G., Alvarez, H., and Charnov, E. L. 2000 The Grandmother Hypothesis and Human Evolution. In *Human Behavior and Adaptation: An Anthropological Perspective*, edited by L. Cronk, N. A. Chagnon, and W. Irons, pp. 371–395. Aldine, New York.

Hewlett, B. 1991. *Intimate Fathers: The Nature and Context of Aka Pygmy Paternal Infant Care*. University of Michigan Press, Ann Arbor.

Hewlett, B. and M. Lamb 2005 Emerging Issues in the Study of Hunter-Gatherer Children. In *Hunter-Gatherer Childhoods: Evolutionary, Developmental, and Cultural Perspectives*, edited by B. S. Hewlett and M. E. Lamb. Aldine, New Brunswick and London.

Hewlett, B., M. Lamb et al. 2000 Internal Working Models, Trust and Sharing among Foragers. *Current Anthropology* 41(2):287–296.

Hewlett, B. L. 2005 Vulnerable Lives: The Experience of Death and Loss among the Aka and Ngandu Adolescents of the Central African Republic. In *Hunter-Gatherer Childhoods: Evolutionary, Developmental, and Cultural Perspectives*, edited by B. S. Hewlett and M. E. Lamb, pp. 322–343. Aldine, New Brunswick and London.

Hirasawa, A. 2005 Infant Care among the Sedentarized Baka Hunter-Gatherers in Southeastern Cameroon. In *Hunter-Gatherer Childhoods: Evolutionary, Developmental, and Cultural Perspectives*, edited by B. S. Hewlett and M. E. Lamb. Aldine, New Brunswick and London.

Hirschfeld, L. A. 2002 Why Don't Anthropologists Like Children? *American Anthropologist* 104(2):611–627.

Howell, S. 1984 *Society and Cosmos: Chewong of Peninsular Malaysia*. Oxford University Press, Oxford.

Howell, S. 1988 From Child to Human: Chewong Concepts of Self. In *Acquiring Culture: Cross Cultural Studies in Child Development*, edited by G. Jahoda and I. M. Lewis, pp. 147–168. Croom Helm, London.

Ingold, T. 2000 *The Perception of the Environment: Essays in Livelihood, Dwelling, and Skill*. Routledge, London and New York.

James, A., C. Jenks et al. (editors) 1998 *Theorizing Childhood*. Polity Press, Cambridge.

Jenks, C. 1996 *Childhood*. Routledge, London and New York.

Katz, R. 1982 *Boiling Energy: Community Healing among the Kalahari Kung*. Harvard University Press, Cambridge.

Konner, M. 2005 Hunter-Gatherer Infancy and Childhood: The !Kung and Others. In *Hunter-Gatherer Childhoods: Evolutionary, Developmental, and Cultural Perspectives*, edited by B. S. Hewlett and M. E. Lamb, pp. 19–65. Aldine, New Brunswick and London.

Lakoff, G., and M. Johnson 1982 *Metaphors We Live By*. University of Chicago Press, Chicago.

Lee, R., and R. Daly (editors) 1999 *The Cambridge Encyclopedia of Hunters and Gatherers*. Cambridge University Press, Cambridge.

Lee, R. B. and I. DeVore (editors) 1968 *Man the Hunter*. Aldine, Chicago.

LeVine, R. A., and R. S. New (editors) 2008 *Anthropology and Child Development: A Cross-Cultural Reader*. Blackwell, Oxford.

Marshall, J. 1969 *N/um Tchai: The Ceremonial Dance of the !Kung Bushmen*, Documentary Ediucational Resources.

Mead, M. 1955 *Theoretical Setting. Childhood in Contemporary Cultures*. M. M. a. W. Martha. University of Chicago Press, Chicago and London.

Naveh, D. 2007 Continuity and Change in Nayaka Epistemology and Subsistence Economy: A Hunter Gatherer Case from South India. Department of Sociology and Anthropology. PhD thesis. University of Haifa, Haifa.

Pandya, V. 1993 *Above the Forest: A Study of Andamanese Ethnoanemology, Cosmology, and the Power of Ritual*. Oxford University Press, Delhi.

Strathern, M. 1992 *After Nature: English Kinship in the Late Twentieth Century*. Cambridge University Press, Cambridge.

Tucker, B., and A. G. Young 2005 Growing up Mikea: Children's Time Allocation and Tuber Foraging in Southwestern Madagascar. In *Hunter-Gatherer Childhoods: Evolutionary, Developmental, and Cultural Perspectives*, edited by B. S. Hewlett and M. E. Lamb, pp. 147–171. Aldine, New Brunswick and London.

Turnbull, C. M. 1965 *Wayward Servants: The Two Worlds of the African Pygmies*. Greenwood Press, Westport, Connecticut.

Turner, M. 1987 D*eath is the Mother of Beauty: Mind, Metaphor, Criticism*. The University of Chicago Press, Chicago and London.

Van Esterik, P. 2002 Contemporary Trends in Infant Feeding Research. *Annual Review of Anthropology* 31:257–278.

Woodburn, J. 1968 An Introduction to Hadza Ecology. In *Man the Hunter*, edited by R. B. Lee and I. DeVore. Aldine, Chicago.

Woodburn, J. 1982 Egalitarian Societies. *Man* 17(3):431–451.

Woodburn, J. 1982 Social Dimensions of Death in Four African Hunting and Gathering Societies. In *Death and the Regeneration of Life*, edited by M. Bloch and J. Parry. Cambridge University Press, Cambridge.

Woodburn, J. 1998 "Sharing Is not a Form of Exchange": An Analysis of Property-Sharing in Immediate-Return Hunter-Gatherer Societies. In *Property Relations: Renewing the Anthropological Tradition*, edited by C. M. Hann, pp. 48–63. Cambridge University Press, Cambridge.

PART II

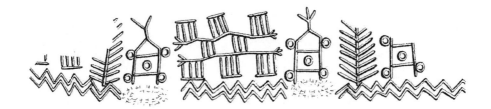

Interdisciplinary and Archaeological Approaches to Studying Children and Childhood in the Past

CHAPTER SIX

Grown Up

Adult Height Dimorphism as an Archive of Living Conditions of Boys and Girls in Prehistory

Eva Rosenstock

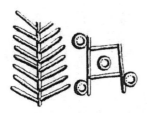

Abstract   *Burials of children are an excellent source for both the archaeology and the physical anthropology of childhood. The information that they provide, however, is only part of the picture: while the biological age can be assessed quite precisely, the determination of sex is difficult for infants unless high-cost analyses on ancient DNA are undertaken. For this reason, so far gender- and sex-related questions pertaining to prehistoric times have hardly been resolved. Moreover, children's burials represent only those individuals who did not survive childhood and thus are to be regarded as a biased sample. Adult burials, on the other hand, represent the survivors and therefore complement our sample. They also preserve a variety of physical information on living conditions during childhood and youth, because the growth of bony structures only lasts until the fusion of the dia- and epiphyses. Some of this information, such as enamel hypoplasia, is precisely datable within an individual's childhood, while other information, such as body height, represents the net nutrition throughout childhood and youth of an individual. Drawing on concepts of the biological standard of living and anthropometric history that have been developed in the field of economic history, this chapter examines the value of adult skeletons as an archive of prehistoric childhood and youth in a long-term perspective, extending from the Palaeolithic period up to ca. 1000 B.C. and using multivariate models. Thereby, special attention is paid to the fact that the sex of adult skeletons can—provided that the diagnostically relevant skeletal areas are preserved—be easily distinguished using morphological criteria, thus enabling us to explore possible sex and gender differentiations in childcare and nutrition as reflected in body height dimorphism.*

ADULT BURIALS AS AN ARCHIVE OF LIVING CONDITIONS IN CHILDHOOD

To have a look at the anthropological, archaeological, iconographical, and textual evidence of children is the first thing that comes to our minds when we are asked how to solve questions regarding childhood in archaeology, and many of the papers presented in this volume use this approach. It must be kept in mind, however, that children's burials represent only those children who did not survive childhood. The remains of deceased children (as in, e.g., Brown, this volume) are thus to be regarded as a highly biased sample, or the "losers." If we wish to make our sample complete, however, we should have a look at the "winners," that is, the adult burials, as well. In addition, sex determination of children of the *infans* I and II stages is very problematic unless high-cost analyses on ancient DNA can be undertaken, whereas adult burials can be sexed using morphological methods, allowing us to view their childhood in terms of the childhood of girls and boys.

Archaeologically, however, it is very difficult to decide which time period in the life span of an individual is represented in the attributes found in an adult burial, such as grave location or grave goods (e.g., Burmeister 2000; Steuer 1968). There might be items of wealth gained through inheritance and wealth gained by achievements in adulthood. We should also contemplate wealth that represents the prestige held by an individual at the time of his/her death, but also about wealth accumulated until the time of death. Moreover, the archaeology of a burial may represent the status that the surviving community wished to bestow upon the deceased. Anthropologically, on the other hand, the health of an individual can be viewed as a measure of wealth, except of course in the case of congenital diseases. Whereas many traces of accidents and violence such as fractures, or of malnutrition and sickness, which can be diagnosed by Harris lines, heal again after some time and are not precisely datable within the individual's growth period (Haidle 1997:75–76; Martin et al. 1985:253–255), specific traces of childhood life remain archived and unchanged in the adult body. And as far as they are conserved in the hard tissues and therefore visible to today's physical anthropologists, these traces were, with the exception of enamel hypoplasia and body height, unknown to the respective person. That is to say the information stored in bones is more objective than, for example, grave goods that could be easily falsified anytime.

We can examine enamel hypoplasia or the less severe Wilson's bands on the second set of teeth. As the teeth crowns are formed during well-defined time slots in the development of an individual and, unlike bone, not restructured during later life, the time period during which a lack of nutrients or diseases occur, the possible reasons for enamel hypoplasia, can be determined as well as its severity—given the fact that a long-lasting undersupply of nutrients leaves a more marked malformation of the enamel (Haidle 1997:63–74; Rose et al. 1985).

Tooth enamel, which mostly consists of inorganic apatite, can also be used to extract samples of certain trace elements, as it conserves the intake during childhood, whereas the intake in the years before death can be derived from the apatite of the long bones. This situation is now mostly used to identify migrations, as the intake of trace elements such as strontium (Sr) and barium (Ba) depends on the content of these elements in the geology of the region. If comparison of the two reveals a difference and large-scale trade with food can be excluded, the individual must have moved at some point in time between formation of the enamel and its death. Yet, needless to say, we must examine children's skeletons in order to identify migrations in childhood, and, therefore, this topic will be left aside in this chapter. But Sr/Ca and Ba/Ca ratios can also mirror the trophic level that an individual had during the formation of the respective tissue, with low ratios being a sign of a rather carnivorous lifestyle. Certain methodological biases in this approach, however, are still debated (Grupe et al. 2005:133–134 vs. Schutkowski 2000; Knipper 2005) and are a reason why the determination of the trophic level by quantifying the relative content of the nitrogen isotope ^{15}N (δ^{15}N) in the organic collagen component of bones is regarded as more reliable today. While δ^{15}N informs us about how much protein came from animal resources, δ^{13}C in addition mirrors plant protein in nutrition (Grupe et al. 2005:126–127). Like milk-drinking and meat-eating herders, completely breastfed babies appear very carnivorous, thus providing a good method for tracing the weaning age in burial remains of children (Dittman and Grupe 2000; see below). The only chance to find out about δ^{15}N and δ^{13}C during the childhood of the "winners," however, could be to take samples from the collagen contained in primary dentine of the tooth roots (Hujić, in prep.). It should be kept in mind, however, that the question has not yet been completely resolved as to whether it is indeed possible to sample this collagen separately from the secondary dentine formed during later life, and whether primary dentine is definitely not subject to life-long reformation (Rummel et al. 2007:392–393; Salamon et al. 2008).

Irrespective of the potential that trace elements and isotope evidence from adult teeth have in identifying childhood nutrition of the "winners" to a precision of a few years, it is very expensive and not likely to become a standard procedure in the near future for large samples. Also, the comparability between populations remains an important and yet unresolved issue. Harris lines and enamel hypoplasia, on the other hand, are very sensitive indicators and, thus, might overemphasize short-term problems in health, work, and nutrition. Body height, however, mirrors the nutrient supply for the skeleton over the complete growth period of an individual within its genetically determined potential body height and, hence, will be the approach of this chapter.

SEXUAL DIMORPHISM IN BODY HEIGHT
AND ITS POTENTIAL FOR CHILDHOOD STUDIES

The systematic difference in form between the two sexes of a species, or sexual dimorphism, is a well-known phenomenon in zoology. In accordance with the parental investment theory (Trivers 1972), primates with their long investment in offspring show a relatively small sexual dimorphism in comparison with other species. Also the assumed correlation with the degree of monogamy seems to hold true for most *Hominidae*, but *Homo sapiens sapiens* shows rather subtle differences.

Among the qualitative primary and secondary sex characteristics, such as genital organs, body shape, and facial and body hair, the difference in height is one of the most prominent secondary characteristics (Stini 1985). A variety of world mean values

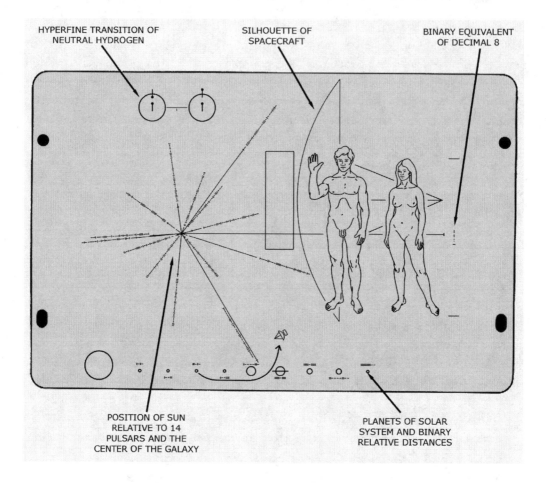

FIGURE 6.1 The Pioneer Plaque (National Aeronautics and Space Administration 2010).

have been published, ranging between circa 11 cm in a worldwide sample collected by Gaulin and Boster (1985) and 15 cm (Gustafsson and Lindenfors 2004). The latter is supported by the ideal as defined by the Pioneer Plaque in 1972 (Figure 6.1). Since the woman's height is indicated as 168 cm, the man must be 183 cm tall—a figure that is quite high given the average height of United States citizens today: 162.2 cm for females and 176.5 cm for males, a difference of 14.3 cm (Deaton 2008). However, if we express the differences in terms of the index:

$$I = \frac{S_m - S_f}{S_m} \times 100$$

with S_f being the female and S_m being the male stature (Lalueza-Fox 1998), we arrive at 8.2 and 8.1. These are very high values in comparison to the world average, which is 6.8 according to the Gaulin and Boster (1985) sample. However, before jumping to the quick conclusion that society in the United States shows a much higher degree of height inequality than the world average, it must be noted that some scholars claim that men obviously grow proportionately taller than women if the whole population is taller (Lalueza-Fox 1998:269; Stini 1985). However, this notion is not supported by a sample of 216 modern societies (Figure 6.2), collected by Gray and Wolfe (1980).

The maximum height that an individual can reach is determined genetically, and there is a considerable debate about the relative degree of genetic and environmental factors on body height. Estimates derived from studies of twins vary between less than 60 percent and more than 95 percent heritability (Knußmann 1980:61–62; Silventoinen et al. 2000; Susanne 1977; for a review of the polygenic nature of growth see Weedon and Frayling 2008), and the question of genetic differences between populations for both maximum height (Eveleth and Tanner 1976:222; Hur et al. 2008) and height dimorphism (Eveleth 1975; Gray and Wolfe 1980) is not yet resolved either, "pygmies" being the only genetically smaller populations securely identified so far (Bozzola et al. 2009).

The most prominent environmental factor for height development within the genetic potential is nutrition. As most parts of our body mass are formed by means of amino

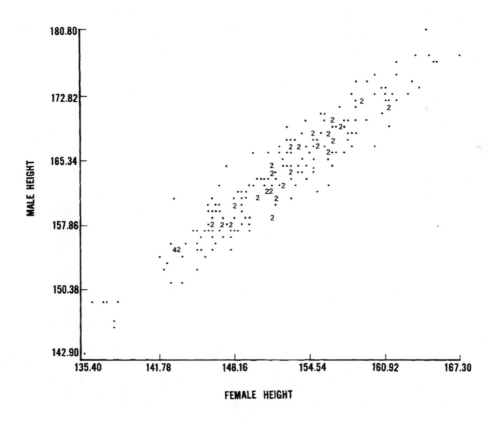

FIGURE 6.2 Height dimorphism in cm in 216 modern populations (Gray and Wolfe 1980:447, Figure 1).

acids, of which some are essential and cannot be synthesized by the body itself, the body height attained thus mainly represents the protein fraction of our net nutrition. Net nutrition is the amount of nutrition that remains available for the production and maintenance of tissue once any energy that is required for keeping the body temperature stable, moving the body, and fighting diseases has been subtracted from the food intake (Komlos 1989:27). This mechanism could be ascertained experimentally in rats and so far has only been viewed in humans by retrospective studies using oral or textual records on childhood nutrition (Wurm 1982:21–22). Improving net nutrition in protein through an increasingly protein-rich diet, a decreased workload, and better medical care is thus to be regarded as the main reason for the increase in body height during the late nineteenth and twentieth centuries in Western industrialized nations (Cole 2003:161), although a direct influence of physical workload on growth is also debated (Ambadekar 1999).

Body height, therefore, has been used in econometry since the late 1980s as an alternative key figure called "biological standard of living." It is often applied for times when and regions where other economic indicators such as the gross national product or per capita income are unreliable or not available, or as a control of these figures; John Komlos (1989) has termed this procedure "anthropometric history." Interesting applications of this method include the care for slaves in the antebellum United States (Margo and Steckel 1992) or the diverging height trends in the two German states from 1945 to 1989 (Komlos and Kriwy 2003). Needless to say, due to the uncertainties of the genetic component, large sample numbers are needed to cancel out these differences, and studies across populations have to control population differences as a possible disruptive factor.

As noted above, long bone length and body height are a cumulative result of net nutrition over the whole growth period of an individual and, thus, cover a variety of stages within an individual's social life. In the following, some physical signs of the maturation process, the modern normal curve of growth development (Figure 6.3) (Eveleth and Tanner 1976; Stini 1985), and certain social markers are contrasted in order to illustrate that some of these rhythms are synchronous but some not at all. Long bone growth starts during pregnancy and at that time is completely dependent upon the nutritional status of the mother. The same holds true as long as the infant is nursed, with gradually increasing importance of other sources of food. The weaning age varies between one and five years in most traditional societies (Stuart-Macadam 1995), being completed by the time of the eruption of the first permanent molar (M_1). This is not only the time of weaning in all nonhuman primates (Dettwyler 1995:55–56; Henke and Rothe 1994:33–36) and the end of the *infans* I stage in anthropological research, but also marks the end of childhood, or *infantia* for the Romans (for an overview of the definition of ages in Europe since Antiquity see Arnold 1993; Bastl 1993; Stahlmann 1993). The weaning age could indeed be pinned down to the third and fourth year for the early medieval period in southern Germany using stable isotope data from children's burials, coinciding well with other signs of ill health and malnutrition, as outlined above, and mortality peaks (Dittmann and Grupe 2000). It should also be kept in mind that in some cultures girls are weaned earlier than boys (McKee 1984; see Dettwyler 1995 for a critical discussion emphasizing natural thresholds such as relative weight rather than sex discrimination).

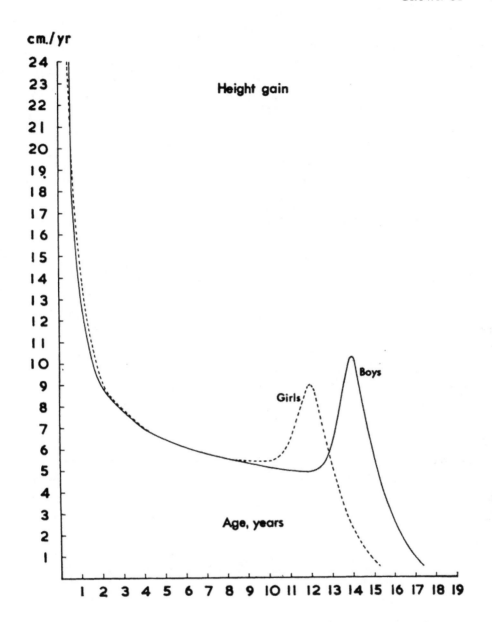

FIGURE 6.3 Human postnatal growth (Tanner et al. 1966:466, Figure 8).

Infans II, lasting until the eruption of the M2 at around age 12, largely overlaps with the Roman *pueritia*, which ends at age 12 to 14. It is characterized by a slowdown in growth until the pubertal growth spurt makes girls taller than their male peers around age 12. At age 14, however, they are outrun by boys, so their growth spurt falls completely within the following *juvenis* stage, or Roman *adolescentia*. During this time span, important and osteologically invisible changes such as menarche, spermarche, and the breaking of the voice occur, thus marking—although earlier exceptions are common—the "sensible" marriageable age and age of consent (Diddle Uzzi, this volume) not only in the Roman and European medieval sources, but also in most modern societies, where it lies somewhere between 12 and 18 years. Therefore, it must be noted that at least for boys a large proportion of growth occurs in a time span that is already denoted as early adulthood by several legally and socially defined markers. Given historical information from the Old World and ethnographic evidence from other regions, we have reason to believe that, especially for participation in daily labor, young individuals were considered able much earlier in past societies than today by the International Labor Organization, which defines child labor as lasting until age 14 or 15. Rather, children increasingly take part in household and farm-level work from age four onward, although it is difficult to distinguish between play and serious tasks. Capacity in business is conceded between seven and 18 years, marriage is usually legal after age 16 for women and 18 for men, and the age of maturity is sometime between ages 18 and 21.

Nevertheless, it should be kept in mind that biological and social developments are not independent: rather, there appears to be a complex network of interaction that is not yet fully understood and still subject to research. Weaning, as noted above, may be a major disruption in health and, thus, diminish net nutrition, leading to slower growth. An early start of workload that is not compensated by more food intake may lead to the same result. Signs of sexual maturity, such as the menarche, the onset of ejaculation, and the breaking of the voice in males, seem to be correlated with certain growth thresholds (Brooks-Gunn and Reiter 1990:31), but they might also be social events that change the individual's access to food. For example, Margo and Steckel (1992) noted a much slower growth in the children of slaves in the southern United States during the eighteenth and nineteenth centuries in comparison to the children of whites of the same time and in the same region. This was followed by a so-called "catch-up growth" after the young slaves started to work, a phenomenon that may even include a prolonged growth period beyond age 20 (Komlos 1989:27; Wit and Boersma 2002), during which in today's Western societies the epiphyseal gaps of the long bones obliterate (Szilvássy 1998:424ff). Thus, under conditions in which the amount of food an individual is entitled to get depends on her or his contribution to the community, we must bear in mind the possibility that children could have been somewhat underfed as long as they did not participate in society as adults, whereas the onset of social adulthood might have drastically increased growth during the last years before the closure of the diaphyseal gaps. But we also should think about practices such as the Bedouin feast called *manzaf*, where only the leftovers of the men's meal are eaten by rest of the household, thus allowing juvenile men free access to the available protein, while young women are often deprived of it.

THE DEVELOPMENT OF HEIGHT DIMORPHISM
IN ARCHAEOLOGY: AN INITIAL SKETCH

The fact that information on body height is not only archived in major sources of historical anthropometry, such as military conscripts or prisoner lists, and also in human skeletal remains, has led to a number of studies by economic historians, anthropologists, and archaeologists in which the development of body height using archaeological data is investigated (e.g., Angel 1984; Bach et al. 1985 and similar Jaeger et al. 1999; Bennike 1985; de Beer 2004; Formicula and Giannecchini 1999; Güleç 1989; Haidle 1997; Helmuth 1965; Hiramoto 1972; Huber 1968; Köpke 2008 and similar Köpke and Baten 2005; Kunitz 1987; Lalueza-Fox 1998; Schröter 2000; Siegmund 2010; Steckel 2004; Waldron 2001; Wurm 1982; cf. the list in Köpke 2008:2). Several of these studies have also discussed aspects of sex dimorphism (Köpke 2008; Lalueza-Fox 1998). However, there are some methodological differences between height data collected on living individuals and on skeletons, which should be noted.

First of all, the stature or measurement "S" as defined by Knußmann (1998:259–260) cannot be assessed directly, but must be calculated from the lengths of long bones. A variety of regression formulae have been developed during the past one hundred years by making regressions between long bone or limb lengths of dead or live bodies and their heights. All of the formulae thus derived have the same linear structure as, for instance,

$$S = a \times R1 + b$$

with R1 being the maximum length of the radius. The differences in these formulae—"a" (slope) and "b" (y-intercept)—are due to different reference populations, ranging from late-nineteenth-century anatomy corpses in Lyon to female students of the 1960s in the German Democratic Republic (for an overview see, e.g., Krogman 1962; Rösing 1988; Siegmund 2010; Wurm 1985). For this reason, it is actually neither possible to directly compare body heights reconstructed using different methods, as made by Lalueza-Fox (1998), nor to compare reconstructed body heights with body heights measured on living individuals (made by, e.g., Jaeger et al. 1998). Instead, reconstructed body height has to be regarded as a virtual figure, which the individual would have had under the assumption that she or he had belonged to the reference population (Röhrer-Ertel 1978:123; Rösing 1988:588f)—but which she or he in fact never did. Hence, a formula fitting best for all prehistoric populations cannot be identified, and ways have to be found to establish comparability: the first steps in this direction have been taken by, for example, Wurm and Leimeister (1986) or Köpke and Baten (2005). As the spine is not used in most formulae, skeletons of elderly individuals can be included in the sample: as long as the joints do not show excessive loss of tissue due to arthritic diseases, the long bones of even a senile individual whose back is bent by old age can inform us about the original adult body height (Trotter and Gleser 1951), whereas, oppositely, individuals who are already mature must be excluded from studies on living heights because of the shrinking of the intervertebral discs. Determining an individual's sex, however, is in most cases straightforward in living persons, whereas the sex of skeletal remains can only be assessed with a certain amount of uncertainty. This information is not only necessary for tracing sex differences in height development, as in this chapter, but also because all the aforementioned regression formulae are sex-specific. As only methods based on ancient DNA provide full security about the sex (see above), this is the most important source of error in studying skeletal remains, although it is still possible to determine the individual's sex with some certainty. If the pelvis is preserved, its traits, which are mainly qualitative, genetically determined and related to the pelvis' functions during pregnancy and birth, make the morphological determination of sex fairly reliable (Sjøvold 1988). Besides some approaches using the inner ear canal (Graw et al. 2005) and the supraorbital margin (Graw et al. 1997), some of the quantitative criteria on the skull (Acsádi and Nemeskéri 1970), such as the external occipital protuberance, are partly dependent upon the strength of the muscles attached, which, however, react to workload and thus environmental factors and render them less reliable. Problems such as these can be dealt with, for example, by giving such individuals less weight in statistical analyses. Thus, those cases in which sex is determined by the length of the long bones or the degree of muscle traces (as in, e.g., Angel 1971; Çiner 1964), must be excluded from the sample.

Given the statistical dispersion of genetically determined body height, sound conclusions can only be drawn from a sufficient database. So far, 789 partially aggregated datasets of 1,348 individuals from 214 sites dating between the Palaeolithic and the Urnfield periods have been collected in collaboration with the Chair of Economic History at the University of Tübingen. The sample thus forms a "prequel" to previous studies investigating Iron Age and later periods (Köpke 2008; Köpke and Baten 2005). Data on individuals with insecure sexing and subadult age were excluded, and it should be noted here that the sample—with 532 females in 355 datasets and 820 males in 434 datasets—has a very uneven sex distribution. It is still largely unclear as to whether the reasons for this well-known phenomenon are biases in the anthropological sexing method or in the archaeological record (Kemkes-Grottenthaler 1997).

Figure 6.4 shows the rather uneven spatial and chronological distribution of the sample. The relative lack of data from before the sixth millennium and of data from the fourth millennium B.C. in Europe renders all conclusions drawn from this sample as still preliminary.

This chapter uses reconstructed body heights according to the following procedures. Instead of using corrections for the two sides of the body, side differences were ignored (Rösing 1988:589), and the arithmetic mean was used if both measurements were available. If, for example, instead of F1 solely F2, namely, the total length in natural position (all measurements according to Martin 1928:1037; cf. Bräuer 1998:216), Rösing's (1988:595) correction was used. When femur lengths were missing, but other long bone lengths were available, the correlation formulae published by Trotter and Gleser (1952:489) for American "white" soldiers were used to calculate an approximation. If only calculated body heights were published, a virtual F1 was calculated using the formula given in the source and then recalculated into Trotter/Gleser 1952 heights. If no formula was indicated, or the length was taken from a complete skeleton, the Trotter and Gleser formula of 1952 was used.

With mean women's and men's heights of 155 cm and 168 cm, our samples shows a sex dimorphism index of 8.7. The fact that this is even higher than the index of the Pioneer Plaque couple seems satisfying at first, but it should be kept in mind that the average male in the sample is 15 cm shorter than the Pioneer Plaque man and that morphological sexing of the skeletons in the sample might be biased by body height. After all, such a dimorphism is relatively high in comparison with the modern world average.

The time trend in the sample is drawn in Figure 6.5 and shows that the Palaeolithic and Epipaleolithic were times of a good biological standard, a time when the girls and boys in our sample reached body heights of ca. 160 cm and 172 cm respectively.

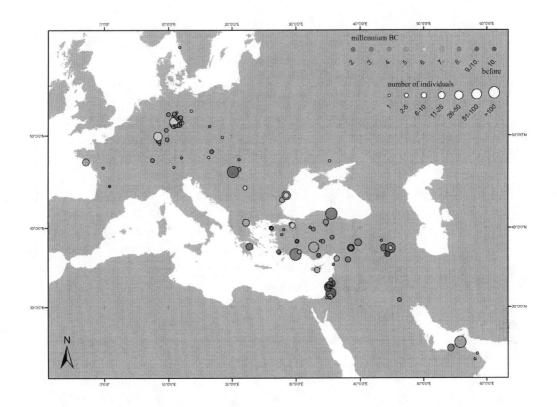

Figure 6.4 Spatial and chronological distribution of the sample. For a list of sites and references, see Rosenstock (2014: 155–157).

time trend in body height with 95% confidence intervals

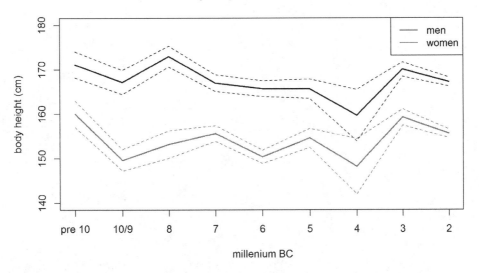

Figure 6.5 Time trend of male and female body height in the sample. For details to reconstruction according to Trotter and Gleser (1952), see text.

The taphonomic conditions of Palaeolithic skeletal finds, however, illustrate how much factors such as social status might have influenced the selection and probability of preservation of burials, a status that again might have been the result of better nutrition during childhood. The tenth and ninth millennia B.C., however, are characterized by the process of Neolithization in the Near East, on the one hand, and the continuation of the Mesolithic hunter-gatherer lifestyle, on the other; they show that time cannot be used as the only explanatory variable. However, some trends in our sample, such as the decline of body height between Palaeolithic and Mesolithic can be seen in other studies, too (Angel 1984; Formicula and Giannecchini 1999). In addition, the clear negative trend during the Neolithic is also visible in Greece and Denmark and was only counteracted in the third millennium B.C., exactly as in the Early Bronze age in Greece and the Late Neolithic in Denmark (Angel 1984; Bennicke 1985). At the same time, body height rises in Central Europe with the Beaker and Corded Ware cultures (Brothwell 1973:290; Jaeger et al. 1998; Jörgensen 1973; Menninger 2008). To properly reflect the various economic strategies coexisting until the fourth millennium B.C., such as hunter-gatherers, farmer-stockherders, and pure herdsmen, methods such as the Multiple Linear Regression Analysis (MLRA) should be used, since they have the potential to evaluate a number of explaining variables in one single model.

Of the variables listed in Table 6.1, a geographic factor, two dummies for economy and millennia as categorical variables could be used in a linear regression model. More precisely, a linear mixed model (LMM) with latitude, sex, economic factors, as well as the interaction term of the latter two as fixed effects, was fitted to the data. The millennium variable was introduced as a random effect to cover the heterogeneity not explained by the fixed effects. The coefficients can be interpreted as deviations from body height predicted by the coefficients of the fixed effects only (Table 6.2). With an adj. R^2 of 43 percent, its explanatory potential is relatively high.

TABLE 6.1
LIST OF VARIABLES USED IN THE REGRESSION MODEL

Name	Explanation
Constant	Constant, for dependent variable F1, when all independent variables = 0
Sex	Dummy for sex, 0 = female, 1 = male
Reliability	Reliability of F1, ordinal scale from 1 to 3, s. Table 1
Latitude	Degree of northern latitude
Domplant	Dummy for cultivation, 0 = not present, 1 = present
Domanimal	Dummy for animal husbandry, 0 = not present, 1 = present
Millenium	Factor Variable for dating with categories: before 10th millennium B.C., 10th or 9th millennium B.C., 8th millennium B.C., 7th millennium B.C., 6th millennium B.C., 5th millennium B.C., 4th millennium B.C., 3rd millennium B.C., 2nd millennium B.C.

TABLE 6.2
MULTIPLE LINEAR (MIXED EFFECTS) REGRESSION.
THE CONSTANT REFERS TO A FEMALE INDIVIDUAL LIVING UNDER HUNTER-GATHERER CONDITIONS (AVERAGED OVER MILLENNIA)

	Coeff	std. Error	p-value
Fixed effects:			
Constant	155.28	2.58	0.000
Sex	11.35	1.76	0.000
Latitude	0.06	0.05	0.226
Domplant	−5.15	2.50	0.040
Domplant: men	5.76	2.52	0.015
Domanimal	2.00	2.35	0.428
Domanimal: men	−5.15	1.82	0.012
Random effects:			
Pre 10	−2.45		
10/9	−1.92		
8	3.50		
7	0.78		
6	−3.36		
5	−0.98		
4	−4.62		
3	3.66		
2	0.50		
R^2	0.43		
N (underlying)	1348		

Males are 13 cm taller than females in the sample, and the negative correlation between plant domestication and biological standard of living seems to be a problem predominantly among females, whereas there is a clear negative relationship between body height and animal domestication in males. Interestingly, latitude does not have any notable effect on body height. This confirms that the chronological development is not only an effect of a linear relationship with the position of the sites and, thus, a result of the uneven distribution of the sample. It might, moreover, be a hint that the so-called Bergmann and Allen rules—which claim that endo- and homoiothermal animals are larger in the northern regions of their habitat (Blackburn et al. 1999)—are not applicable to humans.

CHANGES IN HEIGHT DIMORPHISM:
A PRELIMINARY DISCUSSION OF SOME POSSIBLE REASONS

In this last section, I would like to discuss some mechanisms that may underlie the trends outlined above (cf. Wolfe and Gray 1982 for a modern sample). The good biological standard of living in the Palaeolithic supports the idea of an "original affluent society" invoked by the Bible, archaeology, and ethnology with low populations, but self-sufficient economics in hunter-gatherer societies (Gen. III:17–19; Gen. XXV:27–28; Eaton et al. 1988; Sahlins 1972), who ate high proportions of animal protein. So far, geochemical data derived from Palaeolithic skeletons support this for adult diet (Richards 2002). The very low height dimorphism seems to indicate that girls were entitled to get their share of the prey, while the findings from Sungir (Richards et al. 2001:Table 3) might even suggest an earlier onset of self-supply for young boys who were not yet skilled as hunters and, thus, had lower $\delta^{15}N$-values (Bahn, this volume).

Given the assumption that plant cultivation in prehistory was mainly the domain of females, we can interpret its significant negative correlation with female height as evidence for a high workload of girls and young women, reducing their net nutrition, whereas young men did not participate as much in cultivation. Given the contrary assumption that it was men's work, modern examples show that the high physical demands, particularly on the strength of the upper arm, in cultivation make boys the better investment regarding food for the welfare of the community (Klasen 1998; Ogilvie 2003). Similar mechanisms seem to work in modern societies, such as India (Deaton 2008), and are often expressed also in cultural habits like the bride price to be paid by the bride's parents to compensate for the additional eater in the groom's family. Interestingly, animal domestication appears to be a significant detrimental factor for men's body height in our model, while no significant effect can be seen for women; reasons have yet to be explored, but it can be noted that especially in dealing with small livestock like sheep and goats, men have no physical advantage over women. Moreover, a gendered way of milk consumption as an additional protein source has to be considered given that the care for milk livestock, dairy activities, and milk products consumption is mainly the domain of women in cross-cultural samples today (Badran 1982; Murdock and Provost 1973: 207; Sandgruber 2004). Milk use is first attested as early as the seventh millennium B.C. in the archaeological record (Craig et al. 2005; Evershed et al. 2008).

The drop of femur lengths of both sexes in the sixth millennium B.C. can perhaps be explained by an increase in population during the expansion of the Neolithic, so that the available protein had to be distributed to more people and, thus, children. The body height rise along with a decreasing height dimorphism in the third and second millennia B.C. prompts questions as to which changes led to an improvement in overall gross nutrition (Scheibner, in prep.) and net nutrition of girls. We could think of a reduction in the workload and better applicability of women in cultivation by the introduction of less demanding technologies such as slash-and-burn agriculture (Schier 2009), or animal traction starting to become prominent during the second half of the fourth millennium B.C. (Fansa and Burmeister 2004). In view of the evidence that milk use also becomes denser in the fourth and third millennia B.C. (Rosenstock et al. in press), and that the onset of lactase persistence has not yet been securely dated (Burger et al. 2007; Itan et al. 2009), we could argue for an onset of more intense or even qualitatively different milk use as the reason for this trend as well.

Because of the distortions in the sample as well as the small number and plumpness of the explaining variables, these preliminary results are further scrutinized in a project titled "Living Conditions and Biological Standard of Living in Prehistoric Southwest Asia and Europe: Anthropometric, Cliometric and Archaeometric Approaches (LiVES)" at the Institute of Prehistoric Archaeology in the Free University Berlin (Rosenstock 2014) and funded by the German Research Foundation (DFG). Not only more anthropometric data and more sophisticated statistical techniques to circumvent biased samples (Groß, in prep.), but also more and better proxies for economy, protein supply, work- and disease-load, population density, climate, etc. have to be defined. As climatic events are very precisely datable, higher dating precision for the archaeological data is a main task besides the control of further modifying factors such as social status and migrations. Although the results achieved so far are very encouraging, it should be kept in mind that all anthropometric approaches use in fact biological childhood net nutrition as a proxy for adult nutrition. And as biological childhood and the socially constructed childhood are by no means synchronous phenomena, the proportion of child- and adulthood reflected in the adult body height might vary through time and space in prehistory.

ACKNOWLEDGMENTS

I thank Jörg Baten (chair of Economic History, University of Tübingen) and Nikola Köpke (Departament d'Història i Institucions Econòmiques, University of Barcelona) for their support in methodology and data collection. Thanks are also due to Alisa Hujić (Emmy-Noether-Group LiVES, Free University Berlin) for her advice on physical anthropology, and special thanks are due to Marcus Groß (Emmy-Noether-Group LiVES and Statistical Counseling Unit, Free University Berlin) for doing the statistical parts of this chapter.

REFERENCES CITED

Acsádi, G., and J. Nemeskéri 1970 *History of Human Life Span and Mortality*. Akadémiai Kiadó, Budapest.

Ambadekar, N. N., S. N. Wahab, S. P. Zodpey, and D. W. Khandait 1999 Effect of Child Labour on Growth of Children. *Public Health* 113(6):303–306.

Angel, J. L. 1971 *The People of Lerna. Analysis of a Prehistoric Aegean Population*. American School of Classical Studies at Athens, Washington, D.C.

Angel, J. L. 1984 Health as a Crucial Factor in the Changes from Hunting to Developed Farming in the Eastern Mediterranean. In *Paleopathology at the Origins of Agriculture*, edited by M. N. Cohen and G. J. Armelagos, pp. 51–73. Academic Press, Orlando.

Arnold, K. 1993 Lebensalter: Mittelalter. In *Europäische Mentalitätsgeschichte. Hauptthemen in Einzeldarstellungen*, edited by P. Dinzelbacher, pp. 248–254. Alfred Kröner, Stuttgart.

Bach, H., U. Jaeger, and K. Zellner 1985 Die säkulare Akzeleration der Körperhöhe. In *Medizinische und gesellschaftliche Probleme der Humangenetik*, edited by W. Göhler, pp. 63–72. Verlag Volk und Gesundheit, Berlin.

Badran, M. 1981 Women and Production in the Middle East and North Africa. *Trends in History* 2:59–88.

Bastl, B. 1993 Lebensalter: Neuzeit. In *Europäische Mentalitätsgeschichte. Hauptthemen in Einzeldarstellungen*, edited by P. Dinzelbacher, pp. 255–264. Alfred Kröner, Stuttgart.

Bennicke, P. 1985 *Paleopathology of Danish Skeletons*. Akademisk Forlag, Kopenhagen.

Blackburn, T. M., K. J. Gaston, and N. Loder 1999 Geographic Gradients in Body Size: A Clarification of Bergmann's Rule. *Diversity and Distributions* 5:165–174.

Bozzola, M., P. Travaglino, N. Marziliano, C. Meazza, S. Pagani, M. Grasso, M. Tauber, M. Diegoli, A. Pilotto, E. Disabella, P. Tarantino, A. Brega, and E. Arbustini 2009 The Shortness of Pygmies is Associated with Severe Under-expression of the Growth Hormone Receptor. *Molecular Genetics and Metabolism* 98(73):310–313.

Bräuer, G. 1998 Osteometrie. In *Anthropologie: Handbuch der vergleichenden Biologie des Menschen (= ⁴Lehrbuch der Anthropologie) Band I/1: Wesen und Methoden der Anthropologie. Wissenschaftstheorie, Geschichte, morphologische Methoden*, edited by R. Knußmann, pp. 160–232. Gustav Fischer, Stuttgart and New York.

Brooks-Gunn, J., and E. O. Reiter 1990 The Role of Pubertal Processes. In *At the Threshold: the Developing Adolescent*, edited by S. S. Feldman and G. R. Elliott, pp. 16–53. Harvard University Press, Cambridge.

Brothwell, D. R. 1973 The Human Biology of the Neolithic Population of Britain. In *Die Anfänge des Neolithikums vom Orient bis Nordeuropa VIIIa: Anthropologie Teil 1*, edited by I. Schwidetzky, pp. 280–299. Böhlau, Köln-Wien.

Burger, J., M. Kirchner, B. Bramanti, W. Haak, and M. G. Thomas 2007 Absence of the Lactase-Persistence-Associated Allele in early Neolithic Europeans. *Proceedings of the National Academy of Sciences* 104(10):3736–3741.

Burmeister, S. 2000 *Geschlecht, Alter und Herrschaft in der Späthallstattzeit Württembergs*. Tübinger Schriften zur ur- und frühgeschichtlichen Archäologie 4. Waxmann, Münster.

Cole, T. J. 2003 The Secular Trend in Human Physical Growth: a Biological View. *Economics and Human Biology* 1:161–168.

Craig, O. E., J. Chapman, C. Heron, L.H. Willis, L. Bartosiewicz, G. Taylor, A. Whittle, and M. Collins 2005 Did the First Farmers of Central and Eastern Europe Produce Dairy Foods? *Antiquity* 79:882–894.

Çiner, R. 1964 Evdi Tepesi ve Civarından Çıkarılan İskelet Kalıntıların Tetkiki. *Antropoloji* I:78–98.

Deaton, A. 2008 Height, Health, and Inequality: The Distribution of Adult Heights in India. *American Economic Review* 98:468–474.

de Beer, H. 2004 Observations on the History of Dutch Physical Stature from the Late Middle Ages to the Present. *Economics and Human Biology* 2(1):45–55.

Dettwyler, K. A. 1995 A Time to Wean: The Hominid Blueprint for the Natural Age of Weaning in Modern Human Populations. In *Breastfeeding: Biocultural Perspectives*, edited by P. Stuart-Macadam and K. Dettwyler, pp. 39–73. Aldine de Gruyter, New York.

Dittmann, K., and G. Grupe 2000 Biochemical and Palaeopathological Investigations on Weaning and Infant Mortality in the Early Middle Ages. *Anthropologischer Anzeiger* 58:345–355.

Eaton, S. B., M. Shostak, and M. Konner 1988 *The Paleolithic Prescription*. Harper and Row, New York.

Eveleth, P. B. 1975 Differences between Ethnic Groups in Sex Dimorphism of Adult Height. *Annals of Human Biology* 2(1):35–39.

Eveleth, P. B., and J. M. Tanner 1976 *Worldwide Variation in Human Growth*. Harvard University Press, Cambridge.

Evershed, R. P., S. Payne, A. G. Sherratt, M. S. Copley, J. Coolidge, D. Urem-Kotsu, K. Kotsakis, M. Özdoğan, A. E. Özdoğan, O. Nieuwenhuyse, P. M. M. G. Akkermans, D. Bailey, R.-R. Andeescu, S. Campbell, S. Farid, I. Hodder, N. Yalman, M. Özbaşaran, E. Bıçakcı, Y. Garfinkel, T. Levy, and M. M. Burton 2008 Earliest Date for Milk Use in the Near East and Southeastern Europe linked to Cattle Herding. *Nature* 455:528–531.

Fansa, M., and S. Burmeister 2004 *Rad und Wagen: der Ursprung einer Innovation*. Wissenschaftliche Begleitschrift zur Sonderausstellung vom 28. März bis 11. Juli 2004 im Landesmuseum für Natur und Mensch, Oldenburg (= Archäologische Mitteilungen aus Nordwestdeutschland Beiheft 40). Von Zabern, Mainz.

Formicula, V., and M. Giannecchini 1999 Evolutionary Trends of Stature in Upper Paleolithic and Mesolithic Europe. *Journal of Human Evolution* 36:319–333.

Gaulin, S., and J. Boster 1985 Cross-Cultural Differences in Sexual Dimorphism: Is There any Variance to be Explained? *Ethology and Sociobiology* 6:219–225.

Graw, M., H.-T. Haffner, and A. Czarnetzki 1997 Methode zur Untersuchung des Margo supra-orbitalis als Kriterium zur Geschlechtsdiagnose—Reliabilität und Validität. *Rechtsmedizin* 74:121–126.

Graw, M., J. Wahl, and M. Ahlbrecht 2005 Course of the Meatus Acusticus Internus as Criterion for Sex Differentiation. *Forensic Science International* 147:113–117.

Gray, J. P., and L. D. Wolfe 1980 Height and Sexual Dimorphism of Stature among Human Societies. *American Journal of Physical Anthropology* 53(3):441–456.

Groß, M. in press Spatio-temporal Bayesian Error-in-Variables-Models in Application to Prehistoric Anthropolocial Data. *Annals of Applied Statistics*.

Grupe, G., K. Christiansen, I. Schröder, and U. Wittwer-Backofen 2005 *Anthropologie. Ein einführendes Lehrbuch*. Springer, Berlin.

Gustafsson, A., and P. Lindenfors 2004 Human Size Evolution: No Allometric Relationship between Male and Female Stature. *Journal of Human Evolution* 47:253–266.

Güleç, E. 1989 Paleoantropolojik verilerer göre eski Anadolu bireylerinin boy açısından incelenmesi. *Arkeometri Sonuçları Toplantısı* 5:147–160.

Haidle, M. N. 1997 Mangel—Krisen—Hungersnöte? Ernährungszustände in Süddeutschland und der Nordschweiz vom Neolithikum bis ins 19. Jahrhundert. Urgeschichtliche Materialhefte 11. Mo Vince, Tübingen.

Helmuth, H. 1965 Über die Körpergröße Kieler Männer vom Mittelalter zur Jetztzeit. *Anthropologischer Anzeiger* 29:90–95.

Henke, W., and H. Rothe 1994 *Paläoanthropologie*. Springer, Berlin.

Hiramoto, Y. 1972 Secular Change of Estimated Stature of Japanese in Kanto District from the Prehistoric Age to the Present Day. *Journal of the Anthropological Society of Nippon* 80(3):221–236.

Huber, N. M. 1968 The Problem of Stature Increase: Looking from the Past to the Present. In *The Skeletal Biology of Earlier Human Populations*, edited by D. R. Brothwell, pp. 67–102. Pergamon Press, Oxford.

Hujić, A. in press. Das Kind in uns unter der Lupe der Isotopie, Allometrie und Pathologie: Zusammenhang zwischen δ15N und δ13C als Ernährungsproxies und longitudinalem Knochenwachstum bei adulten, prähistorischen Skelettindividuen unter Berücksichtigung weiterer Indikatoren für Nährstoffversorgung.

Hur Y. M., J. Kaprio, W. G. Iacono, D. I. Boomsma, M. McGue, Karri Silventoinen, N. G. Martin, M. Luciano, P. M. Visscher, R. J. Rose, M. He, J. Ando, S. Ooki, K. Nonaka, C. C. Lin, H. R. Lajunen, B. K. Cornes, M. Bartels, C. E. van Beijsterveldt, S. S. Cherny, and K. Mitchell 2008 Genetic Influences on the Difference in Variability of Height, Weight, and Body Mass Index between Caucasian and East Asian Adolescent Twins. *International Journal of Obesity* 32:1455–1467.

Itan, Y., A. Powell, M. A. Beaumont, J. Burger, and M. G. Thomas 2009 The Origins of Lactase Persistence in Europe. *Public Library of Science Computational Biology* 5, 2009. Electronic document, http://www.ploscompbiol.org/article/info:doi%2F10.1371%2Fjournal.pcbi.1000491; accessed January 18, 2010.

Jaeger, U., H. Bruchhaus, L. Finke, K. Kromeyer-Hauschild, and K. Zellner 1998 Säkularer Trend bei der Körperhöhe seit dem Neolithikum. *Anthropologischer Anzeiger* 56:117–130.

Jörgensen, L. B. 1973 Anthropologie des skandinavischen Neolithikums. In *Die Anfänge des Neolithikums vom Orient bis Nordeuropa VIIIa: Anthropologie Teil 1*, edited by I. Schwidetzky, pp. 280–299. Böhlau, Köln-Wien.

Kemkes-Grottenthaler, A. 1997 Das Frauendefizit archäologischer Serien: ein paläodemographisches Paradoxon? *Anthropologischer Anzeiger* 55:265–280.

Klasen, S. 1998 Marriage, Bargaining, and Intrahousehold Resource Allocation: Excess Female Mortality among Adults during Early German Development, 1740–1860. *Journal of Economic History* 58(2):432–467.

Knipper, C. 2005 Mobility, Diet, and Diagenesis: Trace Elemental Analyses of Faunal Remains from Southern Germany. In *Proceedings of the 33rd International Symposium on Archaeometry, 22.–26. April 2002, Amsterdam*. Geoarchaeological and Bioarchaeological Studies 3, edited by H. Kars and E. Burke, pp. 471–475. Institute for Geo- and Bioarchaeology, Vrije Universiteit, Amsterdam.

Knußmann, R. 1980 *Vergleichende Biologie des Menschen. Lehrbuch der Anthropologie und Humangenetik*. Fischer, Stuttgart.

Knußmann, R. 1988 Somatometrie. In *Anthropologie: Handbuch der vergleichenden Biologie des Menschen (= ⁴Lehrbuch der Anthropologie) Band I/1: Wesen und Methoden der Anthropologie. Wissenschaftstheorie, Geschichte, morphologische Methoden*, edited by R. Knußmann, pp. 232–285. Fischer, Stuttgart and New York.

Komlos, J. 1989 *Nutrition and Economic Development in the Eighteenth-Century Habsburg Monarchy: An Anthropometric History*. Princeton University Press, Princeton.

Komlos, J., and P. Kriwy 2003 The Biological Standard of Living in the Two Germanies. *German Economic Review* 4:493–507.

Köpke, N. 2008 *Regional Differences and Temporal Development of the Nutritional Status in Europe from the 8th century B.C. until the 18th century A.D.* Dissertation. Tübingen 2008. Electronic document, http://nbn-resolving.de/urn:nbn:de:bsz:21-opus-35638>; accessed January 11, 2009.

Köpke, N., and J. Baten 2005 The Biological Standard of Living in Europe during the Last Two Millennia. *European Review of Economic History* 9(1): 61–95.

Krogman, W. M. 1962 *The Human Skeleton in Forensic Medicine*. Charles C. Thomas, Springfield, Illinois.

Kunitz, S. J. 1987 Making a Long Story Short: A Note on Men's Height and Mortality in England from the First through the Nineteenth Centuries. *Medical History* 31(3):269–280.

Lalueza-Fox, C. 1998 Stature and Sexual Dimorphism in Ancient Iberian Populations. *Homo* 49(2):260–272.

Margo, R. A., and R. H. Steckel 1992 The Nutrition and Health of Slaves and Antebellum Southern Whites. In *Without Consent or Contract. Conditions of Slave Live and the Transition to Freedom*, edited by R. W. Fogel and S. L. Engerman, pp. 508–521. W. W. Norton, New York.

Martin, R. 1928 *Lehrbuch der Anthropologie in systematischer Darstellung*. 2nd edition. Fischer, Jena.

Martin, D. L., A. H. Goodman, and G. J. Armelagos 1985 Skeletal Pathologies as Indicators of Diet. In *The Analysis of Prehistoric Diets*, edited by R. I. Gilbert Jr. and J. H. Mielke, pp. 227–279. Academic Press, Orlando.

McKee, L. 1984 Sex Differentials in Survivorship and the Customary Treatment of Infants and Children. *Medical Anthropology* 8(2):91–103.

Murdock, G. P., and C. Provost 1973 Factors in the Division of Labor by Sex: A Cross-Cultural Analysis. *Ethnology* 12(2):203–225.

National Aeronautics and Space Administration (NASA) 2010 The Pioneer Missions. Electronic document, http://www.nasa.gov/centers/ames/missions/archive/pioneer.html; accessed July 3, 2010.

Ogilvie, S. 2003 *A Bitter Living. Women, Markets, and Social Capital in Early Modern Germany*. Oxford University Press, Oxford.

Richards, M. P. 2002 A Brief Review of the Archaeological Evidence for Palaeolithic and Neolithic Subsistence. *European Journal of Clinical Nutrition* 56. Electronic document, doi:10.1038/sj.ejcn.1601646; accessed January 26, 2011.

Richards, M. P., P. B. Pettitt, M. C. Stiner, and E. Trinkaus 2001 Stable Isotope Evidence for Increasing Dietary Breadth in the European Mid-Upper Paleolithic. *Proceedings of the National Academy of Sciences* 98:6528–6532.

Rose, J. C., K. W. Condon, and A. H. Goodman 1985 Diet and Dentition: Developmental Disturbances. In *The Analysis of Prehistoric Diets*, edited by R. I. Gilbert Jr. and J. H. Mielke, pp. 283–305. Academic Press, Orlando.

Rosenstock, E. 2014 Eiweißversorgung und Körperhöhe: zur Übertragbarkeit anthropometrischer Ansätze auf die Archäologie. In *Vom Nil bis an die Elbe. Forschungen aus fünf Jahrzehnten am Institut für Prähistorische Archäologie der Freien Universität Berlin (=Internationale Archäologie—Studia honoraria 36)*, edited by W. Schier and M. Meyer, pp. 147–163. Leihdorf, Rahden, Westfalen.

Rosenstock, E., M. Groß, and A. Hujić in press Back to Good Shape: Biological Standard of Living in the Copper and Bronze Age. In *"Setting the Bronze Age Table": Production, Subsistence, Diet, and Their Implications for European Landscapes. Proceedings of the International Workshop "Socio-Environmental Dynamics over the last 12.000 Years: The Creation of Landscapes III (15th to the 18th of April 2013)" in Kiel (= Universitätsforschungen zur Prähistorischen Archäologie)*, edited by J. Kneisel, W. Kirleis, N. Taylor, M. dal Corso, and V. Tiedtke. Habelt, Bonn.

Röhrer-Ertl, O. 1978 *Die neolithische Revolution im Vorderen Orient. Ein Beitrag zu Fragen der Bevölkerungsbiologie und Bevölkerungsgeschichte*. Oldenbourg, München-Wien.

Rösing, F. W. 1988 Körperhöhenrekonstruktion aus Skelettmaßen. In *Anthropologie: Handbuch der vergleichenden Biologie des Menschen (= ⁴Lehrbuch der Anthropologie) Band I/1: Wesen und Methoden der Anthropologie. Wissenschaftstheorie, Geschichte, morphologische Methoden*, edited by R. Knußmann, pp. 586–600. Gustav Fischer, Stuttgart and New York.

Rummel, S., S. Hölzl, and P. Horn 2007 Isotopensignaturen von Bio- und Geo-Elementen in der Forensik. In *Biologische Spurenkunde Band 1: Kriminalbiologie*, edited by B. Herrmann and K.-S. Saternus, pp. 381–407. Springer, Berlin and Heidelberg.

Sahlins, M. D. 1972 *Stone Age Economics*. Aldine-Atherton, Chicago.

Salamon, M., Coppa, A., McCormick, M., Rubini, M., Vargiu, R., and N. Tuross 2008 The Consilience of Historical and Isotopic Approaches in Reconstructing the Medieval Mediterranean Diet. *Journal of Archaeological Science* 35(6):1667–1672.

Sandgruber, R. 2004 Das Geschlecht der Esser. In *Geschichte des Konsums. Erträge der 20. Tagung der Gesellschaft für Sozial- und Wirtschaftsgeschichte 23–26 April 2003 in Greifswald*, edited by R. Walter, pp. 379–408. Franz Steiner, Stuttgart.

Scheibner, A. in press Changes after the Revolution: Uniformity or Diversity in Late Neolithic and Bronze Age Diets? In *"Setting the Bronze Age Table": Production, Subsistence, Diet, and Their Implications for European Landscapes. Proceedings of the International Workshop "Socio-Environmental Dynamics over the Last 12.000 Years: The Creation of Landscapes III (15th to the 18th of April 2013)" in Kiel (=Universitätsforschungen zur Prähistorischen Archäologie)*, edited by J. Kneisel, W. Kirleis, N. Taylor, M. dal Corso, and V. Tiedtke. Habelt, Bonn.

Schier, W. 2009 Extensiver Brandfeldbau und die Ausbreitung der neolithischen Wirtschaftsweise in Mitteleuropa und Südskandinavien am Ende des 5. Jahrtausends v. Chr. *Praehistorische Zeitschrift* 84:15–43.

Schröter, P. 2000 Anthropologie zur Römerzeit. In *Die Römer zwischen Alpen und Nordmeer: Zivilisatorisches Erbe einer europäischen Militärmacht. Ausstellungskatalog Rosenheim 2000*, edited by L. Wamser, C. Flügel, and B. Zieghaus, pp. 177–181. Von Zabern, Mainz.

Schutkowski, H. 2000 Neighbours in Different Habitats—Subsistence and Social Differentiation in Early Mediaeval Populations of the Eastern Swabian Alb. *Anthropologischer Anzeiger* 58:113–120.

Siegmund, F. 2010 *Die Körpergröße der Menschen in der Ur- und Frühgeschichte Mitteleuropas und ein Vergleich ihrer anthropologischen Schätzmethoden*. Books on Demand, Norderstedt.

Silventoinen, K., J. Kaprio, E. Lahelma, and M. Koskenvuo 2000 Relative Effect of Genetic and Environmental Factors on Body Height: Differences across Birth Cohorts among Finnish Men and Women. *American Journal of Public Health* 90:627–630.

Sjøvold, T. 1988 Geschlechtsdiagnose am Skelett. In *Anthropologie: Handbuch der vergleichenden Biologie des Menschen (= ⁴Lehrbuch der Anthropologie) Band I/1: Wesen und Methoden der Anthropologie. Wissenschaftstheorie, Geschichte, morphologische Methoden*, edited by R. Knußmann, pp. 444–480. Gustav Fischer, Stuttgart and New York.

Stahlmann, I. 1993 Lebensalter: Antike. In *Europäische Mentalitätsgeschichte. Hauptthemen in Einzeldarstellungen*, edited by P. Dinzelbacher, pp. 239–247. Alfred Kröner, Stuttgart.

Steckel, R. H. 2004 New Light on the "Dark Ages." The Remarkably Tall Stature of Northern European Men during the Medieval Era. *Social Science History* 28(2):211–229.

Steuer, H. 1968 Zur Bewaffnung und Sozialstruktur der Merowingerzeit. *Nachrichten aus Niedersachsens Urgeschichte* 37:18–87.

Stini, W. A. 1985 Growth Rates and Sexual Dimorphism in Evolutionary Perspective. In *The Analysis of Prehistoric Diets*, edited by R. I. Gilbert Jr. and J. H. Mielke, pp. 191–226. Academic Press, Orlando.

Stuart-Macadam, P. 1995 Breastfeeding in Prehistory. In *Breastfeeding: Biocultural Perspectives*, edited by P. Stuart-Macadam and K. Dettwyler, pp. 75–99. Aldine de Gruyter, New York.

Susanne, C. 1977 Heritability of Anthropological Characteristics. *Human Biology* 49(4):573–580.

Szilvássy, J. 1998 Altersdiagnose am Skelett. In *Anthropologie: Handbuch der vergleichenden Biologie des Menschen (= ⁴Lehrbuch der Anthropologie) Band I/1: Wesen und Methoden der Anthropologie. Wissenschaftstheorie, Geschichte, morphologische Methoden*, edited by R. Knußmann, pp. 421–443. Gustav Fischer, Stuttgart and New York.

Tanner, J. M., R. H. Whitehouse, and M. Takaishi 1966 Standards from Birth to Maturity for Height, Weight, Height Velocity, and Weight Velocity: British Children, 1965. *Archives of Disease in Childhood* 41:454–471, 613–635.

Trivers, R. L. 1972 Parental Investment and Sexual Selection. In *Sexual Selection and the Descent of Man, 1871–1971*, edited by Bernard Campbell, pp. 136–179. Aldine, Chicago.

Trotter, M., and G. Gleser 1951 The Effect of Ageing on Stature. *American Journal of Physical Archaeology* 9:311–324.

Trotter, M., and G. Gleser 1952 Estimation of Stature from Long Bones of American Whites and Negroes. *American Journal of Physical Anthropology* 10:463–514.

Waldron, T. 2001 *Shadows in the Soil: Human Bones and Archaeology*. Tempus, Stroud and Charleston, South Carolina.

Weedon, M. N., and T. M. Frayling 2008 Reaching New Heights: Insights into the Genetics of Human Stature. *Trends in Genetics* 24(12):595–603.

Wit, J.-M., and B. Boersma 2002 Catch-up Growth: Definition, Mechanisms, and Models. *Journal of Pediatric Endocrinology & Metabolism* 15:1229–1241.

Wolfe, L. D., and J. P. Gray 1982 Subsistence Practices and Human Sexual Dimorphism of Stature. *Journal of Human Evolution* 11(7):575–580.

Wurm, H. 1982 Über die Schwankungen der durchschnittlichen Körperhöhe im Verlauf der deutschen Geschichte und die Einflüsse des Eiweißanteiles der Kost. *Homo* 33:21–42.

Wurm, H. 1985 Zur Geschichte der Körperhöhenschätzung nach Skelettfunden (Körperhöhenschätzungen für Männer). Die vorgeschlagenen Ansätze zur Körperhöhenschätzung nach Skelettfunden seit der Mitte des 20. Jahrhunderts. *Gegenbaurs morphologisches Jahrbuch* 131:383–432.

Wurm, H., and H. Leimeister 1986 Ein Beitrag zur spezifischen Auswahl von Vorschlägen zur Körperhöhenschätzung nach Skelettfunden, zur Vergleichbarkeit von Schätzergebnissen und zur allgemeinen Problematik realistischer Lebendhöhenschätzungen. *Gegenbaurs morphologisches Jahrbuch* 132:69–110.

CHAPTER SEVEN

Placing Children in Society

Using Ancient DNA to Identify Sex and Kinship of Child Skeletal Remains, and Implications for Gender and Social Organization

Keri A. Brown

Abstract *Ancient DNA—DNA preserved in ancient biological material—has the potential to provide basic information about archaeological specimens that is not available by any other method. With children, ancient DNA can address questions about sex and biological parentage. Osteological methods for identifying the sex of prepubertal skeletal remains are problematical, as the sexual dimorphism seen in the adult skeleton has not been developed. DNA-based methods for sex identification can therefore provide information on the biological sex—but not the gender—of pre-adult remains. Most examples of the use of ancient DNA in this context have concerned cases where infanticide has been suspected, the DNA typings being used to identify skewed sex ratios among child burial groups that might indicate selective culling of male or female children. Kinship relationships between child skeletons and with associated adult burials can be addressed by genetic profiling methods, but this work is technically difficult and so far there have been few case studies where DNA-based approaches have been used to study kinship in archaeological or historical burial groups. One successful study, from a Neolithic cemetery in Eulau, Germany, has emphasized the importance placed on the family during this period.*

Ancient DNA extracted from archaeological child remains has the potential to provide basic information about these individuals that is simply not available by any other methods. With ancient DNA, questions about the sex and biological parentage of subadult skeletal material can be posed, and, where DNA preservation conditions permit, answered. But ancient DNA is not a panacea. It cannot "reveal" the presence of children in the archaeological record. It can, however, help to elucidate their identity by establishing their biological sex and their kinship relationships with other individuals—children and adults—with whom they lived and with whom they are buried. In this chapter, I attempt to explain how DNA can be used by archaeologists in the study of children, illustrating these possibilities with examples of the research that has been published to date.

THE SOCIAL ROLES OF SEX, GENDER, AND KINSHIP IDENTITY

From the moment of birth, humans are placed into one of two social categories for which the identification of biological sex is paramount—is it a boy or a girl? This categorization is based on the appearance of the genitalia of the child. Another equally important item of information is the identity of the biological parents of the child. Most of human society seems to be concerned with placing children according to these two criteria. Parentage of the child, especially the acknowledgment of the paternity of the offspring (on the grounds that you can identify the mother via childbirth) remains an important concern in many societies. The knowledge of the parentage enables the rest of the community to "place" the child in a complex web of kinship and status. The knowledge of one's parentage is considered to be so important that UK law allows adopted children and children conceived through sperm and/or egg donation, once they reach the age of 18, to have access to the identities of their biological parents.

Archaeological child skeletal remains lack this social placement. It has been said by many anthropologists that children maybe were not full members of a society, that they lacked the status necessary for full burial rituals, but the fact that children were buried as inhumations at all shows that many societies considered them worthy of this consideration. This suggests that even in prehistory, parents loved their children and were heartbroken by their deaths.

In the twenty-first century, biological sex still remains an important determinant of future life possibilities. But about one in 4,000 babies in the UK has ambiguous genitalia and is thus difficult to categorize simplistically. Until recent years these anomalous infants would be operated on to "turn" them into boys or girls. This attitude has had disastrous consequences in the past, and the policy now is to leave well alone, and let the child decide on its sexual identity when older. The famous case study of a boy turned into a girl by the surgeon John Money springs to mind. We now know that sexual identity is hardwired in the brain and can rarely be altered successfully. A number of syndromes exist that, while comparatively rare, occur at regular frequencies in human populations, and can give rise to various genital anomalies and intersex conditions. These include androgen insensitivity syndrome, Klinefelter's syndrome, and congenital adrenal hyperplasia (see Tables 7.1 and 7.2). Another rare disorder is called 5α-reductase deficiency, a hormonal condition where the infant at birth appears to be female, but at puberty "becomes" male. These conditions must also have existed in the past, and societies then also had the same problems in categorizing infants. However, we cannot assume that past societies were rigidly confined to a choice of two social states or genders (Brown 1998).

Gender is a cultural construction, a system of cultural categorization that uses biological sex differences as a way of structuring thought and practice, but is not determined by them. An important consequence of this definition is that there is a high degree of correlation between biological sex and social gender, but not always a one to one correlation. There are various societies around the world that have more than two genders, and there are documented examples of societies with third genders, or even more, from anthropology and from history. It is important to keep in mind the distinction between biological sex and social gender and not use these words interchangeably, for they have different meanings. A further complication is that sex identification is often referred to as sex determination in many scientific and archaeological articles (Pearson 1996). Sex determination refers solely to the complex chain of events involved in the development of the embryo into a male or female fetus. Sex identification involves assigning the status of female or male to a sample of unknown sex—the sex has already been determined in utero.

OSTEOARCHAEOLOGY AND CHILDREN

Osteological methods for identifying the sex of prepubertal skeletal remains are problematical, as the sexual dimorphism seen in the adult skeleton has not been developed. Morphological and morphometric techniques of sex identification have been developed using modern population skeletal data, which means that the standard data against which archaeological specimens are compared are representative only of modern populations. Not all modern populations show the same degree of sexual dimorphism, and even past populations in, for example, medieval Britain, may show very little dimorphism. Criteria developed for sex identification on one population cannot and should not be applied to other populations. These factors must be taken into account not just for sexing adult remains, but also children. Some attempts have been made to devise methods of sex identification for fetuses and infants based on the pelvis (Krogman and Iscan 1986), but the level of accuracy is only about 70 percent. For prepubertal remains the accuracy is in the order of 75–80 percent, and this level of accuracy depends on the presence of an almost complete skeleton. Without the presence of an intact pelvis, identification of the correct sex of juveniles is only 50–50; in other words, an informed guess (Krogman and Iscan 1986:259). While there is measurable sexual dimorphism in the sciatic notch at an early age (seen in fetuses and infants), there is too much overlap in measurements for this to be used as a reliable sex indicator (Holcomb and Konigsberg 1995) and is soon lost with the subsequent growth of the infant. Schutowski (1993) claimed 70–90 percent accuracy when sexing childrens' skeletons from Spitalfields, a large post-Medieval cemetery in London. The sex of the remains used in his analysis were known in advance by the anthropologist, so this could not be said to be a scientifically controlled test of accuracy of the sex identification criteria used. It is generally considered that the methods currently used in human osteology do not allow sex identification of infants and juveniles based on pelvic morphology with a high degree of confidence. The possibility of using the skull to identify the sex of juveniles has been explored (Molleson et al. 1998).

This method had a 78 percent success rate with juvenile remains of documented sex, and the males thus identified also had larger canine teeth. It has been suggested that the larger dimensions of permanent teeth in adult males is due to the presence of the Y chromosome, which promotes the growth of tooth enamel and dentine, while the X chromosome promotes only enamel growth (Alvesalo 1997). It is known that the gene for amelogenin, a tooth enamel protein, is found on both sex chromosomes, and in fact several DNA-based methods of sex identification target this gene (see below). With the lack of a reliable osteological method for identifying the sex of children, DNA analysis is the only way forward.

Identification of kinship among a group of burials is not possible with osteological methods. An adult and a child buried together are often assumed to be parent and child, especially if the adult is female, but of course, without firm evidence of biological relatedness, this has to remain in the realm of speculation. Small morphological variations in the skeleton, called nonmetric traits, have been used in the past by osteoarchaeologists to infer close kinship within burial groups, and to identify families. The assumption was that nonmetric traits were genetically inherited in a Mendelian fashion, so that offspring would inherit the traits seen in the parents' skeletons. Some 400 nonmetric traits have been catalogued in the human skeleton (including dentition). A brave attempt was made to use nonmetric traits to identify kinship patterns at the megalithic tomb of Chausee-Tirancourt, near Amiens, France (Scarre 1984). But despite much research and statistical analysis, there seems to be no simple correlation between genes and nonmetric traits (Tyrrell 2000). They are usually recorded as standard practice by osteoarchaeologists and even field archaeologists, but there may be differences in observer recognition of these traits. But it is now suspected that many other factors, such as environment and diet, play a significant part in the appearance of nonmetric traits in populations, and they therefore cannot be used to assign kinship or family groupings in burials. Again, DNA-based methods are in fact the only way to show kinship within burial groups.

DNA AND HOW IT IS STUDIED

The molecular structure of DNA (deoxyribose nucleic acid) was discovered by Watson and Crick in 1953. Since then, the double helix has become an icon of our scientific times and the molecular mechanisms of genetic inheritance, the transmission of biological information from one generation to the next, has been unraveled. Genes code for proteins such as enzymes, receptors, immunoglobins, and so on. There are also large tracts of DNA that do not appear to have any known function. They do, however, contain a vast amount of repetitive DNA, more of which when we come to analyze kinship. DNA in humans is packaged into 23 pairs of chromosomes, which are found in the nucleus of every cell except red blood cells. There are 22 pairs of autosomal chromosomes and one pair of sex chromosomes, called X and Y. Normally, females have two X chromosomes and males have an X and a Y chromosome. One chromosome in each pair is inherited from each parent—the genetic sex of the offspring is therefore determined by whether it receives an X or a Y chromosome from the male parent. Biological sex is more complex and many more factors come into play, so that it is possible for genetic sex to differ from biological sex.

In addition to nuclear DNA, human cells possess another type of DNA called mitochondrial DNA (mtDNA). This is a tiny piece of DNA compared to the chromosomes, found in the mitochondria of cells, which are small organelles found in the cytoplasm. These organelles make energy for us. MtDNA is inherited maternally—males do not transmit this DNA to their offspring. MtDNA has been a very useful tool for studying human evolution and migrations out of Africa as it does not undergo recombination and thus mtDNA sequences represent lineages going back into deep time. Single nucleotide mutations in mtDNA have been classified into haplogroups. At least 90 haplogroups are known in human populations around the world, as well as many thousands of haplotypes (individual mtDNA types). The concept of the *molecular clock* has been used to date the emergence of new haplogroups, and the timings of human evolutionary events, such as the movement out of Africa by *Homo sapiens*. The molecular clock assumes that the single nucleotide mutations used for classifying haplogroups occur at a constant rate over time, so by counting the number of base changes it is possible to estimate dates for the origins of mitochondrial lineages. Of course, this is a highly simplified explanation—it is highly complex to do these calculations, and the dates have very wide confidence limits. Nevertheless, mtDNA coalescence dates have tended to correlate very well with archaeological dates for the same events.

Similarly, the Y chromosome has also been classified into haplogroups, but the markers used are more complex, not just single base changes. As the Y chromosome is passed from father to son, it can be used to study paternal lineages over times, thus complementing the maternally inherited lineages of the mitochondrial DNA. Dating the emergence of Y chromosome haplogroups is more complex than with mtDNA, as the markers involved comprise different types of DNA motifs with different genetic histories. There is also the factor to consider that fewer males may have more input into the next generation and thus skew the distribution and frequency of Y chromosome haplogroups, leading to misleading estimates of the emergence of Y chromosomal lineages.

Ancient DNA is defined as DNA obtained from preserved biological material—this may be thousands of years old, or even from a week-old banana skin. Immediately after death, DNA starts degrading through enzymatic, hydrolytic, bacterial, and environmental radiation onslaughts. The complex repair mechanisms in the cell no longer work to maintain the integrity of the DNA sequence information. Ancient DNA thus is fragmented into very small pieces, with chemical damage to the bases, and survives in minute amounts, if it survives at all. There is little difference between *forensic* DNA and ancient DNA. Forensic DNA is defined as DNA retrieved from material up to 75 years old from the present time—this means that there is the possibility of testing this DNA against living relatives. Because it is younger, the hydrolytic scissioning of the DNA strands and the exposure to environmental radiation are less severe, so more information may be recovered from this DNA. The successful reopening of "cold cases"—DNA from crimes committed more than 30–40 years ago—also shows the results of improved DNA techniques. But age is not the only factor in determining ancient DNA preservation.

Environmental temperature is of huge importance. A concept called *"thermal history"* explains how DNA can survive in extremely cold, dry conditions for thousands of years, while DNA from material found in hot, damp conditions rarely survives (Smith et al. 2003). Soil pH also plays a part—acidic pH destroys DNA, while neutral to alkaline pH seems to be helpful for DNA survival. Bacterial activity in the soil can also be destructive—anoxic conditions inhibit bacterial growth, so cold, waterlogged, or otherwise oxygen-free environments are also favorable for DNA survival.

The first ancient DNA study was carried out in 1984 using a sample taken from a museum skin of a quagga, an extinct type of zebra. This was more than 140 years old, but enough DNA was retrieved and used to place the quagga into a phylogenetic tree along with zebras and horses. In 1985, the first human ancient DNA was extracted from an Egyptian mummy. Unfortunately, this has now been realized to be contaminating modern human DNA. At this time ancient DNA was seen as more of a scientific curiosity rather than having any real applications, and it was thought that a high degree of biological and structural integrity was necessary for DNA survival, the sort of biological preservation that is rarely found. It was the invention of the *polymerase chain reaction* (PCR) in the mid-1980s that allowed ancient DNA to emerge as a field of study in its own right. In this method (whose inventor, Kary Mullis, was awarded the Nobel Prize for Chemistry) a short DNA sequence can be targeted and copied many times over so that there is then enough to read the DNA sequence (Figure 7.1). The first PCRs used with ancient DNA

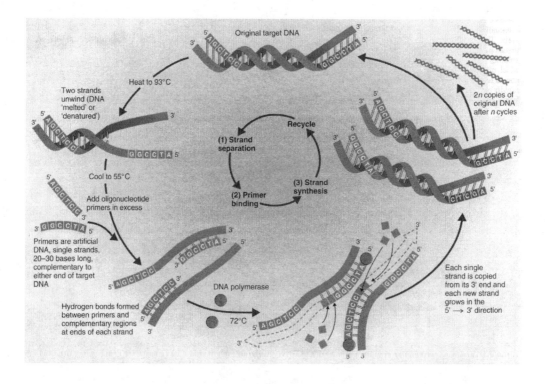

FIGURE 7.1 The Polymerase Chain Reaction (published by permission of Biological Sciences Review)

extracted from archaeological bone material was published in 1989 (Hagelberg et al. 1989), and this showed that it was possible to obtain ancient DNA from ordinary archaeological remains, not just the exceptionally preserved material such as mummies and bog bodies.

DNA-Based Methods of Sex Identification

At the genetic level, there is very little difference between human males and females. The human female has two X chromosomes, the human male has an X chromosome and a Y chromosome. It is the presence of the Y chromosome that determines maleness in humans. When only one X chromosome is present (XO as in Turner's syndrome) the phenotype is female (YO never occurs and is assumed to be lethal). But there are always exceptions to every rule (see below for more detail), but these are very rare. With modern DNA samples, the identification of sex is straightforward and usually involves targeting a multiple repeat sequence on the Y chromosome. Ancient DNA is damaged, fragmented, and survives in picogram amounts, so that the failure of a PCR directed at a Y chromosome locus could be interpreted as indicating a female (for example, Brown 2001; Hummel and Herrmann 1991). A more satisfactory experimental approach is one that gives unambiguous results for both male and female. The presence of the amelogenin gene on both X and Y chromosomes means that a PCR experiment directed at this gene can be designed that will give a product from each sex chromosome (Nakahori et al. 1991b). The complete sequence for the X and Y versions of the amelogenin gene was published by Nakahori et al. (1991a), and the sequence shows a number of differences, in the form of *indels* (*in*sertions and *del*etions of the DNA sequence), between the male and female versions. PCR systems have been designed to take advantage of these indels, so that the products from the two chromosomes show a difference in length that can be visualized on an electrophoresis gel. When using template DNA from a female, only one band is seen, whereas two bands are seen for a male DNA sample, one for the X and one from the Y chromosome. Of the various PCR systems that have been published for sex identification based on the amelogenin gene (Faerman et al. 1995; Götherstrom et al. 1997; Stone et al. 1996), the one that is now used routinely in ancient and forensic DNA work was devised by the Forensic Science Service in the UK (Sullivan et al. 1993) (Figure 7.2 on page 136).

PCR-based sex identification may use targets other than the amelogenin gene. Other loci on the X and Y chromosomes have been used by other groups, such as the ZFX and ZFY genes (zinc finger proteins; Stacks and Witte, 1996) and the alphoid satellite repeat sequences found in the centromeric regions of the X and Y chromosomes (Hanaoka and Minaguchi 1996), but in both examples further experiments are needed to confirm the PCR results. The amelogenin PCR is elegant and simple and remains the method of choice for sex identification with ancient DNA templates.

Complications in Sex Identification

There are rare scenarios where genetic sex (the genotype) can differ from biological sex (the phenotype) (Tables 7.1 and 7.2 on page 137). In humans, the absence of the Y chromosome usually results in a female (XX and XO). Turner's syndrome occurs in indi-

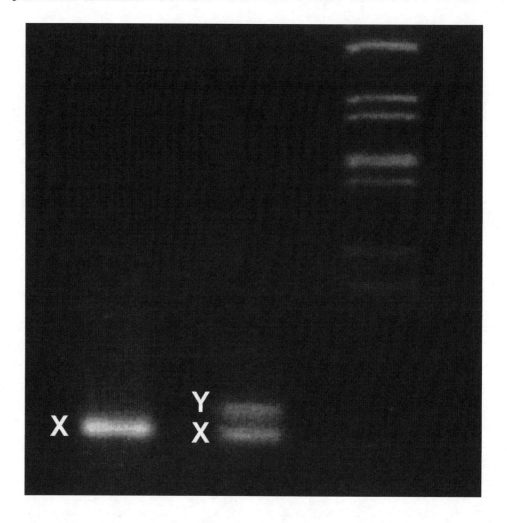

FIGURE 7.2 Electrophoresis gel of PCR products from the amelogenin gene in human DNA. The single band is from the X chromosome and is 106 bp long. The two bands are from the Y chromosome, the upper band is 112 bp long. One band means that DNA originated from a female; two bands show a male. The multiple bands represent a DNA marker for checking the size of the PCR products.

viduals with one X chromosome. However, XX males are known to occur, 80 percent of these individuals possessing the male-determining SRY gene, probably because of a rare transfer from a Y chromosome. These are phenotypically male, but the amelogenin-based sex identification would identify them as female. There are also instances of XX males who lack the SRY gene, so some other unknown cause must be responsible in these cases. Conversely, XY females are also known, but only 15 percent of these have an SRY-deleted version of the Y chromosome. Other XY reversals occur because of the presence of two copies of the DAX gene on the X chromosome. DAX is antagonistic to SRY, therefore an extra copy of DAX results in the female phenotype (Swain et al. 1998). One in

TABLE 7.1
SEX IDENTIFICATION ANOMALIES: SEX REVERSALS AND SIMILAR ANOMALIES

Sex chromosome complement	Anomaly	Frequency in population	Biological sex	Amelogenin PCR result
XX	Sex reversal	1:25,000	Male	Female
XY	Sex reversal	1:20,000	Female	Male
XY	Androgen insensitivity syndrome	1:20,000	Female	Male
XX	Congenital adrenal hyperplasia	1:15,000	Male	Female
XY	Amelogenin deletion	1:2500?	Male	Female

20–25,000 males is XX, and one in 20,000 females is XY. Other causes of sex reversals in humans are hormonal in origin, such as congenital adrenal hyperplasia, androgen insensitivity syndrome, and 5α-reductase deficiency (Imperato-McGinley et al. 1979).

As well as these rare sex-reversed individuals, other phenomena involving the sex chromosomes may occur more frequently in human populations. Invariably, these involve abnormal sex chromosome numbers. The XXY male (Klinefelter's syndrome) is often an *intersex* in phenotype (because of the presence of the second X chromosome), while XO (Turner's syndrome) and XXX females are *infrafemales,* which are sexually underdeveloped. The presence of abnormal chromosome numbers has no effect on the validity of

TABLE 7.2
SEX IDENTIFICATION ANOMALIES: SEX CHROMOSOME ANEUPLOIDIES

Sex chromosome complement	Frequency in live births	Biological sex	Amelogenin PCR result
XO[a]	1:3000	Female	Female
XXX	1:1000	Female	Female
XXY[b]	1:800	Male or intersex	Male
XYY	1:700	Male	Male
XXXX	?	Female	Female
XXXY	?	Male	Male
XXYY	?	Male	Male
XXXXX	?	Female	Female
XXXXY	?	Male	Male
XXXYY	?	Male	Male

[a]Turner's Syndrome
[b]Klinefelter's Syndrome

the amelogenin PCR test, as the presence of the Y chromosome always indicates a male phenotype. Originally, the amelogenin PCR test devised by Sullivan et al. (1993) was quantitative, and so could be used to identify the numbers of X and Y chromosomes present in a modern DNA sample; however, due to the degradation and fragmentation of ancient DNA, it would probably not be possible to identify sex chromosome aneuploidy in ancient DNA samples.

The above examples emphasize that biological sex is not a simple male/female dichotomy. Instead, there are many variations in the biological status of maleness or femaleness in humans, these variations are reflected in the enormous plasticity of phenotypic expression. Some of the varieties of human sexual phenotypes are not merely physical, but also psychological, in their effects. Some societies are able to accommodate these variations better than others, and may indeed allow "third genders" to exist.

APPLICATIONS OF SEX IDENTIFICATION IN ARCHAEOLOGY

It so often seems to be the case in archaeology that the most interesting human remains are the most fragmentary, or disarticulated, or cremated, or juvenile and therefore unidentifiable as to whether they belong to a male or a female. Although the osteological methods of sex identification described above serve well for the vast majority of cases, there are always some instances where a molecular-based method would be appropriate. DNA methods of sex identification have now been applied to many assemblages of human archaeological remains; however, few of these studies have addressed archaeological hypotheses, with most being concerned with methodology. What follows is a brief survey of some of the most interesting applications, where insights about gender roles, construction, and behavior may be obtained.

While there have been various papers describing the use of molecular methods of sex identification on human bone samples, there are very few where an archaeological question to do with gender has been addressed. The work by Faerman et al. (1997) on the infant remains from the Roman bathhouse at Ashkelon is a good example that addresses the question of sex-selective infanticide in a historical society. It seemed likely that the infant remains were the victims of infanticide, a widespread practice in the ancient world (but also not uncommon, unfortunately, in some countries today), usually involving the disposal of unwanted female offspring. Of the 43 specimens tested by amelogenin PCR, 19 yielded PCR results. These included 14 males and five females. The results are significant at the 5 percent level of confidence and they would have been significant at the 1 percent level of confidence with just one more male result. The conclusion reached from this study was that male infanticide was practiced at this site. As they were thought to be the offspring of the prostitutes that serviced the baths, there would have been more economic sense in keeping the female infants. In the ancient world, female slaves were considered to be more valuable that male slaves, especially if virgins. It was more likely to be poorer families unwilling or unable to pay expensive dowries for their daughter's marriages who resorted to female infanticide.

The possibility that the Romans in Britain practiced infanticide was investigated by Mays and Faerman (2001) with DNA-based sex identification of infant remains from Roman villas. Out of 31 specimens, 13 yielded PCR products enabling biological sex to be assigned. Nine were male, and four were female, more than twice the number of males to females, and the discussion points out that these results would seem to offer little support for the practice of female infanticide. But the numbers are too small to come to any firm conclusions about selective infanticide in Roman Britain.

Another archaeological site where infanticide was suspected is that of the late Roman infant cemetery at Lugnano in Teverina, approximately 70 miles northwest of Rome in the Tiber valley (Sallares et al. 2003). The excavator suspected that a malarial epidemic had caused the deaths of fetuses, neonates, and infants. The first question to be addressed with DNA was whether selective infanticide was taking place, which would account for the neonates and infants. Amelogenin-based sex identification was carried out. Nine out of fifteen samples could be identified, which consisted of five females and four males. This was interpreted as representing a normal sex ratio in this cemetery assemblage, and helping to strengthen the malarial epidemic interpretation.

Recently our lab has carried out DNA analysis of the human remains from the Grave Circles at Mycenae (Bouwman et al. 2008; Brown et al. 2000). It was important to establish whether DNA survived and that useful information about the burials could be obtained. With this in mind, sex identifications were carried out on bone samples from Grave Circle B, the most recently excavated set of shaft graves. Twenty-two samples from different individuals were obtained, DNA extracted and amplified with primers directed at the amelogenin locus. The biological sex of most of these burials had already been established by osteological methods, except for a child aged between two and three years old. PCR products were obtained for nine individuals, a success rate of 41 percent (comparable with the rate of success obtained by other groups). Six of these results correlated with the biological sex obtained via osteology; the child was identified as a definite male.

A New World example of sex identification of children with DNA comes from Mexico (De La Cruz et al. 2008). At the site of Temple R, at Tlatelolco, Mexico City, the remains of human sacrifices were recovered in the late 1990s. They consisted of six adults and 37 subadults; two-thirds of the latter were less than three years old. They have been interpreted as sacrifices to the Aztec god of wind and rain, Ehecatl-Quetzalcoatl, and carried out at a time of great drought and famine between A.D. 1454–57, which is when Temple R itself was founded. The human sacrifices are thought to have been made in a single ceremony. Many valuable objects accompanied the remains, and 17 infants and one adult were buried in urns, while others were buried directly in the ground. Only one adult was complete, the others were fragmentary, with only vertebrae and ribs being found for four adults and a fragmented skull and all of the vertebrae found for another adult. The sex identification of these remains could not be assessed by osteoarchaeological methods because of the age and/or fragmentary state of the remains. A DNA-based approach was used employing PCR of the amelogenin gene. MtDNA and Y chromosome haplotyping were also attempted. The mtDNA haplotyping showed that 14 out of the 15 individuals who were tested belong to the mtDNA haplogroups found in the New World. Six out of the 15 individuals gave results for Y haplotyping, four or possibly five of these having New World haplotypes. Sex identifications were carried out on 38 individuals, including the six adults and 32 subadults. Two research groups did these experiments in parallel, one of the criteria of authenticity proposed for ancient DNA analysis by Cooper and Poinar (2000). One group obtained results for 26 individuals, 24 of which were male. The other group, obtained nine results, eight of which were male. It could well be that all the individuals in this study are males. It seems probable that males were chosen as sacrificial victims because the god they were being sacrificed to was also male, the children being chosen to represent the Tlaloque, the little gods who were supposed to be the helpers of the rain god. The Tlaloque were also deities of various diseases, and it has been suggested that the children chosen for sacrifice may have been suffering from diseases and were thus selected by the gods for this ritual. Ancient DNA analysis has supported the archaeological interpretation of the events of 1454–57.

GENETIC PROFILING OF MODERN HUMAN REMAINS

Forensic DNA scientists in Britain, America, and elsewhere have developed methods to identify criminals from traces of DNA left at crime scenes, and these methods can be applied to archaeological human remains with varying degrees of success. The questions in archaeology are different, however—not so much the identification of individuals but to identify kinship among a group of individuals.

Genetic profiling techniques have their origins in the 1980s with the discovery of repetitive DNA sequences called STRs (short tandem repeats) or microsatellites. These STRs do not appear to have any obvious function—they do not code for proteins and some have called them "junk" DNA. Although their function is largely unknown, STRs have proved valuable to forensic scientists because the length of an STR is variable, meaning that within the population as a whole there are several or many different versions of each STR. These versions are called alleles, and the number of repeated DNA motifs is called the allelic number. The variability of STRs is such that no two humans alive have the same combination of alleles. If enough STR loci are examined, then a unique genetic fingerprint can be established for every individual in the world (except, of course, for monozygotous identical twins). At the moment it is not possible to analyze all 10,000+ STRs in the human genome to obtain a complete genetic fingerprint, nor is it necessary. CODIS (Combined DNA Index System) consists of 12 STRs plus the amelogenin gene and was developed in the United States. It is sufficient to give enough variability to provide a genetic profile such that there is only a one in 10^{15} chance that two individuals will have exactly the same combination of STR alleles—this is higher than the planet's current human population of six billion. STRs are inherited in Mendelian fashion, one allele from each parent, thus by comparing the allele numbers between putative parents and offspring it is possible to identify related individuals.

Some STRs are on the Y chromosome. The use of these sequences enables the genetic profiling of Y chromosomes, in much the same way as mtDNA haplotyping or genetic profiling via autosomal STRs. Determination of the allelic lengths of a sufficient number of STR loci can therefore identify paternal lineages as well as provide additional confirmation of genetic sex. Y chromosomal STRs are used routinely in forensics and paternity testing, and they are employed in evolutionary and population studies.

KINSHIP ANALYSIS IN ARCHAEOLOGY

So far, there have been few case studies where DNA-based approaches have been used to study kinship in archaeological or historical burial groups. However, where DNA preservation is good, as in historical burial groups, the information recovered shows why kinship analysis is worth persevering within archaeological scenarios.

Nearly ninety years ago the last tsar of Russia and his family, doctor, and servants were executed by the Bolsheviks and their remains buried in a shallow grave at Yekaterinburg in the Urals. The burials were exhumed in 1991 and showed signs of violence; the presence of porcelain, platinum, and gold fillings in the teeth of some individuals suggested that they were aristocrats. With the fall of communism the new Russian leaders wished to give the Romanovs a state funeral, but before they could do so they had to be sure that these were the right bodies. Nine skeletons had been found in the grave—six adults and three subadults—and examination by Russian forensic scientists established the sex and age at death, and used computer-aided facial reconstruction. The scientists thought that the remains were probably those of Tsar Nicholas II, his wife Alexandra, and three of their daughters, as well as three servants and the family doctor. The question was how to confirm this identification and to distinguish between the royal family members and the servants and doctor, and DNA preserved in the bones was extracted and analyzed in order to answer this question (Gill et al. 1994). This work was carried out by the Forensic Science Service in Birmingham, UK, the pioneers of forensic DNA analysis. The focus of the DNA analysis was to establish the presence of a family group among the burials and to use mtDNA from maternally descended present-day relatives of the Romanovs to confirm or disprove the identity of the burials. Sex identification of the remains was first carried out which correlated with the identifications from osteological evidence, showing four males and five females (including all three subadults) in the burial group.

If a family group was present, then we should expect to see that two of the adults are the parents of the three subadults. STR analysis was used to test whether any of the burials were related. The loci used and the allelic lengths obtained are shown below (Table 7.3a). Although five loci were used, the parentage of the three subadults can be identified by the results from just two loci, HUMVWA/31 and HUMTH01. This genetic profiling showed that the skeletons were a family group of mother, father, and three offspring, plus four unrelated adults, which tied in with them being the royal family, three of their daughters, the doctor and three servants, with one daughter and the son

TABLE 7.3
AUTOSOMAL STR ANALYSIS OF THE ROMANOVS

	STR				
Skeleton	VWA/31	TH01	F131A1	FES/FPS	ACTBP2
a) Identification of a Family Group					
1 Male adult	14,20	9,10	6,16	10,11	ND
2 Male adult	17,17	6,10	5,7	10,11	11,30
3 Child	15,16	8,10	5,7	12,13	11,32
4 Male adult	15,16	7,9.3	7,7	12,12	11,32
5 Child	15,16	7,8	5,7	12,13	11,36
6 Child	15,16	8,9.3	3,7	12,13	32,36
7 Female adult	15,16	8,8	3,5	12,13	32,36
8 Male adult	15,17	6,9	5,7	8,10	ND
9 Female adult	16,17	6,6	6,7	11,12	ND
b) The Last of the Romanovs					
Alexei	15,16	8,9.3			
Anastasia/Maria	15,16	7,8			

Each entry is the pair of allelic lengths possessed by each individual for each STR. The parents of the three children are skeleton 4 and skeleton 7—the Tsar and Tsarina. Skeleton 3 is thought to be that of Olga, skeleton 5 is Tatiana, while skeleton 6 is Maria or Anastasia. Skeletons 1, 2, 8, and 9 are those of the servants and doctor.

missing from the burial (some historical accounts suggest that two bodies were buried separately). To conclusively prove that the family group was indeed that of the Romanovs, mtDNA from the skeletons was compared with mtDNA from matrilineal descendants of Tsar Nicholas's grandmother (men do not transmit mtDNA to their offspring) and Tsarina Alexandra's sister. The sequence from four of the skeletons—the putative mother, Alexandra, and the three offspring—was exactly the same as Prince Philip's. Prince Philip is maternally descended from the Tsarina's sister. Two lines of matrilineal descent were traced from Tsar Nicholas's grandmother, Louise of Hesse-Cassel. The DNA tests would appear to be conclusive, identifying the remains of the Romanovs and distinguishing them from those of the servants and doctor. All remains were given a state funeral in 1998 at St. Petersburg.

That two offspring were missing from the burial has led to various claims from individuals, but with the availability of DNA evidence these claims will be much harder to sustain in the future. DNA has been used to disprove the claim of Anna Anderson to be Anastasia, who legend says escaped the massacre—Anna Anderson had died, but an archived tissue sample was tested and the mtDNA obtained indicated a person of Polish origins (Gill et al. 1995). There have also been various people claiming to be descended from Tsarevich Alexei, the only son. Again, DNA can prove or disprove the claims.

However, the missing Romanovs have now been identified by DNA analysis (Coble et al. 2009). They had been buried in a second grave located in 2007 c.70 m from the main burial. MtDNA, autosomal STRs, and Y chromosome STRs were targeted by PCR on the DNA extracted from these highly fragmented remains. The results confirmed that these remains came from two siblings—the mtDNA haplotypes matched those previously established for the Tsarina, while 15 autosomal STR alleles were in accordance with their being the offspring of the Tsar and Tsarina. Table 7.3b shows only those STRs that were common to both sets of DNA typing. Sex identification with the amelogenin gene confirmed that one male and one female were present, while the Y chromosomal analysis showed that the male child shared the same Y haplotype as that of Tsar Nicholas and a living paternally descended relative. It is still not known whether the female child in the second grave was Anastasia or Maria—this is beyond the abilities of ancient DNA analysis.

Before this second comprehensive analysis by Coble et al. (2009) doubt had been cast on the authenticity of the Romanov DNA results by Knight et al. (2004). They analyzed mtDNA extracted from a preserved finger purported to come from Grand Duchess Elisabeth, the sister of Tsarina Alexandra, who was murdered in 1918, some months after the Romanovs. This finger had been removed from the remains of Elisabeth in 1982. However, the mtDNA obtained did not match that of Alexandra. Knight et al. (2004) cast doubt on the authenticity of the Romanov remains and the DNA tests, but to my mind there is just as much doubt over the authenticity of any human remains venerated as holy relics. The DNA results for the Romanovs make a completely convincing case for their identification, and the finger thus comes from an unrelated individual.

The testing of ancient DNA against samples of living relatives is highly unlikely for prehistoric burial groups. Here one can test for relatedness among the individuals, but we cannot find their identities. An example is provided by the excavation of a Neolithic (4,600 years old) cemetery near Eulau, Germany (Haak et al. 2008), which revealed four groups of burials, containing a total of 13 individuals in total, males, females, and children. It is thought that the burials were victims of a single violent event, as skeletal trauma could be seen and even a stone arrowhead was found in a vertebra of one individual. Grave 99 contained four individuals: a female aged 35–50 years, a male aged 40–60 years and two children of four to five years and eight to nine years old. Grave 98 held one adult female 30–38 years old and three children of six months to one year old, four to five years old, and seven to nine years old. Grave 93 held three individuals, a male 25–40 years old, and two children four to five and five to six years old. Grave 90 contained two burials—a female 25–30 years old and a child of four to five years old. The burial groups appear to be contemporaneous according to the radiocarbon dates. There were no burials of adolescents or young adults. The positioning of the individuals in the graves suggested family groups—some of the individuals were placed face to face, while others were closely intertwined. Ancient DNA was extracted from teeth and bone samples and PCRs directed at mtDNA, Y chromosome STRs, and autosomal STRs. Ancient DNA preservation was such that nine out of 12 individuals could be haplotyped with mtDNA (75% success rate) to haplogroups H, I, K, U, and X, all of European origin. Three individuals from Grave 99 shared the same unusual haplotype K1b, indicating maternal relatedness between the female adult and the two children. The male in this grave had a U5B haplotype, but was found to share the same Y chromosomal haplogroup R1a with the two children, who were therefore shown to be males. These were the only individuals at this site whose Y chromosomal DNA was sufficiently preserved for PCR. In this grave, ancient DNA has revealed a family group of adult male, female, and two offspring, and this biological kinship is reflected in the positioning of the bodies in the grave.

In Grave 98, two of the three children (age seven to nine and four to five) shared the same mtDNA haplogroup of X2, so are probably siblings or maternally related in some way. But the adult female in this grave was not their mother, as she belonged to haplogroup H. This is thought to be reflected in the positioning of the bodies, as the two children were spatially separated from the female. Unfortunately, no mtDNA results were obtained from the youngest child (six months to one year old), so its maternal kinship with the adult female could not be established, although its position in the grave close to the adult female might suggest one. The seven to nine-year-old child was found to be a male, while the four to five-year-old was female. The sex of the youngest could not be identified with ancient DNA. Interestingly, the male child was buried with a stone axe, which might give it an adult status in the Corded Ware culture this cemetery belongs to.

The other burials in Grave 90 and Grave 93 were not so well preserved, and less ancient DNA information could be obtained. Only one individual from Grave 90 gave mtDNA results and belonged to haplogroup I, and only one individual from Grave 93 could be haplotyped and belonged to haplogroup K1a2. There was some limited STR data from the same two individuals, but it was not possible to identify relationships within these two graves because of the lack of ancient DNA. It must be remembered that the dead do not bury themselves—it seems that survivors of the violent event returned to bury the dead and place them in their final positions in the graves so as to reflect the biological relationships they shared in life.

CONCLUSIONS

Ancient DNA extracted from archaeological child remains has the potential to provide basic information about these individuals that is simply not available by any other methods. With ancient DNA, questions about the sex and biological parentage of sub-adult skeletal material can be posed, and, where DNA preservation conditions permit, answered. In this type of research, it is important that the right questions are asked, framed in such a way that archaeological hypotheses can be tested with the outcome of DNA analysis. We cannot elucidate an individual's identity unless there is a line of descent connecting to living relatives, as was the case with the Romanovs. Most archaeological scenarios would be like that at Eulau for example, where burial groups can be analyzed for kinship among the burials. However, it must be remembered that ancient human DNA research is time consuming, costly, and beset by problems with modern human DNA contamination (Brown and Brown 1992). This can take place at the point of excavation, by archaeologists handling human remains with bare hands, and washing bones in buckets of water on site. Further contamination can take place via osteoarchaeologists handling human remains with bare hands. In the laboratory, we do our very best to remove this contamination and identify authentic ancient DNA from human remains. Archaeologists should play their part by keeping on-site and postexcavation contamination to a minimum (Brown and Brown 1992)—this would then help the biomolecular archaeologist in the lab obtain good results, which may shed light on those archaeological orphans of the past, children.

NOTE

This article was submitted for publication in early 2011. Due to circumstances beyond the author's control, publication has been delayed for several years. Readers should be aware of this and realize that the article and bibliography may therefore be slightly out of date, as later relevant publications may have appeared.

REFERENCES CITED

Alvesalo, L. 1997 Sex Chromosomes and Human Growth, a Dental Approach. *Human Genetics* 101:1–5.

Bouwman, A. S., K. A. Brown, A. J. N. W. Prag, and T. A. Brown 2008 Kinship Between Burials from Grave Circle B at Mycenae Revealed by Ancient DNA Typing. *Journal of Archaeological Science* 35:2580–2584.

Brown, K. A 1998 Gender and Sex—What Can Ancient DNA Tell Us? *Ancient Biomolecules* 2:3–15.

Brown, K. A., and T. A. Brown 2001 Identifying the Sex of Human Remains by Ancient DNA Analysis. *Ancient Biomolecules* 3:215–225.

Brown, T. A., and K. A. Brown 1992 Ancient DNA and the Archaeologist. *Antiquity* 66:10–23.

Brown, T. A., K. A. Brown, C. F. Flaherty, L. Little, and A. J. N. W. Prag 2000 DNA Analysis of Bones From Grave Circle B at Mycenae: a First Report. *Annual of the British School at Athens* 95:115–119.

Coble, M. D., O. M. Loreille, M. J. Wadhams, S. M. Edson, K. Maynard, C. E. Meyer, H. Niederstätter, C. Berger, B. Berger, A. B. Falsetti, P. Gill, W. Parson, and L. N. Finelli 2009 Mystery Solved: The Identification of the Two Missing Romanov Children Using DNA Analysis. *PloS One* 4:4838.

Cooper, A., and H. Poinar 2000 Ancient DNA: Do it Right or Not at All. *Science* 289:1139.

De La Cruz, I., A. González-Oliver, B. M. Kemp, J. A. Román, D.Glenn Smith, and A. Torre-Blanco 2008 Sex Identification of Children Sacrificed to the Ancient Aztec Rain Gods in Tlateloco. *Current Anthropology* 49:519–526.

Faerman, M., D. Filon, G. Kahila, C. L. Greenblatt, P. Smith, and A. Oppenheim 1995 Sex Identification of Archaeological Human Remains Based on Amplification of the X and Y Amelogenin Alleles. *Gene* 167:327–332.

Faerman, M., G. Kahila, P. Smith, C. Greenblatt, L. Stager, D. Filon, and A. Oppenheim 1997 DNA Analysis Reveals the Sex of Infanticide Victims. *Nature* 385:212–213.

Gill, P., P. L. Ivanov, C. Kimpton, R. Piercy, N. Benson, G. Tully, I. Evett, E. Hagelberg, and K. Sullivan 1994 Identification of the Remains of the Romanov Family by DNA Analysis. *Nature Genetics* 6:130–136.

Gőtherstrom, A., K. Lidén, T. Ahlström, M. Källersjő, and T. A. Brown 1997 Osteology, DNA, and Sex Identification: Morphological and Molecular Sex Identifications of Five Neolithic Individuals from Ajvide, Gotland. *International Journal of Osteoarcheology* 7:71–81.

Haak, W., G. Brandt, H. N. de Jong, C. Meyer, R. Ganslmeier, V. Heyd, C. Hawkesworth, A. W. G. Pike, H. Meller, and K. W. Alt 2008 Ancient DNA, Strontium Isotopes, and Osteological Analyses Shed Light on Social and Kinship Organisation of the Later Stone Age. *Proceedings of the National Academy of Sciences USA* 105:18226–18231.

Hagelberg, E., B. Sykes, and R. Hedges 1989 Ancient Bone DNA amplified. *Nature* 342:485.

Hanaoka, Y., and K. Minaguchi 1996 Sex Determination from Blood and Teeth by PCR Amplification of the Alphoid Satellite Family. *Journal of Forensic Science* 41:855–858.

Holcomb, S. M. C., and L. W. Konigsberg 1995 Statistical Study of Sexual Dimorphism in the Human Fetal Sciatic Notch. *Journal of Physical Anthropology* 97:113–125.

Hummel, S., and B. Herrmann 1991 Y-Chromosome–Specific DNA Amplified in Ancient Human Bone. *Naturwissenschaften* 78:266–267.

Imperato-McGinley, J., R. E. Peterson, T. Gautier, and E. Sturla 1979 Androgens and the Evolution of Male-Gender Identity among Male Pseudohermaphrodites with 5α-Reductase Deficiency. *New England Journal of Medicine* 300:1233–1237.

Knight, A., I. A. Zhivotovsky, D. H. Kass, D. E. Litwin, L. D. Green, P. S. White, and J. L. Mountain 2004 Molecular, Forensic, and Haplotypic Inconsistencies Regarding the Identity of the Ekaterinburg Remains. *Annals of Human Biology* 31:129–138.

Krogman, W. M., and M. Y. Iscan (editors) 1986 *The Human Skeleton in Forensic Medicine.* 2nd edition. Charles Thomas, Springfield.

Mays, S., and M. Faerman 2001 Sex Identification in Some Putative Infanticide Victims from Roman Britain Using Ancient DNA. *Journal of Archaeological Science* 28:555–559.

Molleson, T., K. Cruse, and S. Mays 1998 Some Sexually Dimorphic Features of the Human Juvenile Skull and Their Value in Sex Determination in Immature Skeletal Remains. *Journal of Archaeological Science* 25:719–728.

Nakahori, Y., K. Hamano, M. Iwaya, and Y. Nakagome 1991a A Human X-Y Homologous Region Encodes "Amelogenin." *Genomics* 9:264–269.

Nakahori, Y., K. Hamano, M. Iwaya, and Y. Nakagome 1991b Sex Identification by Polymerase Chain Reaction Using X-Y Homologous Primer. *American Journal of Medical Genetics* 39:472–473.

Pearson, G. A. 1996 Of Sex and Gender. *Science* 274:328–329.

Sallares, R., S. Gomzi, A. Bouwman, C. Anderung, and T. Brown 2003 Identification of a Malaria Epidemic in Antiquity Using Ancient DNA. In *Archaeological Sciences 1999. Proceedings of the Archaeological Sciences Conference, University of Bristol, 1999, edited by* K. R. Brown, pp. 120–125. BAR International Series 1111, Archaeopress, Oxford.

Scarre, C. J. 1984 Kin-Groups in Megalithic Burials. *Nature* 311:512–513.

Schutkowski, H. 1993 Sex Determination of Infant and Juvenile Skeletons. I. Morphognostic Features. *American Journal of Physical Anthropology* 90:199–205.

Smith, C. I., A. T. Chamberlain, M. S. Riley, C. Stuger, and M. J. Collins 2003 The Thermal History of Human Fossils and the Likelihood of Successful DNA Amplification. *Journal of Human Evolution* 45:203–217.

Stacks, B., and M. M. Witte 1996 Sex Determination of Dried Blood Stains Using the Polymerase Chain Reaction (PCR) with Homologous X-Y Primers of the Zinc-Finger Protein Gene. *Journal of Forensic Science* 41:287–290.

Stone, A. C., G. R. Milner, S. Pääbo, and M. Stoneking 1996 Sex Determination of Ancient Human Skeletons Using DNA. *American Journal of Physical Anthropology* 99:231–238.

Stoneking, M., T. Melton, J. Nott, S. Barritt, R. Roby, M. Holland, V. Weedn, P. Gill, C. Kimpton, R. Aliston-Greiner, and K. Sullivan 1995 Establishing the Identity of Anna Anderson Manahan. *Nature Genetics* 9:9–10.

Sullivan, K. M., A. Manucci, C. P. Kimpton, and P. Gill 1993 A Rapid and Quantitative DNA Sex Test: Fluorescence-Based PCR Analysis of X-Y Homologous Gene Amelogenin. *Biotechniques* 15:636–641.

Swain, A., V. Narvaez, P. Burgoyne, G. Camerino, and R. Lovell-Badge 1998 Dax1 Antagonises SRY Action in Mammalian Sex Determination. *Nature* 391:761–767.

Tyrrell, A. 2000 Skeletal Non-Metric Traits and the Assessment of Inter- and Intra-Population Diversity: Past Problems and Future Potential. In *Human Osteology in Archaeology and Forensic Science*, edited by M. Cox and S. Mays, pp. 289–305. Greenwich Medical Media, London.

Watson, J. D., and F. H. C. Crick 1953 Molecular Structure of Nucleic Acids: a Structure for Deoxyribose Nucleic Acid. *Nature* 171:737–738.

CHAPTER EIGHT

Metaphors for Understanding Children and Their Role in Culture

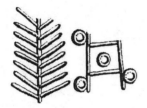

Jack A. Meacham

Abstract *Four primary metaphors—essence, organism, machine, and historical context—are used to introduce four families of theories of children's development. The assumptions, models, and meanings implicit within these four primary metaphors have important implications for how heredity, environment, and children's actions are understood to interact and influence the course of their development. Describing and explaining children's development in terms merely of heredity and environment, while neglecting the influence of children's actions upon the course of their lives, has often led to the invisibility, within our research and scholarly discourse, of the children themselves as actors and their roles in maintaining and changing cultures. These four metaphors also provide alternative frameworks for understanding the involvement of children, parents, and teachers, through various educational processes, in the transmission and adaptive evolution of culture. Some of the metaphors direct our attention toward stability and transmission of culture; others direct our attention toward human creativity and the possibilities for cultural change. The chapter concludes with implications of these disparate ways of thinking about children's development for the disciplines of anthropology and archaeology.*

Descriptions and explanations of how children and adolescents develop have been organized into numerous theories. One textbook of developmental psychology provides a survey of six theories (Miller 1983); two others include comparisons of more than 20 theories, each of which has its strengths and adherents (Crain 1992; Thomas 1979). In short, there are far too many developmental theories to introduce, compare, and contrast. A better approach is to consider these theories not one-by-one but instead in terms of only a few groups or families of similar theories. Awareness of the diversity of approaches to understanding children's development may assist researchers and scholars in disengaging from their personal and contemporary understandings and becoming more open to alternative approaches that might provide a better understanding of how children lived in other, historical cultures.

Communication among our disciplines can be facilitated by setting aside our specialized, technical vocabulary and, instead, building our collaborative discussion around some everyday words that will already be familiar to and readily understandable by parents, teachers, and researchers. In this chapter, I make use of four primary metaphors—essence, organism, machine, and historical context—to introduce four families of developmental theories. These four metaphors and families of theories can be introduced with everyday language: parents, teachers, and researchers commonly believe that each child is special, with unique qualities; or that a child is like a growing and blossoming flower; or that a child is like a machine, with inputs and outputs; or that a child's life is like a story that writes itself.

When the assumptions, models, and meanings that are implicit within the primary metaphors of essence, organism, machine, and historical context are transferred into the four families of developmental theories, they have important implications for how heredity, environment, and children's actions are understood to interact and to influence the course of their development. These four metaphors also provide alternative frameworks for understanding the involvement of children and their parents and teachers, through various educational processes (broadly conceived, as more comprehensive than formal teaching and learning, e.g., enculturation), in the transmission and evolution of culture.

Heredity, Environment, and Children's Actions

Discussions of children's development turn, sooner or later, to a consideration of causes, determinants, factors, or influences in development. Typically, only two categories are considered: heredity, nature, biology, or maturation, on the one hand; and environment, nurture, or culture (including socialization and education), on the other. This often leads to the question, Which is more important in children's development, heredity or environment? Unfortunately, by neglecting the role of children's action as a third cause of their development (Meacham 1981), this question can never lead to a complete and correct answer.

Parents and teachers commonly describe two-year-olds as assertive, four-year-olds as stubborn or unpredictable, middle school children as passionate for sports or music or literature, and adolescents as having a direction or mission in life. From early in life forward, characteristics of children such as these can become functionally autonomous from and at least as powerful as heredity or environment. If such characteristics of children—which can be included together under the term *action*—are of such significance as developmental causes, then why are children's actions so often neglected? One answer is that our implicit, everyday notions about heredity and environment have come largely from agricultural research. In the first half of the twentieth century, new knowledge about genetics was applied to the improvement of vegetables and grains. Agricultural experimentation involves control of heredities through selection of seeds from plants with desirable characteristics and control of environments through variation of soil types, amount of water, and fertilizers. Understanding the interaction of heredity and environment within agricultural science does not require consideration of action, because seeds and plants cannot act upon the environment to change the conditions for their development. Children, on the other hand, continually act upon and introduce multiple changes into their physical and social environments, changes that can in turn powerfully influence the course of their own development.

Another answer is historical, social, and cultural: the mere suggestion that heredity plays a role in development—as it does in all development—has been a convenient rationale for racism, sexism, and other political views that support the maintenance of social inequalities (Meacham 1981). In counteracting these views, one must make clear that while children's development is always under genetic control this does not mean that improving the prospects for children's lives is necessarily difficult. Substantial benefits for children's development can follow from improving physical and social environments and through strengthening societal resources directed toward children's education (consistent with mechanistic approaches to education, described below), and through encouraging and empowering children to act upon the environment and change the course of their own development (as in organismic and contextualist approaches to education, below).

Unfortunately, the tendency within developmental psychology and other disciplines to describe and explain children's development in terms merely of heredity and environment, while neglecting the role of children's actions, has often led to the invisibility, within our research and scholarly discourse, of the children themselves as actors and their roles in maintaining and changing culture: we investigate the biological processes of inheritance and maturation, we measure and catalog the social and cultural environmental forces acting upon children, but we fail to see the children themselves and how their own actions are influencing the course of their lives and lead to changes in the cultures they live in (Baxter 2005, 2008; Kamp 2001, 2006).

If we conceive of children's development as a function merely of heredity and environment, then our research will focus merely on kinship and DNA and on social norms and parenting practices, but not on children. However, if we conceive of children's development as a function of heredity, environment, and children's actions, then our research will focus in addition on children's art, roles, behaviors, personal life stories, and much more.

Given these three causes of children's development—heredity, environment, and children's action—then logically six models can be constructed to represent their interaction, depending on the relative influence of each. In a first model, heredity is most important, followed by environment, followed by action as least important; in a second model, heredity is most important, action is second, and environment is third. The remaining four models can be constructed similarly. How children's actions are conceptualized and what role actions are thought to play along with heredity and environment in children's development can be quite different, depending on whether the place of action is of primary importance (as in the contextualist metaphor, described below) or only secondary or tertiary importance.

FOUR METAPHORS FOR UNDERSTANDING CHILDREN'S DEVELOPMENT

The four primary metaphors of essence, organism, machine, and historical context are loosely derived from a conceptual framework described by the philosopher Stephen Pepper in *World Hypotheses* (1942) (see also Meacham 2004). The assumptions, models, and meanings hidden within these metaphors influence how and what we think about children's development and about the roles that children play in cultural transmission and change. When these metaphorical meanings are transferred into discussions of children's development, they lead to describing and understanding children according to their intrinsic qualities (essentialism), general processes of living systems (organicism), children's behavioral repertoires (mechanism), or children's interpretations of events in their lives (historical context, or contextualism). Furthermore, each of the four metaphors leads to describing and understanding children's action in particular ways and provides less support for other possible understandings. Table 8.1 provides a summary and comparison of the metaphors.

In the sections that follow, each of the four metaphors is described, beginning with (1) an introduction to the metaphor and application of the metaphor to describing children's development, followed by (2) description of children's action from this metaphorical

TABLE 8.1
FOUR METAPHORS FOR UNDERSTANDING CHILDREN'S ACTION AND IDENTITY

Understandings	Essence	Organism	Machine	Historical Context
Children understood primarily by:	Their intrinsic qualities	General processes of living systems	Repertoires of behaviors	Their interpretation of life events
Children's action understood as:	Self-reflecting	Self-organizing	Behaving	Interpreting
Children's identity development understood as:	Discovering who one is	Growing into one's potential, balancing biology and culture	Being made by others	Making oneself

perspective and an illustration of the metaphorical language in describing children; (3) the relative influence of heredity, environment, and action within this family of theories; (4) some developmental theories that fit within this family; and (5) children's identity development from this metaphorical perspective.

THE ESSENTIALIST METAPHOR

Why does an orange taste like an orange and not like a lemon or peach? Well, it just does. It's in the intrinsic, unchanging, indispensable nature of an orange that it tastes like an orange. This is an orange's distinguishing property, attribute, trait, or feature—in short, its essence. Within the essentialist metaphor, the method for describing and understanding children's development is to identify the intrinsic essences—the qualities, attributes, traits, and features—of individual children and groups of children.

From this essentialist perspective, action is self-reflection upon, awareness of, and seeking insight into attributes, traits, and features. A child who is feeling that he or she is, for example, smart, shy, athletic, lonely, or creative is engaging in essentialist action. An adult who uses the essentialist metaphor in thinking and talking about children similarly labels individual children as, for example, intelligent, introverted, masculine, difficult, or of a particular race, ethnicity, or religion. Both the child and the adult are referring to presumably essential, relatively unchanging traits of children.

The essentialist metaphor assumes the importance of heredity in bringing about and maintaining these relatively stable traits and assumes that the environment (including culture) and children's actions have little or no role. In short, heredity is most important, followed next by the environment, and then by the child's actions. Within this essentialist metaphor, what the child experiences or whether the child feels smart or lonely is unlikely to alter the assumption that heredity determines the child's abilities and personality.

The use of essentialist metaphors and theories is increasingly rare among child development professionals. Only a few advocate understanding children merely in terms of inherent and stable traits. And only a few maintain that personality traits, moods, or styles of behavior persist from childhood into adulthood without being substantially modified by the influence of parents, teachers, peers, and the media. One example is the temperament theory of Chess and Thomas (1986), according to which infants' moods and styles persist into later development. By contrast, the essentialist metaphor can frequently be detected in discussions among parents and teachers and in popular media presentations on child and adolescent development.

The four primary metaphors lead to alternative perspectives on the nature and significance of identity in children's lives. A child's sense of identity reflects an understanding of being a unique individual, with relatively stable and enduring characteristics, and the feeling of belonging to a group or community with others who share some or many of these characteristics. From the essentialist perspective, one's identity is simply who and what one is, determined primarily by heredity. Identity development is a process of discovering this inherent identity. The child's actions play little or no role in establishing identity, although the action of self-reflection can be important in discovering one's essential traits. The essentialist metaphor for identity development corresponds well with popular notions of identity, according to which identity development is an individual process of discovering who one truly is, deep inside, at the core. The essentialist perspective on identity is congruent with the vision quest experience of adolescents in some North American cultures, spending time alone with the aim of finding one's true self and direction in life.

The Organismic Metaphor

We are immersed in a biological world of living organisms, both plants and animals, including ourselves. Living organisms are organized, self-regulating, and actively functioning systems. Just as a seed planted in favorable conditions is expected to unfold and mature into a tree, so a child provided with a supportive environment is expected to mature into a productive and responsible adult. Within this organismic (i.e., living organism) perspective we can understand children's development by asking how they maintain an adaptive balance between acting on the environment and being acted upon and supported by the environment.

From this organismic perspective, action is self-organization, coordination, and self-regulation. A child striving to coordinate and balance his or her own needs and desires with the expectations of parents, teachers, peers, society, and culture is engaging in organismic action. The child's coordinating and balancing actions are important in resolving the competition and conflict among multiple desires and needs and between what the child would like and what the adult world expects. An adult who understands children from an organismic perspective focuses on the difficulties, conflicts, and turmoil of childhood and adolescence and how these might be alleviated and resolved.

In this organismic metaphor of living, biological systems, heredity is most important, followed closely by the child's actions, with the child's environment as relatively less important. However, the relative influence of these three is more nearly equal than within the other three perspectives. Heredity and environment can present competing and conflicting demands that can be resolved through the child's own coordinating, mediating, and balancing actions.

The use of the organismic metaphor is evident in many common notions about child and adolescent development. For example, a typical organismic notion is that child development reflects the unfolding of a biological plan, marked by critical periods during which specific learning experiences are important. Examples are Rousseau's conception of children as having innate qualities that unfold naturally and Gesell's theory of development as a natural unfolding of a biological plan (Crain 1992; Thomas 1979), Lorenz's ethological theory and the idea of critical periods when specific types of learning can occur and Chomsky's theory of an innate structure for language acquisition (Crain 1992; Miller 1983), and Ainsworth's (1982) theory of infant attachment to parents.

A second organismic notion is that child development is determined primarily by physical maturation, to which the social environment responds with increasing expectations for the child's actions. An example is Erikson's psychosocial theory of eight stages of physical maturation to which the social environment responds with new expectations for the individual's actions. A third notion is that proper development is a matter of coordination or self-regulation in order to maintain an adaptive balance between heredity and the physical and social environments. An example is Piaget's structural-developmental theory in its emphasis on equilibration (self-regulation) and its description of a series of stages in children's understanding of the logic of their actions upon the physical and social world (Crain 1992; Miller 1983; Thomas 1979; Wadsworth 2003).

From the organismic perspective, a sense of identity emerges gradually as a process of becoming, or of growing into one's potential. Heredity and environment combine to provide opportunities for identity development or, said differently, potential identities toward which the child grows and matures. The child's action in identity development involves the growing into, or unfolding of, a mature identity that is an adaptive balance among the conflicting demands and expectations of heredity and environment, of biology and culture. A concrete example is the adoption by boys and girls of traditional, culturally appropriate gender roles, as they strive to negotiate the tensions and conflicts between their changing bodies, on the one hand, and the expectations of family and community, on the other. Yet within the organismic metaphor, children's actions in support of identity development remain secondary, merely responding to and coordinating the primary, compelling demands of biology and culture.

THE MECHANISTIC METAPHOR

Not surprisingly, given the technology of the nineteenth and twentieth centuries—steam engines, telephone switchboards, internal combustion engines, electric motors, and computers—the machine has frequently been adopted as a metaphor for thinking about children. Machines are typically described in terms of the parts from which they are assembled—for example, gears, transistors, chips, etc. Characteristic of machines is that they remain at rest until energy is supplied from the external environment. Within the machine, or mechanistic, metaphor, we understand children's development by identifying the component parts and processes of childhood and by observing how children's development is a response to stimulation (energy) from the physical and social environments.

From the mechanistic perspective, action is behaving, forming goals and plans, and engaging in self-control. A child who is laughing, running, speaking, studying, or crying is engaging in mechanistic actions. An adult who adopts a mechanistic perspective focuses on the repertoires of children's behaviors—on their actions—that are directly observable and on what motivates children to behave. From the mechanistic perspective, children's action, behaving, and thinking reflect primarily the causal influence of the physical and social environments.

The child's own actions—how the child behaves and what the child believes about the social world and his or her own abilities—have relatively little influence in determining the child's abilities and personality, compared to the strong role played by the social environment. In this mechanistic metaphor, environment is considered to be most important, heredity next, and action least. Examples include Locke's conception of the infant's mind as a blank slate that is written on by the environment; Skinner's theory of operant conditioning, according to which environmental reinforcement of a child's behavior by parents, teachers, and peers increases the likelihood that it will be repeated (Crain 1992; Thomas 1979); and Bronfenbrenner's (1977) ecological theory describing relations among family, school, community, and cultural environments.

A variation of the mechanistic model of development is to maintain the importance of the environment but to view action as next and heredity as least important. Children's mental actions play an important role in Bandura's social-cognitive theory, in which children's beliefs about the social world and their own abilities can be influential, and in Vygotsky's description of scaffolding and the transmission of social and cultural knowledge from adults to children (Crain 1992; Miller 1983; Thomas 1979). Similarly, information-processing theories of development, which seek to understand the child's mind by analogy with computer hardware and software (Miller 1983), provide a greater role for the child's mental actions than did earlier learning theories of development.

From the mechanistic perspective, identity is what one is made to be, as a result primarily of environmental influences. A child's identity develops as a reflection of what significant others—parents, teachers, peers—think about the child and as a consequence of their actions upon the child. The child's own actions play little or no role in establishing identity, for identity is primarily imposed on the child by the social and cultural environment. The child needs merely to be shaped and guided by others and to learn what others believe his or her identity to be. An example of mechanistic identity development is initiation rituals, through which adolescents become members of a group after having been taught certain beliefs and practices by senior group members.

THE HISTORICAL CONTEXT (OR CONTEXTUALIST) METAPHOR

Historical events—for example, an election, revolution, or war—have no significance when considered in isolation. The significance of any particular event depends upon its context—that is, its relationship with other events that precede and follow it in time and the interpretations that people construct and ascribe to this sequence of events. Historians select among many events, contexts, and interpretations and weave these into coherent and significant stories. Within this historical context, or contextualist, metaphor, we understand children by considering how they interpret various events in their lives, as well as the way they weave these events and interpretations into identities and life stories that are meaningful and significant. From the contextualist perspective, children's actions include interpreting events, constructing identities, and making commitments.

Children engage in contextualist action when they are constructing and choosing among alternative identities for themselves, that is, constructing life stories that provide coherent explanations of where they have come from and who they used to be, who they feel and believe themselves to be now, and the trajectory of their aspirations and prospects for the future. Adults who adopt a contextualist perspective when interacting with children focus on being good listeners. When children reveal their emerging identities and life stories, adults try to alert children to potential internal contradictions. Through conversation they try to help children and adolescents understand the importance—indeed, the necessity—of accepting responsibility for the choices they are making in the personal narratives they are constructing.

From a contextualist perspective, action is most important, heredity is intermediate, environment is least important (or, alternatively, first action, then environment, then heredity). To a greater extent than the other three metaphors, the contextualist metaphor incorporates children's actions as a cause of their own development. Neither heredity nor environment constitutes assured opportunities for, or unassailable barriers to, the prospects for children's development. What matters most are children's personally constructed narratives and the significance they ascribe to perceived opportunities, barriers, and prospects in their lives. Discussions of children's development based on the contextualist metaphor focus on children's interpretations of their experiences, as in children's construction, creation, and invention of new knowledge as individuals and in society (e.g., in Piaget's constructivist, structural-developmental theory), and on children's construction of a sense of identity in adolescence and young adulthood, as in Erikson's theory (Crain 1992; Miller 1983; Thomas 1979; Wadsworth 2003). Given its emphasis on action, the contextualist metaphor is far more congruent with, for example, Baxter's (2005, 21, 112) emphasis on children as social actors and Kamp's (2006, 117, 119) highlighting of children's agency, than are the metaphors of essentialism, organicism, or mechanism.

From the contextualist perspective, identity development is a process of making oneself through choices and commitments and through constructing a life narrative about oneself. The child's actions—constructing and choosing among alternative identities, making and maintaining commitments, engaging in social roles in relationship to others, and constructing a coherent and meaningful life story—are fundamental in this creative process of identity development. From an essentialist perspective identity development is a process of discovering one's personal attributes (e.g., a vision quest), while from a contextualist perspective identity development is a process of creating and constructing one's attributes and life course. Whereas from an essentialist perspective identity development is a solitary activity, a looking inward (vision quest), from a contextualist perspective identity development is a social process. It includes considering alternative roles for being in relationship with others in society, choosing among those roles, accepting responsibility for one's choices, and making a commitment to enduring and positive relationships with other people.

The contextualist emphasis on children's agency and social constructivism opens up, more so than within the essentialist, organismic (e.g., traditional gender roles), or mechanistic (e.g., initiation rituals) perspectives, possibilities for the emergence of novel identities that diverge from traditional identities within a society. Examples would be adolescents and young adults choosing to pursue new technologies (e.g., metalworking, farming, computers), or to leave their parents to work in far-off lands (migrant workers and immigrants), or to adopt gender roles that might seem strange to their parents, or to pursue occupations different from those of their parents (e.g., to move from a farm or village to a factory job). Contextualist identity development thus has greater potential as a force for cultural change than essentialist, organismic, or mechanistic identity development, which are more consistent with cultural stability.

FOUR METAPHORS FOR EDUCATION AND CULTURAL TRANSMISSION AND CHANGE

Children live, grow, and develop within cultures, that is, within communities and societies that can be characterized by patterns of relationships among knowledge, beliefs, and values, institutions and organizations, technologies and arts, and customs and behaviors. It would be too simplistic to say merely that how children develop is determined in part by the culture in which they live. At the same time and conversely, the survival and adaptive evolution of cultures is also determined in part by each successive generation of children. The survival of a culture depends on the faithful assimilation, through the process of education (broadly conceived, as more comprehensive than formal teaching and learning, e.g., enculturation), of its core beliefs and practices by each new generation. And the adaptive evolution of a culture depends on permitting and even encouraging each new generation to be open-minded and innovative in constructing solutions to environmental, technological, demographic, and other challenges. In short, the survival and evolution of cultures requires that they be both stable and flexible, that they both resist change and encourage change. And so the education of children should provide

TABLE 8.2
FOUR METAPHORS FOR UNDERSTANDING EDUCATION AND CULTURE

Understandings	Essence	Organism	Machine	Historical Context
Culture understood as:	A minor background influence	Setting expectations for children's development	Transmitted from adults to children	Socially constructed by each generation
How parents and teachers educate:	Draw forth	Provide conditions for growth	Instruct, train	Encourage creativity
How children respond to education:	Discover, express	Solve problems, resolve conflicts	Learn, acquire	Question, create
Main influence of education on culture:	Stability, transmission	Stability, transmission	Stability, transmission	Change, adaptation

a balance between cultural transmission, on the one hand, and openness to changes in cultural beliefs and practices, on the other.

The four metaphors for understanding children readily align with descriptions of processes engaged in by parents, teachers, and communities for educating children, that is, with how we conceptualize the involvement of children, through various educational processes, in the transmission and evolution of culture. These four approaches to education can be contrasted as drawing forth (essentialism), providing conditions for growth (organicism), instructing (mechanism), or encouraging creativity (contextualism). These perspectives can be rephrased into everyday language: parents and teachers commonly call on children to express themselves (essentialism), to solve problems and find solutions (organicism), to study, learn, acquire, and remember (mechanism), or to raise questions, "think outside the box," and create (contextualism). Some of the four metaphors direct our attention toward stability and transmission of culture; others direct our attention more toward human creativity and the possibilities for cultural change and adaptation.

ESSENTIALIST EDUCATION AS DRAWING FORTH

From the essentialist perspective, what the child is capable of knowing and doing is determined primarily by heredity. The process of education—carried out by the social environment—is primarily one of drawing forth or pulling out from the child this inherent knowledge and capability for action. (The English word *education* is derived from the Latin word meaning to draw forth, to draw out.) Children are provided through heredity with differing abilities or talents. One may be a gifted athlete or hunter, another a talented singer or dancer, another excellent at crafts, such as weaving or making tools, or at mathematics or astronomy. The responsibility of parents and teachers is to discover and capitalize on the particular strengths of individual children, for example, by giving a child various objects and noting how the child responds and then following up with similar or different objects. Children become able to engage in differentiated action as a result of education, but the child's actions play only a minor role, relative to heredity, in the educational process of drawing forth the child's inherent strengths. Similarly, the social and cultural environments have relatively minor background roles relative to heredity and they remain stable with little prospect for changing from one generation to the next.

ORGANISMIC EDUCATION AS PROVIDING CONDITIONS FOR GROWTH

From the organismic perspective, a program for education takes into consideration the gradual and sequential unfolding of knowledge and abilities that has been determined in large part by heredity but also by subsequent expectations of the social and cultural environment. What kind of learning a child can engage in successfully will depend on the child's readiness, on his or her stage in development, and on prior knowledge, abilities, and experiences that can be a foundation for further growth. Parents and teachers assist the child in this coordination of biological development with social and cultural expectations by providing an educational environment that includes the optimal conditions for growth of knowledge and abilities and assimilation of family and cultural values. If the educational environment contains appropriate materials and experiences presented in a coherent sequence—materials that correspond to the child's needs, curiosities, and understandings given his or her current point in development—then the child will engage enthusiastically with these materials and experiences and move forward successfully in understanding with relatively little direct adult guidance, instruction, or supervision (in contrast to mechanism, below).

An example of an organismic approach to education is the Montessori method for young children (Crain 1992; Thomas 1979), in which the teacher focuses on providing children with materials that are appropriate for their level of development and then steps aside to observe whether and how the children engage with the materials. From this organismic perspective, the child's own actions do play a significant role, for the child grows through the actions of striving to mediate between and resolve conflicting needs, drives, expectations, experiences, and understandings. A second example of the role of children's actions in education is the construction by children themselves, as a result of counting objects arranged in different ways, of the concept of conservation of number, as Piaget has shown (Crain 1992; Miller 1983; Thomas 1979; Wadsworth 2003). A third example of organismic learning and development is the squabbling and bickering among children and adolescents as they mature physically, intellectually, and emotionally and then renegotiate their positions within their peer groups, seeking friends and allies against potential competitors (and similarly, but more formally, as they learn teamwork and leadership skills as members of competitive sports teams). In these examples of organismic education and learning, it is the children who are actively seeking to solve problems, resolve conflicts, and find an appropriate balance between how they are changing internally versus societal expectations; it is the children who are changing and developing, within social and cultural environments that remain relatively stable.

MECHANISTIC EDUCATION AS INSTRUCTING

From the mechanistic perspective, what the child can know and do is determined primarily by the social and cultural environment. Education is a matter of parents and teachers instructing the child by providing certain information or by training the child in a set of skills or to behave in a certain way. This is education in its most narrow sense, that is, formal teaching and learning. From the mechanistic perspective, relatively little is given by heredity to the child's mind or behavioral repertoire. Displaying knowledge and performing behaviors are actions in which the child can engage as a result of education, but the child's actions play only a minor role, relative to the social and cultural environment, in the educational process. Education is largely under the control of parents and teachers, not the child, as they strive to transmit social and cultural beliefs, values, and skills from their own generation to the younger generation. Within the mechanistic perspective on education, it is children who are expected to learn, acquire, and change, while society and culture remain relatively stable.

Education from the mechanistic perspective is similar to the apprenticeship experience that is organized in many cultures to facilitate children's learning, for example, learning how to make stone tools or ceramics or textiles. In some settings, what the child becomes able to do depends merely on observing others and imitating what they say and do. In other settings, what the child learns depends on parents and teachers directing and guiding the child to act in a specified way and then reinforcing the child's learning through constructive criticism, praise, and threats. Some education from the mechanistic perspective involves repeated training, practice, and testing, as in memorization of information such as religious texts and multiplication tables and acquisition of skilled behaviors such as traditional songs and dances.

CONTEXTUALIST EDUCATION AS ENCOURAGING CREATIVITY

It is from the contextualist perspective that the role of the child's action is greatest in the course of development and in the educational process. Education is a process of creating and constructing new knowledge, a process engaged in primarily by the child. What is learned is not transmitted by parents, teachers, and society to the child, but instead reflects the child's actions in being curious, raising questions, and creating original, innovative knowledge from what is already known. Parents and teachers facilitate the construction of new knowledge by children through presenting questions, issues, and situations that engage children in experimentation and debate and permitting children to do most of the thinking and talking among themselves. Parents and teachers enter into discussions with children through summarizing, clarifying, introducing contrasting arguments, challenging, encouraging children to be responsible for their own learning, acknowledging and showing respect for children's efforts and contributions, and encouraging children to move toward more integrative understandings—but not through providing the answers (as from a mechanistic, apprenticeship, formal educational perspective). The primary work of becoming educated reflects not the parents' and teachers' efforts at drawing out (as in essentialism) or instructing (mechanism), but instead the actions of children working together with their peers as they encounter and struggle with arguments and evidence that challenge their thinking and stimulate them to construct more precise, valid, and comprehensive understandings.

Within the contextualist approach to education, parents, teachers, and communities are concerned not only with the stability and transmission of culture (as from the essentialist, organismic, and mechanistic approaches) but also with enabling the next, younger generation to construct its own understanding of cultural issues (such as freedom versus responsibility) and to respond to conflicts and challenges that arise for the society (for example, between population growth and resources) by constructing creative, adaptive, and entrepreneurial solutions. In this way, communities and societies persist from one generation to the next not merely by transmission of existing cultural beliefs and practices, but also by responding to changing conditions and challenges with creative and adaptive solutions for cultural change and evolution. The contextualist metaphor for understanding children and culture is more congruent with archaeological perspectives on children's initiatives and innovations in cultural change (see, for example, Kamp 2006, 119) than the essentialist, organismic, or mechanistic metaphors.

IMPLICATIONS FOR ANTHROPOLOGY AND ARCHAEOLOGY

When we describe children we implicitly draw upon one of four primary metaphors, the metaphors of essence, organism, machine, and historical context. For example, children's play illustrates how the metaphors can lead to thinking about children in quite different ways. From the essentialist perspective, children's play can be conceived as a solitary pursuit, involving self-movement, expression of emotions, and experimentation with motor actions upon objects. Organismic play, by contrast, involves two or more children engaged cooperatively in games with goals and rules of play, for example, children "playing house" and imitating traditional gender roles, or adolescents participating in team sports such as soccer. Mechanistic play is directed toward mastery of toys and other objects provided by adults (e.g., toy dolls and weapons), whose aim is to encourage children to learn adult skills and behaviors as soon as possible. For example, apprenticeship can involve observation and, at least initially, playful trial and error with tools and materials. Finally, contextualist play involves storytelling, drama, and fantasy, in which children imagine, create, and share possible events, situations, and outcomes. Examples of contextualist play are children adapting objects made for other purposes to be used as toys, or children introducing novel pottery shapes and painted designs that are unfamiliar to adults.

What are the implications of these disparate ways of thinking about children and their development for the disciplines of anthropology and archaeology? Each of the metaphors has the power to frame and guide how we describe and understand the development of children, including children's actions and their role as actors in cultural transmission, stability, and change. For this reason, it is essential that we distinguish among these four metaphors, for if we do not, then as researchers and scholars we will not be speaking, writing, and communicating clearly among ourselves. The challenge is to know which metaphor has been adopted, in describing the lives of children in particular historical cultures, and so which meanings of children, action, education, and culture are intended.

In describing and seeking to understand children, education, and culture, we ought to strive to be internally consistent, that is, to draw upon the same implicit metaphor with its underlying assumptions, models, and hidden meanings, rather than drawing from two or more of these metaphors and mixing them together in our thinking. It would be a mistake, for example, to seek to understand children from an essentialist perspective, cultural stability and transmission from a mechanistic perspective, social and cultural change from an organismic perspective, and the education of children and adolescents from a contextualist perspective.

Researchers and scholars should avoid foreclosing prematurely on only one of these metaphors and families of developmental theories, merely because this is how they feel they were raised or how they view their own adult lives, or this is how they think about the development and education of their own children, or this is a view of children that grows out of their graduate coursework or reflects popular views of children as portrayed in the media. As Kamp (2001, 26) notes, "It is perhaps almost self-evident that the most difficult task will be to cast aside our own perceptions of the meaning of childhood." It is better, at least initially, to consider a wide range of approaches to understanding children, education, and culture and, in particular, the possibility that the approach that was dominant in another, historical culture was very unlike any contemporary approaches to understanding children in our own.

I have not advocated for any particular one of these four metaphors. I've suggested merely that we ought to be more aware of the range of possible approaches to understanding children, of which one we are currently adopting in our research and writing, and of how particular approaches might bring greater visibility in archaeology to the roles and importance of children. For example, a small bone or shell comb found with a child's skeleton might mean that the child had beautiful hair (essentialism); or that the child was wrestling with issues of cleanliness versus uncleanliness (e.g., head lice), or of order versus chaos (organicism); or be an artifact of the parents' efforts to socialize the child to cultural norms (mechanism); or have been support for the child's personal life story of being attractive, getting married, and raising a family (contextualism). Or a small wood or clay sheep, goat, or cow found in a child's grave might reflect this particular child's empathy for all living things (essentialism), or the child's struggle to reconcile his or her small size and weakness with the threat of larger and stronger beasts (organicism), or the parents' intention that the child should continue their traditional family work as herders (mechanism), or the child's personal life story and aspiration of having a large herd of animals and becoming wealthy and self-sufficient (contextualism).

The interpretation of cultural artifacts and the conclusions that are ultimately drawn regarding the lives of children in a historical culture will follow not merely from any one of these four approaches but from the integration of the full range of material and historical archaeological evidence into a coherent narrative about the development and education of children and their roles in maintaining and changing that culture. Similarly, a more complete understanding of children will follow not merely from focusing on childhood as an isolated stage but instead by recognizing that childhood is only one among several stages in an individual's life course that, in turn, is embedded within the development of families, communities, societies, and cultures.

REFERENCES CITED

Ainsworth, M. D. S. 1982 Attachment: Retrospect and Prospect. In *The Place of Attachment in Human Behavior*, edited by C. M. Parkes and J. Stevenson-Hinde. Basic Books, New York.

Baxter, J. E. 2005 *The Archaeology of Childhood: Children, Gender, and Material Culture*. AltaMira Press, Walnut Creek, California.

Baxter, J. E. 2008 The Archaeology of Childhood. *Annual Review of Anthropology* 37:159–175.

Bronfenbrenner, U. 1977 Toward An Experimental Ecology of Human Development. *American Psychologist* 32:513–531.

Chess, S., and A. Thomas 1986 *Temperament in Clinical Practice*. Guilford Press, New York.

Crain, W. 1992 *Theories of Development: Concepts and Applications.* 3rd edition. Prentice-Hall, Englewood Cliffs, New Jersey.

Kamp, K. A. 2001 Where Have All the Children Gone?: The Archaeology of Childhood. *Journal of Archaeological Theory and Method* 8:1–34.

Kamp, K. A. 2006 Dominant Discourses; Lived Experiences: Studying the Archaeology of Children and Childhood. *Archaeological Papers of the American Anthropological Association* 15:115–122.

Meacham, J. A. 1981 Political Values, Conceptual Models, and Research. In *Individuals as Producers of Their Development: A Life-Span Perspective*, edited by R. M. Lerner and N. A. Busch-Rossnagel, pp. 447–474. Academic Press, New York.

Meacham, J. A. 2004 Action, Voice, and Identity in Children's Lives. In *Rethinking childhood*, edited by Peter B. Pufall and Richard B. Unsworth, pp. 69–84. Rutgers University Press, New Brunswick.

Miller, P. H. 1983 *Theories of Developmental Psychology.* Freeman, San Francisco.

Pepper, S. C. 1942 *World Hypotheses.* University of California Press, Berkeley.

Thomas, R. M. 1979 *Comparing Theories of Child Development.* Wadsworth, Belmont, California.

Wadsworth, B. J. 2003 *Piaget's Theory of Cognitive and Affective Development: Foundations of Constructivism.* 5th edition. Allyn and Bacon, Boston.

PART III

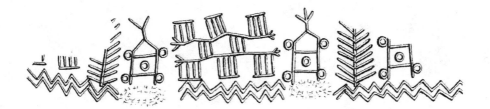

Case Studies in the Archaeology of Childhood

CHAPTER NINE

Children of the Ice Age

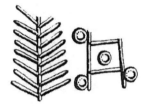

Paul G. Bahn

Abstract   *The subject of children in the Last Ice Age has been a much neglected topic, as in many other periods of the past. In studying the evidence from around the world—but primarily in Eurasia, where the data are most plentiful and varied—there are four major categories to consider: firstly, their burials and skeletal remains, as well as accompanying grave goods; secondly, the traces they have left in caves such as hand stencils, fingermarkings, and footprints—a great deal of research has been done on these in recent years; thirdly, certain artifacts that could conceivably be interpreted as toys, or drawings made by children—although it is, of course, difficult to decide between children or untalented adults as the makers of such images; and finally, actual depictions of recognizable children. The latter category is rare but does exist, although the interpretation of some images is debatable. This chapter will assess each of these categories in turn, and show that the wealth associated with some children suggests status that was inherited rather than achieved.*

BURIALS AND GRAVE GOODS

Burials of children are surprisingly abundant in the Paleolithic, especially in the Middle Paleolithic, the time of Neanderthals. However, with the exception of preserved bodies and artistic depictions showing genitalia, children's remains cannot be sexed with the same degree of reliability as adults, though dental measurements have had some success. Faced with subadult skeletal remains, one can often only guess—though the odds of being right are 50-50! Some progress has been made in sexing them using discriminant function analysis of measurements of juveniles from Spitalfields, London, whose sex and age are known from coffin labels (Renfrew and Bahn 2008:434). Recently, a new technique has been developed of determining the sex of fragmentary or infant skeletal remains from DNA analysis (Stone et al. 1996).

The first probable funerary practices come from the "Pit of the Bones" (Sima de los Huesos) at the site complex of Atapuerca, northern Spain, where the remains of about 30 people have been recovered, dating to more than 430,000—and perhaps even 600,000—years ago. These individuals, representing the species *Homo heidelbergensis*, include one child and 13 adolescents aged between 10 and 16-17 (Cervera et al. 1998). The presence of all parts of the body, and the lack of occupation material or carnivore marks suggest strongly that this was a mortuary ritual, a purposeful disposal of the dead, the oldest known anywhere.

However, it is with the Neanderthals, in the Middle Paleolithic (Mousterian) period of Eurasia, that child burials become not only very clear but also abundant. The type-site of Le Moustier (in Dordogne, France) produced one of the most complete specimens in 1914 from its lower rockshelter, when Denis Peyrony found the remains of a newborn child on its back, together with various Mousterian objects. The skeleton subsequently disappeared, but was rediscovered in a French museum's storeroom in 1996 (Cleyet-Merle and Maureille 2008). The child's age was four months at most according to its teeth, and it is the best-preserved Neanderthal example, along with one found in 1993 in Mezmaiskaya Cave (North Caucasus, Russia). This child was found on its right side. One of its bones has been directly dated to circa 29,000 BP (uncalibrated), but fauna from the same layer has been dated to between 36,000 and 73,000 BP (uncalibrated). If these earlier dates are also valid for the child, it would be the oldest newborn burial known anywhere (Tillier 2008).

The greatest collection of Neanderthal child burials has been found at La Ferrassie, Dordogne (Defleur 1993:79–80; Heim 1976). First, in 1912, in addition to two adults, archaeologists unearthed three children—one newborn and two fetuses. Two pits were found: one contained La Ferrassie 3, a child aged about 10 years; the second contained another youngster, La Ferrassie 4. Both were oriented east-west, and there were exceptionally fine worked flint tools just above the two pits. However, La Ferrassie 4 turned out to be a double burial, containing a newborn child of about eight months as well as another newborn infant of about two weeks (known as La Ferrassie 4b). In 1920, a hollow was found containing La Ferrassie 5, the poorly preserved remains of a fetus of about seven months. It had been buried tightly flexed, and with three fine flint scrapers just above (Defleur 1993:86). The following year produced perhaps the most extraordinary find at this site: La Ferrassie 6, a three-year-old child in a pit. It had been buried flexed, and oriented east-west, with its feet to the west. Only the top of the skull was there, with no teeth or jaw. Once again, three superb flint tools were found, carefully laid out on the human remains. Above the grave was a roughly triangular block of limestone (80 cm per side) with several pairs of cupules carved into its lower face. For a long time, this was considered the only example of Neanderthal artistic activity (Figure 9.1). Finally, in 1973, the fragmentary remains of La Ferrassie 8 were discovered, a child of about two years.

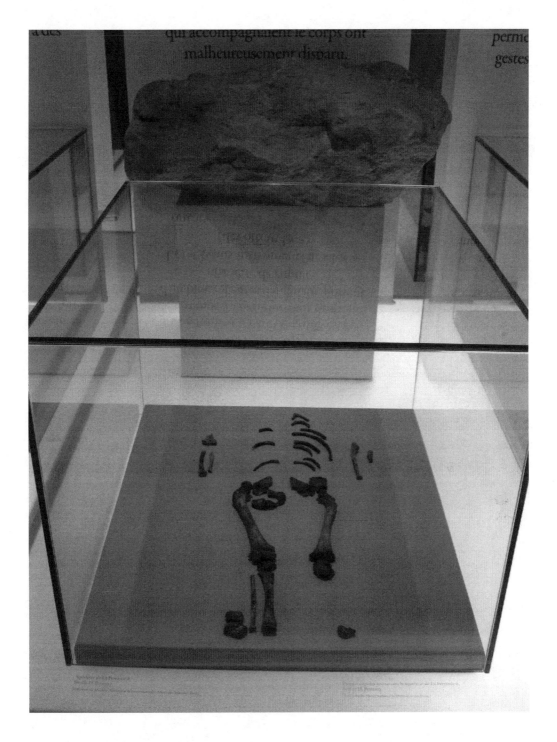

FIGURE 9.1 The limestone rock marked with cupules and the skeletal remains from La Ferrassie 6 (photo P. Bahn).

In short, La Ferrassie shows not only that child burials constitute a very high proportion of the graves of the Neanderthal period, but also that they were sometimes accompanied by high-quality grave goods and even art. This has been confirmed by other finds from totally different areas; for example, the Neanderthal child, aged eight to ten, found buried in the cave of Teshik-Tash (Uzbekistan) seems to have been encircled by five pairs of ibex horn cores (Defleur 1993:188). The Syrian cave of Dederiyeh yielded a first skeleton in 1993; Dederiyeh 1 was an almost complete child, on its back, with a piece of flint on its chest. In 1997 the very fragmentary Dederiyeh 2 was found in a pit, associated with 14 artifacts, knapping debris, and a tortoise shell (Akazawa and Muhesen 2002).

Another major example of this phenomenon is skeleton 11 from the Israeli cave of Qafzeh, which is probably the richest Middle Paleolithic burial yet found. This child was found in a pit, on its back, oriented north-south; it had a large limestone block on its pelvis, was accompanied by numerous lumps of red ochre, and had a big red deer antler in its hands, just below the head (Vandermeersch and Tiller 1976). Like La Ferrassie, Qafzeh also contained many other child burials: No. Q4 (found in 1934) was the skull of a child of six to eight years; Qafzeh 10 (1967) the skeleton of a six-year-old; Qafzeh 11 (1969) the skeleton of a child of 13 to 14; Qafzeh 12 (1969), the skull of a child of five to six; Qafzeh 13 (1969) a fetus skull; Qafzeh 14 (1973), the skull of a fetus or newborn child, scattered in a hearth; and Qafzeh 15 (1973), the upper half of a child's skeleton of eight to 10 years (Defleur 1993:141).

Qafzeh 10 is of particular importance; this child was highly flexed on its left side, with its knees at the thorax, lying at the feet of an adult also flexed on its left side (Qafzeh 9), with lots of ochre around both burials. A double burial, of an adult with child, this phenomenon would become more common in the Upper Paleolithic. Another possible Neanderthal example is that of Kiik-Koba cave (Ukraine), where the lower half of a child aged about one year, buried flexed with its left hand on its knee, was found 30 cm from the head of an adult (Defleur 1993:184).

Among the other noteworthy Neanderthal burials one should mention Skhul VIII (Israel), a child of about eight to 10 years; and Kebara 1 (Israel), a child of about seven months, found in 1965 and dated to about 64,000 years ago (Defleur 1993:174). The little cave of Roc de Marsal (Dordogne) yielded a child of about two to four years, in good condition, lying in a pit, possibly surrounded by limestone blocks, and dating to about 70,000 years ago. Finally, three infants from Shanidar cave (Iraq)—Shanidar IX simply consists of some vertebrae but was first to be buried in a pit, being followed by two adult women and finally an adult male; Shanidar VII, a child of around nine months, flexed with its head to the north, was the first found and the oldest burial in the site (Defleur 1993:166); and finally, Shanidar X comprised some pieces of a child's leg and foot, recently discovered among the faunal remains recovered from the site.

It is therefore clear that a high proportion of Neanderthal burials involved children, often of very low age. Indeed, in one study, out of 47 Neanderthal skeletons that could be aged, 18 (38.3 percent) were youngsters who died before the age of 15; and of these, 55.5 percent were aged one to 10. The next most numerous category was those aged zero to one (Defleur 1993:222–223).

Turning now to the anatomically modern humans—or "Cro-Magnons"—of the Eurasian Upper Paleolithic, we have a wide variety of child burials from this period (circa 33,000 to 11,000 years ago), although we shall start with an individual that may well be a hybrid of Neanderthal and modern human.

It is ironic that the only Ice Age burial we have for the whole of the Iberian Peninsula is that of the "Lapedo child," found at the rockshelter of Lagar Velho, Portugal, in December 1998 (Zilhão and Trinkaus 2002). Although the human remains themselves could not be dated, the animal bones and charcoal found with them place the burial firmly at 24,000 to 25,000 years ago, the "Gravettian period." The evidence indicates that a shallow pit was dug at the back of the shelter, and a branch of Scots pine was burned at the bottom. Then the child was placed in the pit; the fact that red ochre stains both the upper and lower surfaces of the bones, and forms a clear boundary with the surrounding whitish sediment, suggests strongly that the body was wrapped in an ochre-painted shroud. It lay in an extended position, with a young dead rabbit placed across its lower legs, and with two red deer pelvises (perhaps meat offerings) by its shoulder and its feet. Around its neck was a perforated-shell pendant, while on its forehead was some kind of headdress made up of four canines from two different red deer stags and two hinds. Different methods of determining dental age at death give a mean of 4.7 years, and the skeletal age at death corresponds with this assessment.

From the start, it was clear that this was an anatomically modern child—it has a chin and some other modern features—but the bodily proportions, especially those of the legs, suggested some Neanderthal input. Overall, this child is clearly not a normal anatomically modern human, and it displays an unusual mosaic of postcranial characteristics (especially in the lower limbs, but also in some features of the upper limbs). In addition, it has a pitting of the occipital bone in the skull, which some specialists consider virtually diagnostic of Neanderthals. Possible alternative explanations, such as nutritional or climatic factors, have been put forward for the child's odd proportions. However, there is no evidence at all for malnutrition having stunted its growth, and exposure to a far colder climate at Sungir (see below) had no similar effect on the proportions of the youngsters buried there. The excavators' conclusion, therefore, is that no alternative hypothesis has yet been presented that fits the data better than the "hybridization" theory (Zilhão and Trinkaus 2002), that this child is a cross between Neanderthals and Cro-Magnons. Some skeptics, however, still maintain that this is no more than a "chunky modern kid" (cited in Bahn 2003).

The Sungir children constitute the most remarkable burial yet found from the Ice Age (Figure 9.2 on page 172). The site, discovered in 1955 and dated to around 27,000 years ago, also yielded a rich burial of an adult male, but it is the children which concern us here. They are thought to be a boy, aged about 13 based on his teeth (although wisdom teeth seem to have erupted earlier in the Upper Paleolithic); and another child, possibly a girl, of no more than nine or 10. Bone evidence supports these ages (Alexeeva and Bader 2000:64). Their heights are estimated (Alexeeva and Bader 2000:298) as 1.59 m for the boy and 1.19 to 1.21 m for the other child of uncertain sex (Alexeeva and Bader 2000:426–427). The muscular development of both is very advanced, and they

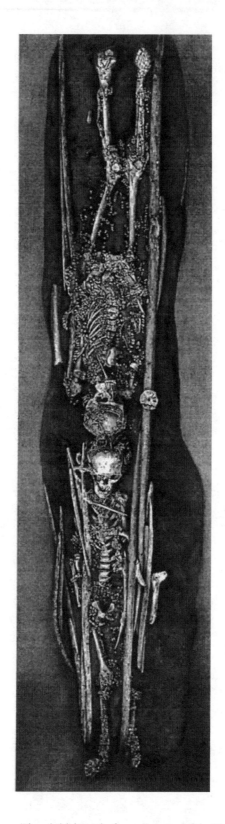

FIGURE 9.2 The child burials from Sungir (after N. Bader).

were clearly very fit. The boy shows a particularly strong development of the right upper arm, perhaps denoting spear throwing. The possible girl displays signs of repeated actions involving the raising and lowering of the collarbone, moving the whole arm and shoulder blade, and the upper arms were also well developed—it is thought that this may have been caused by drilling holes (as in making beads) or geometrical ornaments in stone or bone; this child's bones also have features that indicate that it regularly carried things on its head, unlike the boy and the adult male. Oddly, the boy's diet contained very little meat but lots of different invertebrates and a great deal of plant food, whereas the possible girl's diet was more like the adult's (i.e., meat was the basic food, with plants only of supplementary importance). However, both children underwent some long periods of undernutrition (Alexeeva and Bader 2000:445). Anatomical details and mtDNA indicate that the two children were probably close relatives (Bader and Lavrishin 1998).

The children were buried head to head, with the boy's head to the northeast and the possible girl's to the southwest. The objects buried with them are varied and abundant and quite remarkable. They had batons at their left side, while a human femoral diaphysis filled with ochre lay to the left of the boy. They also had two heavy spears of straightened ivory, 2.4 and 1.6 m long, as well as ivory staves, long bodkins, and small carvings, including a flat, perforated ivory horse (with traces of red coloring on it) and two pierced ivory disks. Finally, each body was adorned with about 3,500 small beads of mammoth ivory, arranged in rows across the forehead, across the body, down the arms and legs and around the ankles. These were probably strung on lengths of sinew which were then attached to items of clothing that have since disintegrated. It has been estimated that it would have taken about 45 minutes to make each bead, if the whole process of cutting the tusk, shaping the bead and drilling the hole is included. This means that each body had 2,625 hours of beadwork buried with it. The standardized and uniform appearance of these objects suggests that they were produced by a limited number of people (Lister and Bahn 2007:134–136). It seems unlikely that these two children could have acquired such wealth and prestige in their lifetimes, so they must have been born into a privileged position, either social or perhaps religious.

The "golden age" of Upper Paleolithic burials is the Gravettian, around 25,000 to 27,000 years ago, and many of its burials, especially in Central and Eastern Europe, are closely associated with mammoth bones. For example, in 1894 at Predmostí (Moravia) eight adults and 12 youngsters lay in an area of 4 by 2.5 m, covered by numerous large mammoth bones including two shoulder blades (Lister and Bahn 2007:132). Were these just convenient covers or do they denote some belief in the mighty mammoth protecting loved ones in the afterlife? Be that as it may, a fragment of a mammoth scapula accompanied the scorched remains of a child at Dolní Vestonice I in Moravia (Oliva 2009:303), numerous large mammoth bones covered a burial pit containing the skeleton of a child and ash at Kostenki XVIII-Chvoikovskaya (Russia), and a mammoth scapula also covered a secondary burial of a child at Kostenki XV-Gorodcovskaya (Oliva 2009:303). Most recently, two child burials at Krems-Wachtberg, Austria, were found overlain by a mammoth scapula supported with a piece of tusk (Einwögerer 2005; Lister and Bahn 2007:132).

There are some particularly poignant burials from the Upper Paleolithic. For example, the Abri Pataud (Dordogne), a huge rockshelter, was used for burials around 20,500 years ago, including four young children (of one month, six months, four years, and seven years) as well as a man and two young women (Billy 1975:250–252). The newborn child was about 59.3 cm tall and had a fetal age of 332 days, so it died aged 1 to 1.5 months. It was found in the arms of a 16-year-old girl who was presumably its mother.

Another probable mother-and-child burial is even more unusual. Excavations in front of the rockshelter of Romito, southern Italy, revealed six Upper Paleolithic skeletons—most notably a grave found in 1963 containing a small middle-aged female together with an adolescent male dwarf: the earliest dwarf known anywhere in the world, since this layer of the site has been dated to 11,150 years ago (Frayer et al. 1987, 1988). That kind of age would also be perfectly acceptable for the site's engravings. This individual, just over a meter tall, was clearly very special within his society, since (on the basis of bone growth and tooth development) he survived to an age of about 17 despite his physical impediments—and it may be no coincidence that he was buried in this very special place, in a decorated shelter (Bahn 2002). Although the pelvis was not found, it is reckoned to be a male on the basis of several features of robustness in muscle attachments. It is likely that that the adult female was his mother, as the two skeletons do display some minor anatomical features in their skulls and teeth that support some kind of link. His condition must have been an impediment to survival, as he could probably not have contributed much to his group's economic life—dwarfs usually have a waddling gait and, although capable of rapid movement, their legs and back tire after walking short distances. In view of the rugged terrain in Calabria, and the probability that Upper Paleolithic groups migrated seasonally, life cannot have been easy for this youth. His limited ability to extend his elbows to more than 130 degrees was a further impediment to his effective participation in hunting activities. Dwarfs of this kind are also usually susceptible to back problems and joint pain. The fact that he survived such physical handicaps into late adolescence must mean that his social group protected and supported him. Indeed, it is likely that his burial in this special place, in front of some rock art, testifies to his important social status.

Some other Upper Paleolithic child burials also contain great quantities of jewelry: at Balzi Rossi (Italy), the Grotte des Enfants got its name from the discovery there in 1874 of a double child burial, on their backs, with a thousand perforated *Nassa neritea* shells on and beneath the pelvis and upper femurs—these are assumed to represent decorated loincloths. In 1901 another double burial was found here, this time of what were thought to be "Negroids," an old woman together with an adolescent (15–17) with four rows of perforated *Nassa neritea* shells on the head (Mussi 2001).

Finally, mention must be made of the extraordinary burial from the rockshelter of La Madeleine (Dordogne) found in December 1926 (Vanhaeren and d'Errico 2001) with its 1,500 pieces of jewelry. The grave was recently dated to 10,190 BP (uncalibrated). Buried in the shelter was a child of two to four, on its back, head to the south, and with its arms along the body. It was so covered with ochre that it stained the soil. Around the head were three limestone slabs forming a kind of protective chest. At all the joints—wrists, knees, elbows, ankles—as well as around the head and shoulders there were strings of shells and teeth. The shells are all seashells, from both the Atlantic and Mediterranean, but some are Miocene fossils from the Bordeaux region or Touraine. More than a thousand shells (*Dentalium, Nerita fluviatilis, Turritella*, etc.) were found, together with some stag canines (Figure 9.3) and fox canines. None of the shells is complete—they have all been sawn into pieces 6–7 mm long. They were sewn onto a garment or support and they seem very worn, so they were clearly not specially made for burial. As with the Sungir children, it seems that this infant had some kind of special hereditary status.

In closing this section, the question of mortality rates needs to be addressed. It is very tempting to use the available data from Upper Paleolithic or Neanderthal burials to construct models about life expectancy among these people, and to speculate about the apparently high incidence of infant mortality. Unfortunately, this cannot be done—one can only calculate an average at death for the skeletons that have survived and been discovered, but this does not—contrary to a frequent practice among archaeologists in

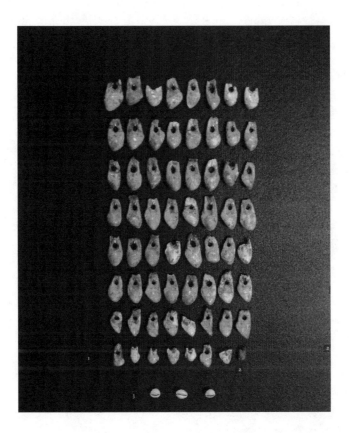

FIGURE 9.3 Stag canines, some of the jewelry from the child-burial of La Madeleine (photo P. Bahn).

the past—provide an accurate guide to the life expectancy and mortality pattern of a particular culture, because that would entail the very considerable assumptions that the sample or cemetery contains all members of the community who died in that place or region during the relevant period; that everyone was buried, or buried there, regardless of age, sex, or status; that nobody died elsewhere; and that all the burials were from roughly the same period. These assumptions cannot realistically be made, especially for the Middle or Upper Paleolithic. We have some disparate samples of these populations, but we have no idea how representative or skewed they might be (Renfrew and Bahn 2008:435–436).

DERMATOGLYPHS

Among the most moving traces of ancient people are the prints left by their fingers, hands, or feet, often made accidentally but sometimes purposely, in caves or other places. It is miraculous that so many of these have survived, although they sometimes look so fresh that they could have been done a few minutes ago.

Almost all Paleolithic footprints known so far have been found in caves in France, and the great majority are from children or adolescents. For example, in the cave of Aldène (Hérault), or that of Pech Merle (Lot) where the dozen or so prints—certainly Upper Paleolithic because the cave was subsequently blocked—belonged to one big child or adolescent (or an adult with very gracile feet) whose feet were approximately 225 mm long (Duday and Garcia 1983). The cave of Montespan (Haute Garonne) contains footprints of a very young child, probably a girl of six to eight years (Garcia and Duday 1993).

In the Grotte Chauvet (Ardèche) the footprints of a child, aged eight or nine, have been found at the back of the cave (Garcia 2001:36–37). They stretch for about 50 m, under a low ceiling. There are also torch wipes (dated to 25,000 to 26,000 years ago) along there, so it is likely that the child was carrying it. It may have been heading for a water source. The youngster was about 1.3 to 1.4 m high, and the width/length ratio of its prints suggests a boy. Two prints of a clay-covered right hand at the bottom of a decorated panel (Garcia 2001:38) seem to have been made by the same child, since their size corresponds well with that of the footprints.

In the Réseau Clastres (Ariège), more than 500 prints have been found—they are not definitely Paleolithic, but it is quite likely that they do date to that period. There are three trails side by side of small feet, 18 to 21 cm long, representing children who were probably eight to ten years old. They were walking normally, not running or jumping. In other caves there is evidence that they were not only totally relaxed in these dark depths, but even played there. At Niaux (Ariège) there is a large group of footprints in clay near the Galerie Profonde (Pales 1976)—24 complete prints and 15 toe or heel marks (Figure 9.4). They represent two children, aged about eight and 11, weighing between 27 and 30 kg, and between 1.33 and 1.39 m tall; they came at least twice to this low muddy area, and they spent some time and effort in carefully making the most perfect prints that they could (Pales 1976).

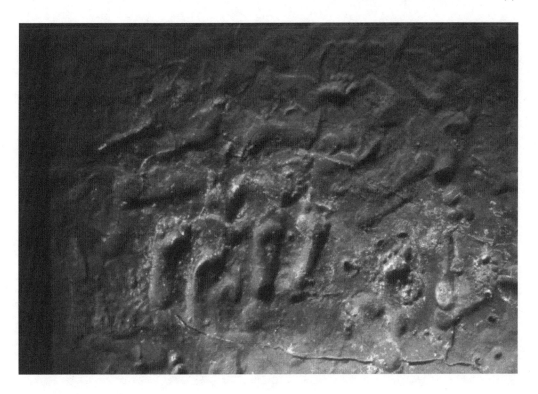

FIGURE 9.4 The carefully made children's footprints from Niaux (photo J. Vertut, P. Bahn collection).

Other indications of play activity can be detected. In the cave of Fontanet (Ariège) a little child of about five—who also left kneeprints and handprints—seems to have pursued a puppy or a fox into the cave's depths, since the animal's tracks are next to its prints (Garcia and Duday 1993). In the same cave there are also traces of adolescents playing together, throwing clay balls at each other. This is reminiscent of the Italian cave of Toirano where, in the innermost chamber, dozens of clay pellets were thrown at the back wall and also at a stalagmitic formation nicknamed the "Sphinx" (Blanc 1957)—many pellets missed and lie on the cave floor; they are three to seven cm in diameter (Figure 9.5 on page 178). In Toirano, the activity dates to around 13,000 years ago (Molleson et al. 1972), which is also the likely date of Fontanet on the basis of its art's style.

Finally, what is also probably play activity can be seen in Le Tuc d'Audoubert (Ariège), where children clearly accompanied the artists who made the famous clay bison at the far end of the cave. Their small footprints can still be seen (Bégouën et al. 2009:256, 272–273)—for example in the Galerie des Petits Pieds where analysis suggested that the prints were those of a four-year-old (Bégouën and Vallois 1928). The Salle des Talons, next to the clay bison, contains at least 183 heelprints, from children or adolescents moving around under a low ceiling (1.2 to 1.5 m high). Bégouën and Vallois (1928; Vallois 1928, 1931) estimated that these were made by five individuals, but the latest studies show that it is

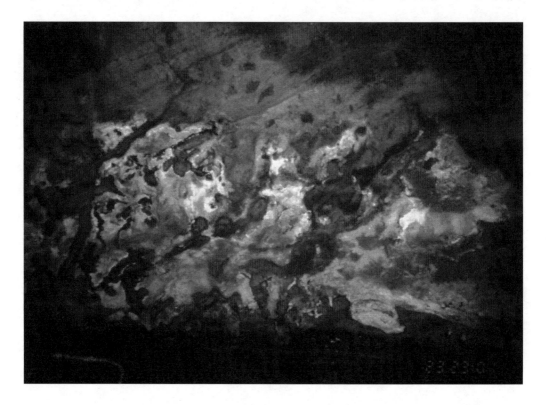

FIGURE 9.5 Some of the clay pellets on the wall of Toirano Cave (photo P. Bahn).

very difficult to tell how many youngsters were present (Bégouën et al. 2009:291). But it is important to note that this chamber also contains a wealth of finger marks and simple drawings on its floor, which could be deeply mystical and significant (just as the heelmarks were long supposed to be some kind of ritual dance), but are perhaps more plausibly seen as the activities of bored children passing time while the adults were making the sculptures.

A different kind of floor marking has been found in the Willandra Lakes region of southeast Australia (Franklin and Habgood 2009) where two crescent-shaped grooves were made in soft clay amid the biggest collection of Pleistocene footprints in the world. They date to between 23,000 and 17,000 years ago. The Pintubi people from central Australia identified these grooves as finger markings made by children playing on the clay surface of a soak (Franklin and Habgood 2009). They also identified some of the hundreds of footprints as being of a four- to five-year-old child; but the crescents could also have been made by a digging stick or a spear end.

Children not only made fingermarks on the ground but also marked the walls and ceilings of caves. For example, on the famous ceiling of Pech Merle (Lot), almost all the markings were made by adults, but on the right of group C there are two bands of lines that were clearly made by two small hands, those of either a woman or an adolescent (Lorblanchet 1992:474). At this point the ceiling was 1.8 m up, and so quite reachable.

Bednarik (e.g., 2008) has claimed that juveniles were responsible for some finger flutings in caves in southern Australia at least 30,000 years ago, but, as has been pointed out (Sharpe and Van Gelder 2006:937), "the case Bednarik makes is more suggestive than definitive, relying on a methodology that requires further refinement with forensics." Bednarik does not say what he means by juveniles, and has not compared his results with measurements of living people of different ages. By contrast, a reliable methodology has indeed been developed by Sharpe and Van Gelder (2004, 2006) and applied to Chamber A1 in the French cave of Rouffignac (Dordogne), located about 300 m from the entrance, where a huge expanse of flutings was made into the thin red clay that coats the white limestone ceiling. Their study was based on the finger widths of people of different ages, and analysis of flutings made by the central fingers held together. They found that there is no perceptible difference between the finger widths of teenagers and adults, but there is a major difference between young children and older people. Very few children younger than two to three years can make fluted lines. Their results for the chamber suggest that some of the flutings here were made by children, and others by teenagers or adults. This is the first case where fluting by children has been truly demonstrated—they found that most of the specimens in this chamber were made by children of two to five, plus one of five to 14, and one of five to 16 (Sharpe and van Gelder 2004, 2006). What is most interesting is that the ceiling in places is just reachable by a man of 1.8 m stretching on his toes, so it is obvious that the children were lifted up to make the fingermarks. Why? Why does not one find adult flutings on high surfaces and children's flutings on lower ones?

Another case of an infant being lifted up has been found in the French cave of Cosquer (Bouches-du-Rhône), where a child's hand was pressed into the soft surface of a wall, 2.2 m up, so it must have been either lifted up or sitting on an adult's shoulders (Clottes et al. 2005:60–61, 215). There is another one nearby, 2.4 m up, with an engraving of a possible sea animal between them. Elsewhere in the cave, traces of a child's four fingers covered in clay (total width 5 cm) can be seen on the moonmilk, in two instances, at a height of 1.9 m. Therefore at least one child—and perhaps several—had access to the deepest parts of this cave.

In the cave of Gargas (Hautes-Pyrénées), a child's or even a baby's hand was held to the wall by an adult while pigment was blown or spat over it (Barrière 1976:59). In the same cave's Pavillon Chinois, a baby's hand, stenciled in black, is well defined at the wrist, but the fingers are more blurred. According to Sahly (1966) the cave also has two intact hand stencils of infants of about three months; two identical intact child hands stenciled in red; and a child's hand stenciled in black in a niche 5 m up. He also claimed to have found a hand print in clay which has its little finger missing—it is a small fine hand, 105 x 60 mm, belonging to a child of 1.3 m, either a boy of 10 to 11 or a girl of 12 to 13.

Children's hand stencils are not limited to France—in the cave of Wargata Mina, Tasmania, some examples occur close to the floor. Preliminary dates from the cave indicate a terminal Pleistocene age, and they are highly unlikely to be more recent.

One child's fingerprint has been detected on the back of the famous fired-clay figurine known as the "Venus of Dolní Vestonice" from Moravia (Czech Republic), dating to about 25,000 years ago. Analysis suggests that the finger belonged to a child aged between seven and 15, most likely around 11 (Králík et al. 2002). But the analysts understandably deny that such a masterful work of art could have been produced by that child.

Bednarik (2008), on the other hand, has expressed the somewhat bizarre belief that, because there are some prints and fingermarks of children in some caves, then much of the figurative art in Europe is by them! He only sees a "possibility" (2008:179) that adults created a certain portion of Paleolithic rock art. Similarly, Guthrie's (2005) conviction that works by youngsters constitute a larger fraction of the Paleolithic art corpus than had hitherto been proposed led to regrettable and sensational newspaper headlines in Britain such as, "Cave paintings are graffiti by prehistoric yobs," and much of the art was attributed to "sexually charged, intoxicated teenagers intent on vandalism." Guthrie's own position is more sober, being based on new analyses indicating that many hand stencils were of young males—but how far can this be extrapolated to figurative art? He identified 201 hands from Spanish and French caves that could be measured for width and length of fingers, and compared the data with measurements taken from 700 children, teenagers and adults at Alaskan schools. Statistically the cave prints matched modern children aged 10 to 16, and he estimates their sex ratio as largely male by three or four to one. He therefore argues that the subject matter of much Paleolithic art is consistent with it being created by adolescent boys, preoccupied with hunting and mating. But unfortunately he grossly exaggerates the ubiquity of sexual imagery, and of hunting—indeed, most of what he considers to be hunting scenes is simple wishful thinking. In fact, out of the tens of thousands of animal images in Paleolithic art we do not have a single clear hunting scene, and not a single clear image of copulation, either animal or human (Bahn and Vertut 1997).

Apart from the prints and markings surveyed above, the only examples of cave art that could plausibly be attributed to children are those in places which only small people could reach—for example, the decorated gallery of Fronsac (Dordogne) is only 35 cm wide; a passage of La Pasiega (Cantabria) filled with geometric motifs is also very difficult for an adult to enter, as is one of the side chambers of Bédeilhac (Ariège); and recently, experienced speleologists managed to push farther into Les Combarelles I (Dordogne) than ever before, and found that Upper Paleolithic people had got through to there and made drawings. If modern adult speleologists find it almost impossible to get through, then it is likely that the Paleolithic explorers were either youngsters or very small and lithe adults. However, the mastery of technique and form displayed in the figures made even in these difficult places strongly suggests that adults were responsible—just as the amazing quality and the depth of knowledge of animal anatomy and behavior displayed so prominently in most Paleolithic art make it clear that experienced adults were responsible.

Why, then, are almost all the footprints in caves those of youngsters? It is highly unlikely that they can all be explained by ideas about initiation ceremonies and the like. Instead, as Garcia (2001) pointed out, it can be far more plausibly explained by the fact that children are always wandering off, away from the main paths, on which the more frequent traffic would obliterate adult footprints.

Be that as it may, children were clearly not afraid to explore the far depths, narrow passages, and tiny chambers of caverns, whether alone (as at Aldène) or with adults (as at Le Tuc d'Audoubert).

ARTIFACTS

It is somewhat ironic that the one object from the Upper Paleolithic that one might have assumed to be a toy—the ivory articulated "doll" found at Brno in Moravia—came from the grave not of a child but an adult male: the puppeteer, perhaps? Other than that, one can only speculate as to whether art objects were dolls or playthings. The very slim ivory female figurine from Laugerie Basse (Bahn and Vertut 1997:16) might be one such, as could the small figurines of women and of birds from Mal'ta and Buret in Siberia, the small crude terracotta figurine from Maininskaya in Siberia (Vasil'ev 1985) (Figure 9.6), or the terracotta statuettes from Afalou Bou Rhummel in Algeria, dating to between 18,000 and 11,000 years ago (Hachi 2003)—but they could also be something more important, meaningful, ritual, or mystical.

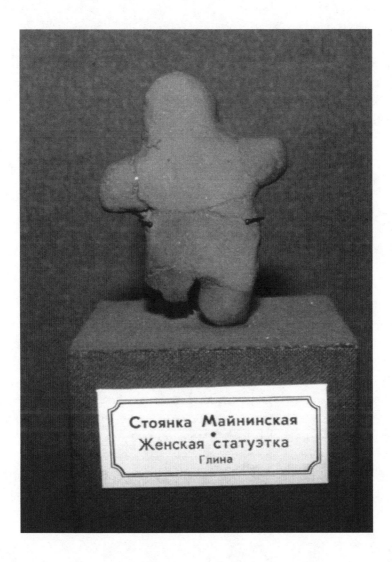

FIGURE 9.6 The Maininskaya terracotta figurine from southern Siberia; 96 mm high, and dating to circa 14,500 B.C. (photo P. Bahn).

The presumably humorous carvings at the end of spearthrowers depicting a fawn or young ibex excreting an enormous turd, with one or two birds perched on it (Bahn and Vertut 1997:98), could also have been playthings—but the amount of skill and effort put into carving antler in this way would argue more for valuable and prestige objects. It is extremely likely that Ice Age toys—which must have existed in great quantities—were primarily made of light and organic materials such as wood and bark and basketry, and so have not survived. We have absolutely no way of deciding which other objects or tools might have belonged to children, unless they are found associated with them in graves—such as the above-mentioned small ivory horse in the Sungir burial; or the little shovel, carved from a mammoth bone, found in a child's grave at Kostenki XV-Gorodtsov (Avant 1979:39), which was covered by a mammoth shoulderblade, and which also contained a smoother and a polished-bone needle, several flint tools, and 150 perforated fox teeth; or at Mal'ta, a child was buried covered with ochre, and wore a necklace of beads and pendants, including a pendant in the form of a bird in flight under its backbone, an ivory belt plaque (Avant 1979:39).

The same applies to other phenomena—for example, in France's Chauvet cave much excitement was caused by the discovery of a cave bear skull placed on a rock in a decorated chamber (Chauvet et al. 1995); but rather than evidence for some kind of cave bear cult (a once-popular notion, especially for the Middle Paleolithic, but long discredited thanks to taphonomic studies) this could again simply be an example of a child playing inside the cave. There is no way of deciding between the two possibilities on present evidence.

Animal bones have occasionally been found stuck deeply into cave floors (e.g., in Chauvet and Enlène), while in Le Tuc d'Audoubert a circle of small stalactites was stuck into the floor (Bégouën et al. 2009). However, even if one assumes that these items were not involved in some kind of game—and one cannot safely make that assumption—this does not necessarily link them to any kind of ritual or religious activity.

DEPICTIONS

Children are very rarely depicted in Paleolithic art (they are perhaps even nonexistent apart from the supposed babies of Gönnersdorf). However, some specialists believe that a few of the humans of La Marche may be infants on the basis of head shape and bodily proportions (Figure 9.7a/b). La Marche (Vienne) is a French rockshelter, dating to 14,280 BP, which yielded hundreds of plaquettes of stone bearing numerous engravings of animals but also of numerous humans, a quite exceptional phenomenon in Paleolithic art. Pales pointed out that in the human on plaquette 35-I the head was "too large in relation to the body" and there are two bulges on the occiput (Pales and de St Péreuse 1968; 1976:Plate 93). Duhard (1993:83) believes that this depicts a newborn child, since it has a very large head, as in babies where the head is a quarter of the height; and he also sees a possible umbilical cord. On plaquette 27, Pales (Pales and de St Péreuse 1976:Plate 58) pointed out that the human heads look like young individuals, either children or teenagers, especially the first one whose face is truly baby-like.

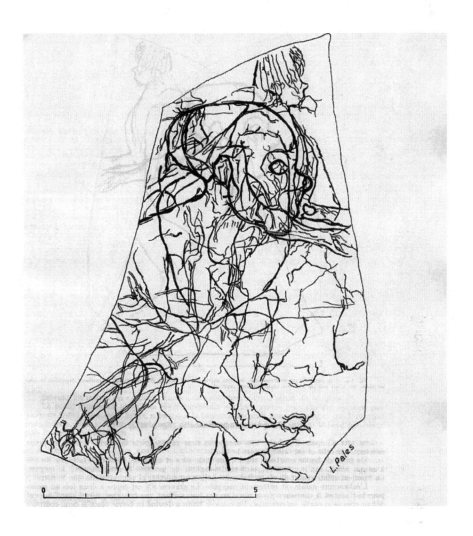

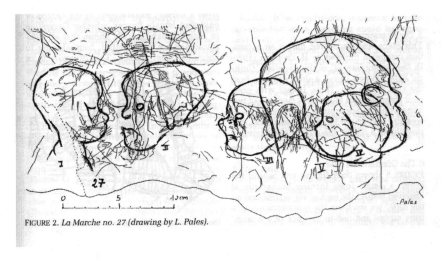

FIGURE 2. *La Marche no. 27 (drawing by L. Pales).*

FIGURE 9.7 A/B The "children" of La Marche (after Pales and de St Péreuse).

Gönnersdorf, an open-air site in Germany of about 12,600 BP, has also yielded hundreds of engraved plaquettes, which mostly depict animals, but also a large number of highly stylized women. On plaquette 87, Bosinski sees four figures, one behind the other, with a small form behind the back of the second one—the representation of a baby carried and tied to the back of a woman (Bosinski and Fischer 1974). Duhard (1993:86) points out that this woman has rounded breasts, while the others have pointed ones. Marshack (1975) saw another plaquette (No. 59) as an anthropomorphous figure linked by lines to a female silhouette (with a flat abdomen and small breasts) as a fetus attached by the umbilical cord. Marshack saw a breast and two upraised arms:

> The microscope revealed what I think is an umbilical cord connecting the female image to the fetus, which is depicted with neither arms nor legs. If so, this is the only image of a human birth ever found from the Ice Age. The engraving, perhaps made by an adult woman living in the camp, may have been related to the monthly periods and eventual pregnancy. (1975:84)

Francesco d'Errico has also studied this plaquette (Bosinski et al. 2001:table 56), and concurs with Marshack's interpretation (d'Errico 2009:104):

> The possible newborn has no traits that are unequivocally and categorically human—apart from a possible head and two eyes. The use of a circle, closed or partially open, to evoke a face, and of two smaller circles inside it to evoke eyes is a phenomenon that has been observed several times at Gönnersdorf . . . which seems to confirm the deliberate and probably human character of this depiction. The resemblance of the tuft close to the head of the possible newborn to the one that decorates the baby-carrier depicted on plaquette 87 is another element which makes one think that we are indeed dealing with a child.

CONCLUSION

While the subject of children in the Ice Age has not received a great deal of attention over the years, there is in fact a wide variety of evidence that can tell us a little about them—although inevitably we have doubtless lost great quantities of toys and other such aspects of their life. The vast majority of what we can glean from the Ice Age archaeological record comes from burials and cave-markings, and what these tell us is that even small children sometimes had considerable wealth and prestige, which were presumably inherited; that numerous infants were accorded full funerary rituals, often with grave goods; and that youngsters were wont to venture into the deepest darkest caves where, far from being fearful, they sometimes engaged in playful activities. So although our knowledge of the children of the Ice Age is limited, it is at least a start—and future discoveries can only improve our knowledge.

REFERENCES CITED

Akazawa, T., and S. Muhesen (editors) 2002 *Neanderthal Burials. Excavations of the Dederiyeh Cave, Afrin, Syria.* International Research Center for Japanese Studies, Kyoto.

Alexeeva, T. I., and N. O. Bader (editors) 2000 *Homo Sungirensis. Upper Paleolithic Man: Ecological and Evolutionary Aspects of the Investigation.* Scientific World, Moscow.

Avant Les Scythes. Préhistoire de l'Art en U.R.S.S. 1979 Catalogue d'exposition. Réunion des Musées Nationaux, Paris.

Bader, N. O., and Y. A. Lavrishin (editors) 1998 [in Russian] *The Upper Paleolithic Settlement of Sungir (Burials and Environment).* Scientific World, Moscow.

Bahn, P. G. 2002 The Romito Dwarf. In *Written in Bones,* edited by Paul G. Bahn, pp. 148–150. Quintet, London.

Bahn, P. G. 2003 A Child in Time. Review of (João Zilhão and Erik Trinkaus, editors) "Portrait of the Artist as a Child. The Gravettian Human Skeleton from the Abrigo do Lagar Velho and its Archeological Context." *Nature* 424, No. 6948, 31 July, p. 490.

Bahn, P. G., and J. Vertut 1997 *Journey through the Ice Age.* University of California Press, Berkeley / Weidenfeld and Nicholson, London.

Barrière, C. 1976 *L'Art Pariétal de la Grotte de Gargas.* BAR Supplementary Series 14, Oxford.

Bednarik, R. G. 2008 Children as Pleistocene Artists. *Rock Art Research* 25(2):173–182.

Bégouën, H., and H. Vallois 1928 Les Empreintes de Pieds Préhistoriques. *Institut International d'Anthropologie* IIIe session, Amsterdam, pp. 323–338.

Bégouën, R., C. Fritz, G. Tosello, J. Clottes, A. Pastoors, and F. Faist 2009 *Le Sanctuaire Secret des Bisons. Il y a 14 000 ans dans la caverne du Tuc d'Audoubert.* Somogy éditions d'art, Paris.

Billy, G. 1975 Etude Anthropologique des Restes Humains de l'Abri Pataud. In *Excavation of the Abri Pataud, Les Eyzies (Dordogne),* edited by Hallam L. Movius, pp. 201–261. Peabody Museum, Harvard University, Cambridge.

Blanc, A. C. 1957 A New Paleolithic Cultural Element, Probably of Ideological Significance: The Clay Pellets of the Cave of the Basua (Savona). *Quaternaria* 4:1–9.

Bosinski, G., and G. Fischer 1974 *Die Menschendarstellungen von Gönnersdorf. Ausgrabung 1968.* Der Magdalenien-Fundplatz Gönnersdorf. Band I. Franz Steiner Verlag GMBH, Wiesbaden.

Bosinski, G., F. d'Errico, and P. Schiller 2001 *Die Gravierten Frauendarstellungen von Gönnersdorf.* Der Magdalenien-Fundplatz Gönnersdorf. Band 8. Franz Steiner Verlag GMBH, Stuttgart.

Cervera, J., J. L. Arsuaga, J. Maria Bermúdez de Castro, and E. Carbonell 1998 *Atapuerca, Un millón de años de historia.* Plot Ediciones, Madrid.

Chauvet, J.-M., E. B. Deschamps, and C. Hillaire 1995 *Chauvet Cave. The Discovery of the World's Oldest Paintings.* Thames and Hudson, London (U.S. edition: *Dawn of Art, The Chauvet Cave: The Oldest Known Paintings in the World.* Abrams, New York).

Cleyet-Merle, J.-J., and B. Maureille 2008 Le Moustier 2. In *Première Humanité. Gestes funéraires des Néandertaliens,* pp. 113–114. Musée National de Préhistoire, Les Eyzies. Editions de la Réunion des Musées Nationaux, Paris.

Clottes, J., J. Courtin, and L. Vanrell 2005 *Cosquer Redécouvert.* Le Seuil, Paris.

Defleur, A. 1993 *Les Sépultures Moustériennes.* CNRS, Paris.

Duday, H., and M. Garcia 1983 Les Empreintes de l'Homme Préhistorique: la Grotte du Pech Merle à Cabrerets (Lot): une Relecture Significative des Traces de Pieds Humains. *Bulletin de la Société Préhistorique Française* 80:208–215.

Duhard, J.-P. 1993 Upper Paleolithic Figures as a Reflection of Human Morphology and Social Organization. *Antiquity* 67:83–91.

Einwögerer, T. 2005 Die gravettienzeitliche Säuglings-Doppelbestättung vom Wachtberg in Krems. *Archäologie Österreichs* 16(2):19–20.

d'Errico, F. 2009 The Oldest Representation of Childbirth. In *An Enquiring Mind. Studies in Honor of Alexander Marshack,* edited by P. G. Bahn, pp. 99–109. American School of Prehistoric Research Monograph series. Oxbow Books, Oxford.

Franklin, N. R., and P. Habgood 2009 Finger Markings and the Willandra Lakes Footprint Site, South-Eastern Australia. *Rock Art Research* 26(2):199–203.

Frayer, D. W., W. Horton, R. Macchiarelli, and M. Mussi 1987 Dwarfism in an Adolescent from the Italian Late Upper Paleolithic. *Nature* 330:60–62.

Frayer, D. W., R. Macchiarelli, and M. Mussi 1988 A Case of Chondrodystrophic Dwarfism in the Italian Late Upper Paleolithic. *American Journal of Physical Anthropology* 75:549–565.

Garcia, M.-A. 2001 Les Empreintes et les Traces Humaines et Animales. In *La Grotte Chauvet. L'Art des Origines*, edited by Jean Clottes, pp. 34–43. Le Seuil, Paris.

Garcia, M., and H. Duday 1993 Les Empreintes de Mains dans l'Argile des Grottes Ornées. In *La Main dans la Préhistoire, Les Dossiers d'Archéologie* 178:56–59.

Guthrie, R. D. 2005 *The Nature of Paleolithic Art*. University of Chicago Press, Chicago.

Hachi, S. 2003 *Aux Origines des Arts Premiers en Afrique du Nord*. Mémoires du Centre National de Recherches Préhistoriques, Anthropologiques et Historiques, Alger, Nlle série No. 6.

Heim, J.-L. 1976 *Les Hommes Fossiles de La Ferrassie (Dordogne)*. Archives de l'Institut de Paléontologie Humaine 35. Masson, Paris.

Králík, M., V. Novotny, and M. Oliva 2002 Fingerprint on the Venus of Dolní Vestonice. *Anthropologie* 40(2):107–113.

Lister, A., and P. Bahn 2007 *Mammoths. Giants of the Ice Age*. 3rd edition. University of California Press, Berkeley.

Lorblanchet, M. 1992 Finger Markings in Pech Merle and Their Place in Prehistoric Art. In *Rock Art in the Old World*, edited by M. Lorblanchet, pp. 451–490. Indira Gandhi National Centre for the Arts, New Delhi.

Marshack, A. 1975 Exploring the Mind of Ice Age Man. *National Geographic* 147(1):62–89.

Molleson, T. I., K. P. Oakley, and J. C. Vogel 1972 The Antiquity of the Human Footprints of Tana della Basura. *Journal of Human Evolution* 1:467–471.

Mussi, M 2001 *Earliest Italy: An Overview of the Italian Paleolithic and Mesolithic*. Kluwer and Plenum, New York.

Oliva, M. 2009 Breaking the Vicious Circle of Mammoth Studies. In *Milovice: Site of the Mammoth People Below the Pavlov Hills*, edited by M. Oliva, pp. 292–308. Moravian Museum, Brno.

Pales, L. 1976 *Les Empreintes de Pieds Humains dans les Cavernes. Les Empreintes du Réseau Clastres de la Caverne de Niaux (Ariège)*. Archives de l'Institut de Paléontologie Humaine 36. Masson, Paris.

Pales, L., and M. Tassin de Saint Péreuse 1968 Humains Superposés de La Marche. In *La Préhistoire. Problèmes et Tendances,* edited by F. Bordes and D. de Sonneville-Bordes, pp. 327–336. CNRS, Paris.

Pales, L., and M. Tassin de Saint Péreuse 1976 *Les Gravures de La Marche II: Les Humains*. Ophrys, Gap.

Renfrew, C., and P. Bahn 2008 *Archaeology: Theories, Methods and Practice*. 5th edition. Thames and Hudson, London.

Sahly, A. 1966 *Les Mains Mutilées dans l'Art Préhistorique*. Privat, Toulouse / Maison tunisienne de l'édition, Tunis.

Sharpe, K., and L. Van Gelder 2004 Children and Paleolithic "Art": Indications from Rouffignac Cave. *International Newsletter on Rock Art* 38:9–17.

Sharpe, K., and L. Van Gelder 2006 Evidence for Cave Marking by Paleolithic Children. *Antiquity* 80:937–947.

Stone, A. C., G. Milner, and S. Pääbo 1996 Sex Determination of Ancient Human Skeletons Using DNA. *American Journal of Physical Anthropology* 99:231–238.

Tillier, A.-M. 2008 L'Enfant de la Grotte Mezmaiskaya. In *Première Humanité. Gestes funéraires des Néandertaliens*, p. 96. Musée National de Préhistoire, Les Eyzies. Editions de la Réunion des Musées Nationaux, Paris.

Vallois, H. 1928 Etude des Empreintes des Pieds Humains du Tuc d'Audoubert, de Cabrerets et de Ganties, in *Congrès International d'Anthropologie et d'Archéologie Préhistoriques III*, Amsterdam. pp. 328–335.

Vallois, H. 1931 Les Empreintes de Pieds Humains des Grottes Préhistoriques du Midi de la France. *Palaeobiologica* 4:79–98.

Vandermeersch, B., and A.-M. Tillier 1976 Les Enfants Moustériens de Qafzeh (Israël). *Comptes rendus de l'Académie des Sciences de Paris* 282, série D:1097–1099.

Vanhaeren, M., and F. d'Errico 2001 La Parure de l'Enfant de la Madeleine (Fouilles Peyrony). Un Nouveau Regard sur l'Enfance au Paléolithique Supérieur. *Paléo* 13:201–40.

Vasil'ev, S. A. 1985 Une Statuette d'Argile Paléolithique de Sibérie du Sud. *L'Anthropologie* 89:193–196.

Zilhão, J., and E. Trinkaus (editors) 2002 *Portrait of the Artist as a Child. The Gravettian Human Skeleton from the Abrigo do Lagar Velho and its Archaeological Context.* Instituto Português de Arqueologia, Trabalhos de Arqueologia 22, Lisbon.

CHAPTER TEN

Children in the Anthropomorphic Imagery of the European and Near Eastern Neolithic

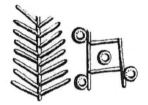

Peter F. Biehl

Abstract *In this chapter I will discuss how studying visual representations of the human body from the southeastern European and Near Eastern Neolithic can aid us in understanding the representation of the human figure in the past and tackle the question of why images of children were so rare in the anthropomorphic imagery of the European and Near Eastern Neolithic from the seventh to fifth millennium B.C. The chapter looks at identity and personhood as well as anthropomorphism, miniaturization, and embodiment in order to better understand and scrutinize corporeal, ideational, and symbolic attributes of the visual body and materializations of identity and personhood in the archaeological record.*

INTRODUCTION

This clay figurine from Hacılar and its imaginative interpretation by the excavator James Mellaart represents vividly the issue of representations of children in the Neolithic (Figure 10.1 on page 190). The figurine shows a mature woman resting on her side or back with a second smaller figure (which is not preserved above the hips) grasping her hips and legs. Mellaart initially saw "the young goddess . . . in the embrace of the adolescent god" but later explained that

> this group does not show a "hieros gamos," but a mother playing with her child. For one thing the sexual act is not depicted, and closer inspection has shown that the goddess is dressed in a painted leopard garment. (Mellaart 1970:170)

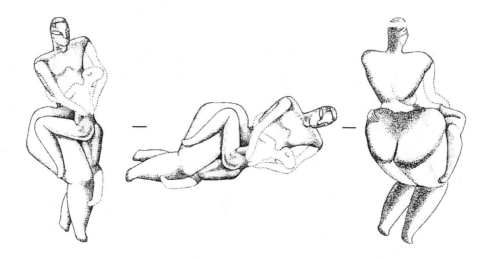

FIGURE 10.1 Clay figurine from Hacılar Level VI House Q5 (after Voigt 2007:Figure 12.10).

Given the position of the smaller figure, its hand shown grasping the hip of the woman, one leg pushed in between her knees and the second wound around her thigh, it has been recently argued that sexual activity seems to be indicated (Voigt 2007:166). Voigt continues that "there is, of course, no indication of the gender of the smaller figure unless one accepts its slim thighs and buttocks as diagnostic for males. Just who the larger figure might represent is another issue," and "if the life course of women is represented in this suite of images, what about pregnancy and childbirth?" (Voigt 2007:166). She convincingly argues that though many figurines from Hacılar have been described as pregnant she rather thinks that "the figures look fat rather than pregnant, but I do not

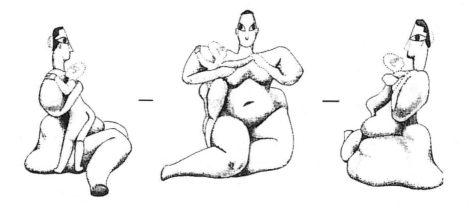

FIGURE 10.2 Clay figurine from Hacılar Level VI House Q5 (after Voigt 2007:Figure 12.10).

think that this is a very important distinction within a society in which most women were probably pregnant for most of their relatively brief adult lives" (Voigt 2007:166). However, Voigt argues that a second figurine from the same site (Figure 10.2) shows a "seated woman holding a small child to her side and is also arguably pregnant."

Only most recently have archaeologists turned to the roles played by figurines as representations of bodies and identities (Bailey 2005; Biehl 2006, 2009; Boric and Robb 2008; Hansen 2007; Joyce 2007, 2008; Lesure 2002, 2011; Meskell 2007; Meskell and Nakamura 2009). The body is a key theme in recent theory—not only in Bourdieu's practice theory and Foucault's cultural analysis, but also in phenomenology, feminism, anthropology, and other strands of recent thought (Robb 2007:11). As John Robb recently formulated, "The body is the locus of experience and social reproduction: human's ability to think and act emerges from the embodied organism. The body is the locus of habituated and routinized action and of much non-discursive action. Moreover, it is through the body that one interacts with, understands oneself, and is understood by other people" (Robb 2007:11).

Representations of the body were undoubtedly complex and important to the people who created them, and analysis that reduces them to a single function-based category should be avoided. By taking the current theories on how figurines represent visual bodies, I will attempt to tackle the question of how a creator's deep understanding of their own body is represented on figurines and why, therefore, representing children's bodies played a marginal part in the worldview and belief system in the Neolithic.

"The link between bodies and thought is well-encompassed in Bourdieu's most enduring contribution, the concept of *habitus*" (Robb 2007:11). John Robb further elaborates that habitus is the deeply instilled generative principles, which provide the cultural logic according to which agents negotiate their way through both old and new situations. Habitus provides the agent's unquestioned tools for thought, the values and oppositions that shape our thinking, the terms of identity and personhood which make us who we are, and the emotional currencies we live through (Robb 2007:11–12).

For Douglass Bailey, the fundamental characteristics of figurines are that "they are miniature, they are representational, and they depict the human form," and "that the ability to make, use, and understand symbolic objects such as figurines is an ability that is shared by all modern humans and this is a capability that connects you, Neolithic men, women, and children, and the Palaeolithic painters of caves" (Bailey 2010: 122).

Rosemary Joyce has pointed out that "universal interpretations of figurines ignore the variety of different ways that images can resemble things they stand for. European [Paleolithic] figurines appeal to us today because we immediately see them as portraits of human beings like us" (Joyce 2008:8). The modern and Western notion of the visual body is a particular cultural and historical product, and not one that can be safely projected into the past. We cannot assume that the creators of Paleolithic or Neolithic figurines viewed their bodies as we have. But which body idea had these people, and how can we approach it archaeologically?

THE CONCEPTION OF THE BODY IN THE NEOLITHIC

When looking at the famous Late Neolithic "couple" from Gumelniţa (Figure 10.3), it is easy to be struck by their alien qualities. As in most cases, a face is absent and a head, featureless but for a ridged nose and clunky representations of breasts and genitalia—in this particular case, both the female pubic triangle and the male penis are represented together with (female) breasts—are the only body parts (except arms and legs) represented. These, as well as the other figurines from Neolithic Southeastern Europe and the Near East, might seem alien because they represent a particular view of a body but not a visual body as we are used to seeing represented today. The figurines from ethnographic records in Western Africa (Biehl 1999) or from archaeological and historic records in Greece or Rome (Green 1998; Voyatzis 1998) are also remarkably different in representing the body. The same is true for the European Bronze Age (Robb 2009) and Iron Age (Huth 2003), which leaves us puzzled with the question: Why are the Neolithic (and to a certain extend the Palaeolithic) "bodies" so similar, and at the same time so different, from later representations?

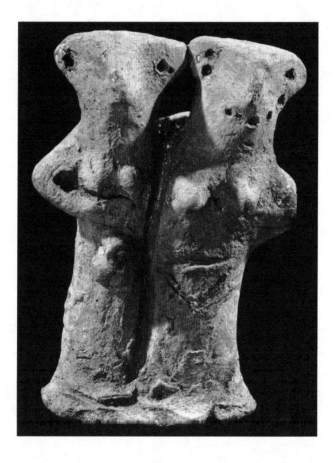

FIGURE 10.3 Figurines from Gumelniţa, Romania (after Biehl 2003:Figure 65).

Even at first glance it seems to be clear that in the shift from the Paleolithic and Neolithic to the Bronze Age and Iron Age, new aesthetic (and symbolic) ideals dictated the way people thought about their bodies, and they constructed anthropomorphic imagery such as figurines accordingly. Douglass Bailey has touched upon this issue in pointing out that figurines are significant in providing southeastern European Neolithic people with a means of comprehending their own identity (Bailey 2005:201), and may have served to unconsciously absorb people into a larger social group (Bailey 2007:124).

Though the ability of figurines to express and shape the notion of "self" may be an intrinsic quality of anthropomorphic representation, abstraction, and miniaturization, the content shared between the maker of a figurine and its user is the product of that material engagement and entanglement that is clearly not universal. Fully excavated Neolithic sites such as Drama in Bulgaria (Lichardus et al. 1996, 2002, 2003) or well-studied and well-published Neolithic sites such as Çatalhöyük in Turkey (Biehl et al. 2009; Meskell 2007; Meskell and Nakamura 2009) indicate the wide spectrum in form, decoration, and possible functions and meaning of anthropomorphic figurines made, used, broken, and discarded in a single settlement layer (Figure 10.4).

Assuming that body and personhood have a single specific material representation imposes a modern conception of agency onto the people in the past (Fowler 2001, 2004). The very diverse and extremely varied workmanship of the visual body and the fact that figurines were not mass produced, but rather made by many different people who expressed their aesthetic freedom in form and decoration, clearly speaks against such an interpretation (Biehl 1996, 2003, 2006).

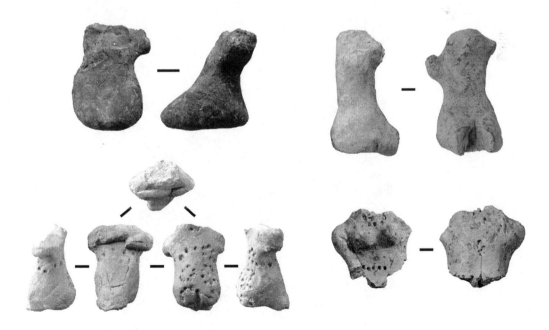

FIGURE 10.4 A selection of figurines from the West Mound in Çatalhöyük, Turkey (after Biehl et al. 2009:Figure 53).

How then do we approach the question of how the Neolithic people might have thought about and represented their own conception of a body, identity, and personhood in the form of clay figurines? And more importantly for this chapter, why are children's bodies only exceptionally represented in the form of—and attached to—clay figurines (Figure 10.5)? In general terms, it seems that sites with figurines representing children are the exceptions and that most well-studied and -published Neolithic sites from Europe and the Near East have no representations of children in the form of figurines at all.

ANALYZING THE VISUAL BODY OF CHILDREN

The human body is a collection of organs and bones united by common psychical and social ideas (Meskell 2000:13). A figurine represents a human body when the same psychical and social ideas are inscribed on other material. It is in this way that figurines fulfill their role as social referents (Hamilakis et al. 2002:4). In the Neolithic period, a sense of a body aesthetic—slender, expressive, and well proportioned—develops and is mirrored in the creation of figurines. The body idea is the subtle and conscious adherence to a

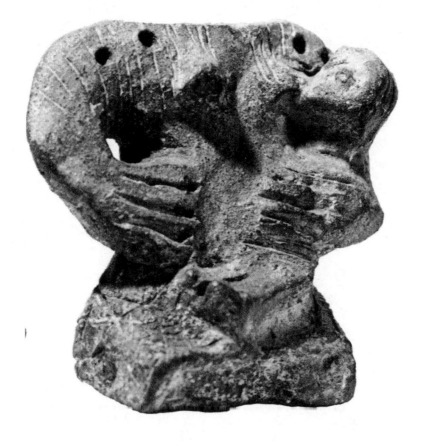

FIGURE 10,5 Figurine from Gradac, Serbia (after Biehl 2003:Figure 70).

corporeal and ideational structure. It is similar to the *habitus* of knowledge surrounding body and *self*, employed toward certain means, sculpting a clay body.

As a result of this development, certain figurine styles that no longer corresponded to body ideas were abandoned, as was the depiction of certain body parts. New body ideas may have been linked to the portrayal of body and person in ritual practices or modulated actions such as dance, which we only can see on one- and two-dimensional representations, as recently argued by Garfinkel (Garfinkel 2003).

It is important to note that it is during the Neolithic that we have the first representations of figurines holding a young child in their arms (Figure 10.6). This iteration of the all too well-known gesture of the "nurturing mother" fits perfectly in the idea of the "figurines in action" (Biehl 2006). Children can be seen as an extension of the adult female body ideationally and symbolically, related to the idea of the "central body" representing life's most pivotal moments (Biehl 2009:104–105).

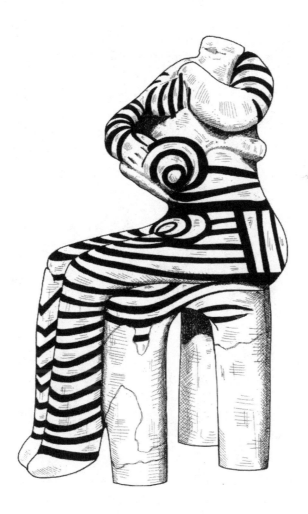

FIGURE 10.6 Figurine from Sesklo, Greece (after Biehl 2003:Figure 96).

The Neolithic figurines also feature the increasing use of masks (Figure 10.7) (Biehl 1996:165; Biehl and Marciniak 2000:186–187). The masks and decorated incisions may indicate a link between the development of a new body idea and new ritual activities, such as dance or transformation rituals including the fragmentation and destruction of the figurine's body (Biehl 1996, 2003, 2006). Such actions were integral processes in defining personhood in many societies; becoming human was not a static identity assumed at birth, but the result of continued specific behavior in the face of exterior risks (Borić 2007:85–86). While concepts of the body would be continually produced or reproduced by forming the body of a figurine, its use in rituals such as transformation and fragmentation provides a manifestation of a central body idea.

It is interesting to note that figurines holding children in their arms are not ritually fragmented and are mostly complete except for accidental breakages at the neck and extremities, which I have elsewhere labeled as "potential breakage/points of fracture" and which represent the structurally weakest parts of the figurine's body (Biehl 1996:167). The same is true for the children's bodies; they are not fragmented and destroyed and do not seem to have played a role in the widely practiced fragmentation ritual with adult figurines (Biehl 1996; 2006). The exception is the figurine from Hacılar (Figure 10.1), where we can see most likely intentional breakage of the bodies of the adult figurine and the embraced "child," or, as I would argue, embraced adolescent.

It is difficult to say whether children played a role in the described transformation ritual in the form of masking the human face (Biehl 1996, 2003). Either the heads of children are not preserved (Figure 10.8), or they are represented in a very schematic, abstract manner (Figure 10.9 on page 198) which makes it almost impossible to recognize and identify the wearing of masks as represented in the figurine from Liubcova-Ornița (Figure 10.11 on page 200).

In sum, children are only rarely represented in clay in three-dimensional form in the European and Near Eastern Neolithic and do not seem to have been actively incor-

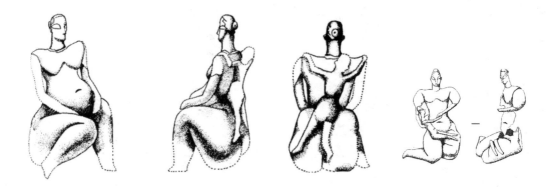

FIGURE 10.7 Figurines from Hacılar, Turkey (after Voigt 2007:Figures 12.10 and 12.7).

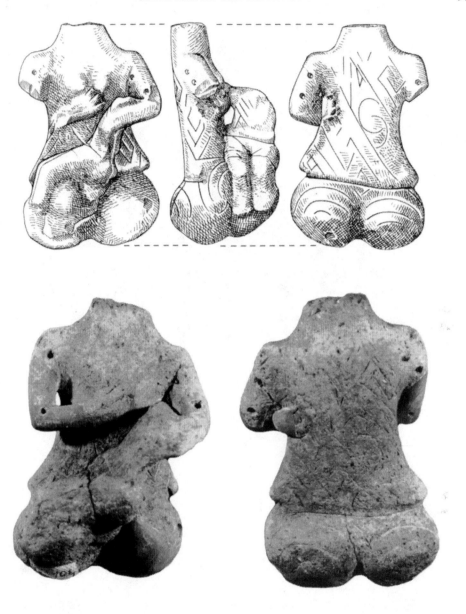

FIGURE 10.8 Figurine from Rast, Serbia (after Biehl 2003:Figure 37).

porated in the rituals involving adult clay figurines. As we can assume that children definitely had a role in Neolithic societies and were inevitably part of everyday life of a Neolithic village, it seems that it is the particular meaning and function of figurines in rituals that excludes them from being represented. Even if children played with figurines as toys occasionally (as they likely did with any other material culture in and outside the Neolithic house), as well as making clay "figurines" themselves, imitating adult figurine makers (though the poorly sculpted figurines with barely recognizable human features

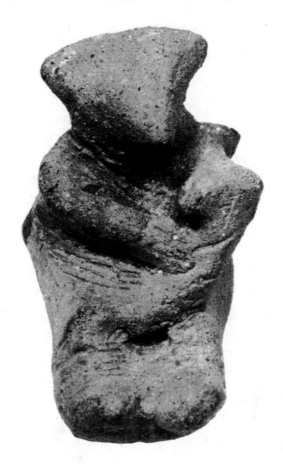

FIGURE 10.9 Figurine from Fafos, Serbia (after Biehl 2003:Figure 38).

could have also been made by unskilled adults), I have argued elsewhere that that they were not made as children's toys (Biehl 1999:175; see also Ucko 1968 and Hutson in this volume). It can be summarized that the represented children are normally held in the arms of a female figurine in a typically nurturing gesture, which most likely represents breastfeeding (Figures 10.5 and 10.6; 10.8–10.10). The figurines from Hacılar (Figures 10.2 and 10.7) are not only different in terms of their elaborate forms, but also in the bodily detail and the positioning of the child on the back or on the lap of the adult figurine, only covertly connected to the female breasts.

By examining specific variations in relation to the larger development of aesthetic and symbolic patterns it is possible to construct a model of representation of the visual body in the Neolithic, which includes all of the styles possible. The term *style* here includes all discernible attributes of a figurine including the representation of children, and the most common choices among them. The process of choosing these styles is culturally charged, and linked to ideas of the body. A person understands their own physical self only through psychical inscription, creating the notion of body (Meskell 2000:13). When

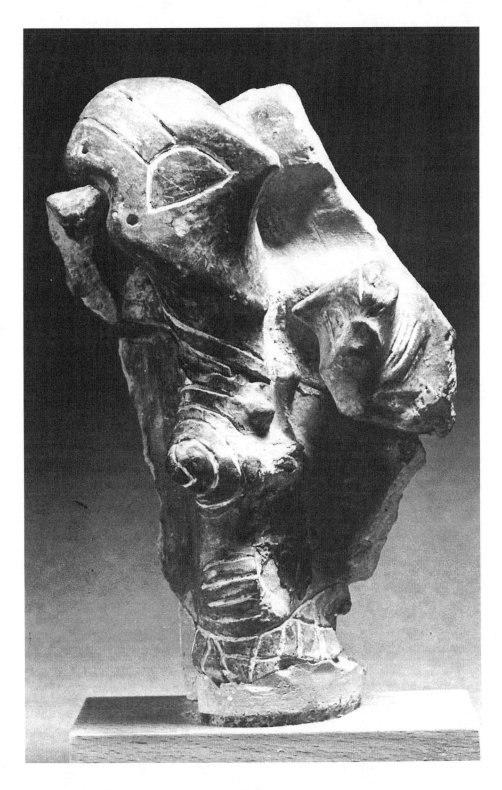

FIGURE 10.10 Plastic decoration of a large vase from Vinča, Serbia (after Biehl 2003:Figure 39).

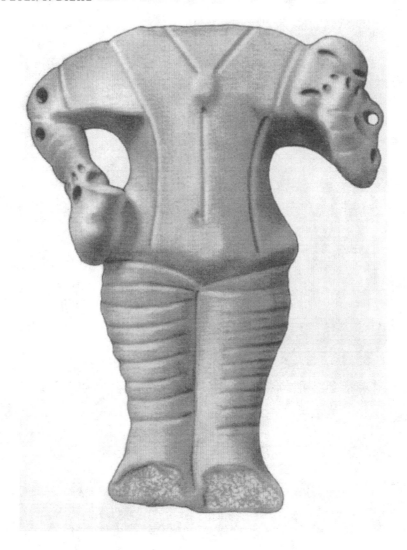

FIGURE 10.11 Figurine from Liubcova-Ornița, Romania (after Biehl 2003:Figure 74).

these inscriptions are present on a figurine, that same notion is called forth and fused with material, creating the medium through which a figurine represents ideas of self that are the basic connection between a people's understanding of their own bodies and of their understanding of the figurine as a body (Meskell 2000).

We are still left with many questions regarding what kinds of meanings these particular representations of the adult and child body hold, and why the people mixed different and often opposing concepts and ideas. But the visual body can be seen to be very significant in terms of the role it plays within these societies. And despite the difficulties in interpreting this role, we must continue to ask new questions of the material and analyze the representation of the body with a sound methodology.

CONCLUSION

In conclusion, I have argued that the Neolithic figurines are linked to central ideas people have about their own bodies, which are recreated on the figurines not as an explicit end product, but as a necessary step in the production of a figurine to be recognized as a body, and the foundation for the identity or function the figurine is meant to have. Suggesting the concept of a *body idea*, and the link between this idea and the creation of figurines with a particular suite of styles and the use of figurines in new rituals, indicates that a new concept of the body emerges resulting in the selection and preference for certain representations of the visual body over others. It seems also very likely that these new body ideas are associated with new ritual practices including dance and transformation and destruction, and therefore are *not* dealing with the idea and meaning of childhood. These Neolithic figurines are dominated by a particular body idea representing an emphasis on particular idealized qualities. This in turn leads to an even more interesting question: Who in society has the ability to manipulate this idea, and, consequently, possesses power over the perception and performance of the body? But this is the starting point of another paper.

REFERENCES CITED

Bailey, D. 2005 *Prehistoric Figurines: Representation and Corporeality in the Neolithic*. Routledge, London.

Bailey, D. 2007 The Anti-rhetorical Power of Representational Absence: Faceless Figurines in the Balkan Neolithic. In *Material Beginnings: a Global Prehistory of Figurative Representation*, edited by C. Renfrew and I. Morley, pp. 117–126. McDonald Institute Monographs, Cambridge.

Bailey, D. 2010 The Figurines of Old Europe. In *The Lost World of Old Europe. The Danube Valley, 5000–3500 BC*, edited by D. W. Anthony and J. Y. Chi, pp. 112–127. Princeton University Press, Princeton and Oxford.

Biehl, P. F. 1996 Symbolic Communication Systems: Symbols of Anthropomorphic Figurines of the Neolithic and Chalcolithic from Southeastern Southeastern Europe. *Journal of European Archaeology* 4:153–176.

Biehl, P. F. 1999 Analogy and Context—A Re-Construction of the Missing Link. In *Ethno-Analogy and the Reconstruction of Prehistoric Artefact Use and Production*, edited by L. R. Owen and M. Porr, pp. 171–184. Urgeschichliche Materialhefte, Tübingen.

Biehl, P. F. 2003 Studien zum Symbolgut des Neolithikums und der Kupferzeit in Südosteuropa. Habelt, Bonn.

Biehl, P. F. 2006 Figurines in Action: Methods and Theories in Figurine Research. In *Festschrift Peter Ucko: A Future for Archaeology—The Past as the Present*, edited by R. Layton, S. Shennan, and P. Stone, pp. 199–215. University College London Press, London.

Biehl, P. F. 2009 Representing the Human Body: Figurines of the Neolithic and Chalcolithic of Southeast Europe. In *Zeiten, Kulturen, Systeme. Gedenkschrift für Jan Lichardus*, edited by V. Becker, M. Thomas and A. Wolf-Schuler, pp. 103–110. Schriften des Zentrums für Archäologie und Kulturgeschichte des Schwarzmeerraumes Bd. 17. Langenweißbach, Beier and Beran.

Biehl, P. F., and A. Marciniak 2000 *The Construction of Hierarchy: Rethinking the Copper Age in Southeast Europe. In Hierarchies in Action: Cui Bono?*, edited by M. W. Diehl, pp. 181–209. Center for Archaeological Investigations, Occasional Paper No. 27. Southern Illinois University, Carbondale.

Biehl, P. F., and E. Rosenstock 2009 West Mound. Çatalhöyük 2009 Archive Report. Electronic document, http://www.catalhoyuk.com/downloads/Archive_Report_2009.pdf; accessed 8 July 2013.

Borić, D. 2007 Images of Animality: Hybrid Bodies and Mimesis in Early Prehistoric Art. In *Image and Imagination. A Global Prehistory of Figurative Representation*, edited by C. Renfrew and I. Morley, pp. 83–100. McDonald Institute Monographs, Cambridge.

Borić, D., and J. Robb 2008 Body Theory in Archaeology. In *Past Bodies. Body-Centered Research in Archaeology* edited by D. Boric and J. Robb, pp. 1–7. Oxbow Books, Oxford.

Fowler, C. 2001 Personhood and Social Relations in the British Neolithic with a Study from the Isle of Man. *Journal of Material Culture* 6(2):137–163.

Fowler, C. 2004 *The Archaeology of Personhood: An Anthropological Approach*. Routledge, London.

Garfinkel, Y. 2003 *Dancing at the Dawn of Agriculture*. University of Texas Press, Austin.

Gimbutas, M. 1974 *The Goddesses and Gods of Old Europe. 6500–3500 BC. Myths and Cult Images*. Thames and Hudson, London.

Green, M. J. 1998 Some Gallo-British Goddesses: Iconography and Meaning. In *Ancient Goddesses: Myths and the Evidence*, edited by L. Goodison and C. Morris, pp. 180–195. University of Wisconsin Press, Madison.

Hamilakis, Y., M. Pluciennik, and S. Tarlow 2002 Introduction. Thinking Through the Body. In *Thinking Through the Body: Archaeologies of Corporeality*, edited by Y. Hamilakis, M. Pluciennik, and S. Tarlow, pp. 1–21. Kluwer, New York.

Hansen, S. 2007 Bilder vom Menschen der Steinzeit. Untersuchungen zur anthropomorphen Plastik der Jungsteinzeit und Kupferzeit in Südosteuropa. *Archäologie in Eurasien* 20. DAI, Mainz.

Huth, C. 2003 *Menschenbilder und Menschenbild: anthropomorphe Bildwerke der frühen Eisenzeit*. Reimer, Berlin.

Jones, A. 2005 Lives in Fragments?: Personhood and the European Neolithic. *Journal of Social Archaeology* 5(2): 193–224.

Joyce, R. A. 2007 Figurines, Meaning, and Meaning-making in Early Mesoamerica. In *Image and Imagination: A Global Prehistory of Figurative Representation*, edited by C. Renfrew and I. Morley, pp. 101–110. McDonald Institute Monographs, Cambridge.

Joyce, R. A. 2008 *Ancient Bodies, Ancient Lives. Sex, Gender, and Archaeology*. Thames and Hudson, London.

Lesure, R. G. 2002 The Goddess Diffracted: Thinking About the Figurines of Early Villages. *Current Anthropology* 43(4):587–610.

Lesure, R. G. 2011 *Interpreting Ancient Figurines. Context, Comparison, and Prehistoric Art*. Cambridge University Press, Cambridge.

Fol, A., and J. Lichardus (editors) 1988 *Macht, Herrschaft, Gold. Das Gräberfeld von Varna (Bulgarien) und die Anfänge einer neuen europäischen Zivilisation*. Saarbrücken.

Lichardus, J., A. Fol, L. Getov, F. Bertemes, R. Echt, R. Katincarov, and I.K. Iliev 1996. Bericht über die bulgarisch-deutschen Ausgrabungen in Drama (1989–1995). *Bericht der Römisch-Germanischen Kommission* 77:5–154.

Mellaart, J. 1970 *Excavations at Hacılar*. British Institute of Archaeology at Ankara Occasional Publications 9–10. Edinburgh University Press, Edinburgh.

Meskell, L. 2000 Writing the Body in Archaeology. In *Reading the Body: Representations and Remains in the Archaeological Record*, edited by A. E. Rautman, pp. 13–24. University of Pennsylvania Press, Philadelphia.

Meskell, L. 2007 Refiguring the Corpus at Çatalhöyük. In *Image and Imagination. A Global Prehistory of Figurative Representation*, edited by C. Renfrew and I. Morley, pp. 137–149. McDonald Institute Monographs, Cambridge.

Meskell, L., and C. Nakamura 2009 Articulate Bodies: Forms and Figures at Çatalhöyük. *Journal of Archaeological Method and Theory* 16:205–230.

Robb, J. 2007 *The Early Mediterranean Village: Agency, Material Culture, and Social Change in Neolithic Italy*. Cambridge University Press, Cambridge.

Robb, J. 2009 People of Stone: Stelae, Personhood, and Society in Prehistoric Europe. *Journal of Archaeological Method and Theory* 16:162–183.

Voigt, M. M. 2007 The Splendour of Women: Late Neolithic Images from Central Anatolia. In *Image and Imagination. A Global Prehistory of Figurative Representation*, edited by C. Renfrew and I. Morely, pp. 151–170. McDonald Institute Monographs, Cambridge.

Voyatzis, M. E. 1998 From Athena to Zeus: An A-Z Guide to the Origins of Greek Goddesses. In *Ancient Goddesses: Myths and the Evidence*, edited by L. Goodison and C. Morris, pp. 133–147. University of Wisconsin Press, Madison.

CHAPTER ELEVEN

From Playthings to Sacred Objects?

Household Enculturation Rituals, Figurines, and Plastering Activities at Neolithic Çatalhöyük, Turkey

Sharon K. Moses

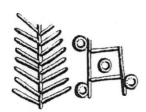

Abstract   *This article examines possible connections between mundane figurine fragments, children's activities in the home, and object transitions from mundane to sacred through a venue of household rituals at Neolithic Çatalhöyük. Previous investigation of household activities at Çatalhöyük, particularly of wall and platform plastering practices, has been the realm of micromorphological and architectural study such as material analyses, technology, frequency, and layering patterns. This article is a departure from that approach and looks instead through the lens of non-Western, oral tradition models toward socialization and identity formation activities within the home. I argue that children would have been involved in household plastering and whitewashing tasks and that some tasks appear to mimic existing household rituals, likely as a means to teach traditional knowledge of the supernatural world. This interpretation may shed some insight into the presence of select figurines and figurine fragments included in some layers of plaster, such as bull figurine horns. I argue that pervasive ritualistic use of horn or bull symbolism in the houses, seen and unseen, carried over into children's material culture. I have applied the model of an oral tradition approach to teaching children traditional symbolism, sacred narratives, and differentiated spaces within the house. Household activities and transformation of mundane objects (figurines) as toys into objects of ritual significance are consistent with the fluidity of children's material culture in such a society.*

A BRIEF BACKGROUND ON ÇATALHÖYÜK AND
INTERNAL HOUSE-RELATED INTERPRETATIONS

Çatalhöyük is situated on the Konya Plain of south central Anatolia. To place it in context with other Neolithic sites to which it is often compared, the earliest levels on its East Mound where the Neolithic settlement is located, coincide with the late PPNB and Final PPNB/PPNC of the Levant; the majority of Çatalhöyük's levels fall within the Pottery Neolithic phase, giving the settlement a date span of 7400 to 6400 cal B.C., or 1,200 years of Neolithic period habitation (Cessford 2007:59–101; Hodder and Cessford 2004:19).

Initial excavations at Çatalhöyük were conducted in the early 1960s by James Mellaart. Houses were constructed in basic Neolithic design found throughout the Near East and Southwestern Asia, that is to say, sun–dried mud brick construction, double width walls and a rectilinear design. Although Çatalhöyük's buildings varied somewhat in size, they were very similar externally in that none to date have been found significantly differentiated from the others. This contributes to the common belief that governance during the Neolithic was still primarily egalitarian despite the size of some settlements such as Çatalhöyük, which was estimated to have had a population of 3,500 to 8,000 at its peak (Hodder and Cessford 2004:21).

James Mellaart, Çatalhöyük's initial excavator, discovered wall paintings (human figures, aurochs, deer, and vultures to name a few), unusual architectural features such as faunal installations in the house (bucrania, vulture beaks, boar mandibles, etc. encased or decorated with plaster and protruding from walls), intramural burials beneath sleeping platforms and floors, and exaggerated female figurines, leading him to believe that Çatalhöyük was a "goddess" cult society. He also surmised that most buildings he excavated were shrines (Mellaart 1967:77–130, 1998:35–41). However, recent excavations and new technologies have changed our understanding of the site and suggest that neither men nor women were privileged and that buildings were not shrines but houses (Asouti 2005:75–29; Hodder 2005:34–41; 2006:208–214).

There is no doubt that Çatalhöyük was a settlement steeped in ritual and symbolism; the Neolithic in general was a time of ritual and symbolic florescence (Verhoeven 2002a, 2002b, 2002c). A discovery in 2004 of a partially plastered skull in an adult female burial suggests a link of some kind to the Levant, where skull plastering in a so-called Skull Cult and ancestor worship thrived for a time. Ritual traditions expressed in burials, material culture, symbolism, and architecture at Çatalhöyük indicate that certain practices endured for hundreds of years. For the purposes of this article, however, I will focus primarily on the frequent replastering and meticulous housekeeping and its impact on the lives of children in the home. Furthermore, it has been previously pointed out that the wall "art" of Çatalhöyük likely functioned as mnemonic devices with spatial significance, and I will not discuss these at length again here (Hodder 2006:119; Hodder and Cessford 2004:17–40; Last 1996:355–378, 2005: 197–208).

In addition to imagery and objects painted or installed as features inside the house, there were also purposely hidden objects incorporated into walls, platforms, and floors, and sometimes deposited at the base of support post holes. Examples of hidden objects include a red painted cone found inserted into a wall and plastered over (Cessford 2007:424–425), and faunal objects such as cattle scapula and horn cores also incorporated into walls or posts, behind mud bricks, and/or plastered over (Russell and Martin 2005:61). Knowledge of them was likely limited to those who constructed the house and the inhabitants. Like burials, these objects suggest magico-religious rituals intended to protect or otherwise benefit the house and family.

Ritually hidden objects can be found in ancient Mesopotamian cultures millennia later. Embedded cones hidden in walls and known only to a few were dedicatory votives—often with the name or seal of individuals who contributed to the building effort or who were recognized as the head of house (Zehren 2006:38). The purpose of these votives was to act as perpetual prayers, bringing good fortune to the house and its inhabitants. While I do not draw direct correlations in meaning between cultures separated temporally and historically, I do believe that the nature of hidden objects as communicative devices in a supernatural sense is not only plausible but likely.

MICROMORPHOLOGY

Micromorphological analyses of the plaster sequences have demonstrated that the inhabitants meticulously cleaned and replastered walls, floors, and platforms regularly over the life span of their houses (Matthews 2005; Matthews et al. 1996). A house inhabited for roughly 70 years could have "up to 700 'washes' and replasterings" applied to its walls (Hodder 2006:09; Hodder and Cessford 2004:22). This is approximately ten whitewash/plastering events per year. In addition, evidence suggests annual treatment and resurfacing on house foundations as well.

Besides plastering and whitewashing, floors were routinely swept and cleaned, so much so that at Çatalhöyük *in situ* floor debris as a means of understanding occupants' degree of daily behaviors and resource use is often limited. Burials can be found beneath platforms along every wall in a house, but the north area and its platform have been called the "clean" area because it is often the least trafficked and also its most meticulously kept (Hodder and Cessford 2004:17–40).

Figurine fragments have been noted in some of the plastered layers of walls, platforms, and other internal features. At first glance, such an observation is often dismissed because figurine bits, obsidian pieces, and faunal chips have also been found in the makeup of construction materials such as mud bricks and fill dirt. The assumption has been that these were inadvertent inclusions; the result of acquiring construction materials from various convenient places around the settlement, including courtyards where refuse and rake out were deposited. For this reason, these observations have not been routinely or systematically documented; at best, they were mentioned intermittently in Mellaart's preliminary reports from the 1960s and again by archaeologists involved in current excavations when these fragments have been obvious enough to attract attention in an otherwise meticulously plastered layer (Hamilton 2005:188; Schiffer 1987).

Mellaart concluded that figurine fragments in plastered surfaces were purposeful rather than inadvertent and represented votive deposits; Naomi Hamilton also stated in her 2005 Çatalhöyük figurine reports that she agreed with Mellaart's evaluation that they were purposeful inclusions but did not elaborate on ritual or social implications (Hamilton 2005:188).

"SCATTERS" AS RITUAL DEPOSITS

Published accounts of ritual scatters tend to be spotty and discussion aimed at deposition, material makeup (bone, ceramics, lithic debitage, etc.), and contextual information. More often than not, scatters are perceived as random discard behavior or natural site formation deposits due to scavengers or environmental events unrelated to ritual. When scatters are correlated to ritual events, they often take the form of ritual feasting debris rather than the material itself as a ritual device. In this article, I am specifically addressing scatters of broken figurine pieces found in household plastering as intentional dedicatory deposits with likelihood of child involvement.

Broken objects as ritual offerings can represent material expressions of thanks, remembrance, apotropaic strategies, or communicative devices in honor of deities, ancestors, spirits, or the deceased (Bell 1992; Metcalf and Huntington 1991). Objects may be purposely broken and used in ritual to remove them from circulation after they have fulfilled their use, as in "wish vehicles," to mark a death and other transitions, or to commemorate some other historic or special event (Cook 1987:49–90; Hamilton 2005:188–189). They may even be viewed as throwaway objects as pointed out by some figurine studies at Çatalhöyük, where a number of figurines were seemingly discarded while the clay was still wet, leading some to believe they were mundane objects with no particular ritual significance (Meskell et al. 2008:139–161).

Ethnographic examples, however, have demonstrated that purposely broken and smashed objects have been associated with termination rituals of structures or to mark the end of their use life upon the death of an individual or as markers in rite of passage ceremonies (McAnany 2000). Broken figurines may also represent healing and curing ceremonies among indigenous communities, when shamans or household members broke small figurines to release healing magic (Rainey 1947).

Although objects may start out as mundane or sacred, in indigenous societies objects are often multivocal and can be transformed. Fragmented, worn-out, or otherwise discarded objects with little or no functional use life left may be collected from previously nonsacred contexts and reenter the world transformed as sacred objects through ritual (Brown 2000:319–333; Walker 1995).

Ritual scatters composed of smashed ceramics, human or animal bones, other organic materials, or articles that human beings have used in the mundane context of daily life may become spiritual objects when used to delineate sacred spaces, floors, altars, or in some way demarcate sacred from mundane spaces. One example is the ancient Maya ritual use of *jute,* a freshwater gastropod that was used for both sacred and secular purposes: as food and as an offering for the dead (Halperin et al. 2003).

A cursory observation of the jute scatters in archaeological sites in Belize was once dismissed as evidence of natural deposits, until it was determined that jute do not naturally inhabit cave floors; secondly, jute has been associated with indigenous sacred landscapes important to the Maya in ancient and contemporary contexts. Ethnographic sources indicate folk beliefs that jute has been a sacred food since ancient times and that the water it is cooked in also becomes sacred; men and women may eat jute in a secular context, but when men take the jute into caves, the shells are transformed into sacred material for ritual use. Some Maya burials have produced remnants of jute shells and other faunal remains, indicating that jute was among the sacred foods given to the dead (Halperin et al. 2003:214).

Besides their association with sacred landscapes, shells in contemporary Maya folk beliefs are symbolic of rain, and are appealing to the rain god. Jute has been associated with fertility in Maya religion because the shape of the shell is phallic-like (Halperin et al. 2003:214).

Understanding the social and sacred context of jute shells suggests that shell material found scattered across ancient Maya ritual caves and on ball courts in the lowlands of Belize are evidence for ritual deposits rather than natural or inadvertent (Halperin 2001).

At the Classic Period Maya village of Joya de Cerén, previously discarded items were found in ritual assemblages in Structure 12 (Brown 2000:319–333). Based upon contemporary ethnographic accounts, small discarded secular objects collected for reuse in rituals transforms them into divination tools. They also serve as "verification" of divine intervention, as people believe finding these objects was made possible by supernatural entities placing them in your path.

Mobile object assemblages in Structure 12 were "*heavily used, broken, or battered items, some well beyond the point of being able to serve any utilitarian function at all*" (Brown 2000:322). Objects such as broken figurines, shell fragments, unmodified crystals, and pot sherds had been stored together inside a niche in a bench. Rounded edges had been found on the broken edges of the objects and suggested that they had either been handled a great deal after they were broken, or that they had been much trampled upon before they were collected. The hypothesis that these were somehow keepsakes or family heirlooms has also been ruled out because of the condition of the pieces. Cherished heirlooms, even when broken, do not normally undergo trampling, abrasion, or further damage, but are put away after they may have been accidentally damaged. Ritual collecting among the contemporary Yucatec, according to Brown (2000:325) is "well documented."

TRADITION, CHILDREN, AND HOUSEHOLD ACTIVITIES

Traditions and rituals in preliterate society are usually learned through observation, mimicry, and participation, and nowhere is this more concentrated in the life of a child than in the home (Child and Child 1992). Children commonly fulfill household labor needs and participate in household-level craft production as well (Baxter 2005:48–49, 50–56, 63–67; Kamp 2002:71–89; Scott 1999).

Children as young as four years old in many Native North American cultures are given the responsibility to assist in household tasks as soon as they are physically or mentally capable. They are entrusted with handling sharp objects, aid with cooking and have to deal with working around fire and boiling liquids, help in daily chores such as cleaning and care of siblings, freeing adults for more demanding or skill-intensive duties (Crown 2002:108–124; Scott 1999; Stearns 2006:13).

In addition, children are often more involved with extended family members, namely, grandparents and elders who are viewed as valuable resources of traditional knowledge and are central in disseminating that knowledge to youth. Very young children and the elderly are often paired together as the two groups are more likely to stay in or closer to the home while parents or older siblings spend time away in planting, harvesting, herding, hunting, and other tasks that require them to be away from the house. Children in an egalitarian, agricultural and herding community the size of Çatalhöyük would have contributed significantly to household labor and participated in all manner of household activities in order for the community at large to have been able to function effectively.

Furthermore, the house would have afforded opportunities to teach children techniques and skills, but also to learn sacred narratives, symbolism, and rituals. Identity formation in indigenous communities is interwoven with learning cosmological knowledge. These concepts are embedded in natural and built environments and the house is a primary confluence of spiritual and secular energies. Learning certain narratives within the context of the home is, therefore, expected. The importance of these principles in identity formation among indigenous and oral tradition peoples cannot be overstated.

Learning and doing are typically accompanied by storytelling when elders are present. Important myths are incorporated in the process of physical participation when teaching the very young, so that mental imagery and physical efforts are paired. Voice inflection, rhythm and eye-hand motor skills (beading, ceramics, sewing, etc.) become a holistic effort. The teaching process can be characterized as a physical application mapped by oral cues and mental imagery, guiding the learner through the stages—a performance.

Most figurines at Çatalhöyük are either partially baked (exposed to heat from an oven or fire) or sun-dried. And while figurines themselves are rarely found in the home at the time of its termination and, to date, never in its burials, it stands to reason at least a percentage of them were crafted in homes. Once again, the degree of skills evident in some of the figurines suggests an adult hand, while others suggest the less adept abilities of children. Crafts of this nature lend themselves to the traditional style of teaching and storytelling. The uniformity of construction in many prehistoric figurines has been noted by Denise Schmandt-Besserat (1997:48–58), who has discerned a uniformity in the step-by-step procedure of figurine construction; many figurines bear the same resemblances to one another, though separated by generations or hundreds of years. This too, is a hallmark of the "storytelling" method of teaching in traditional settings. As each part of an object is crafted together, a story is told about its first creation by an ancestor, or perhaps as part of a mythological story. In any event, an individual growing up learns the "proper" order and manner of creating these objects and, as part of ritual and household life, passes this on to the next generation.

Most traditional communities engage in habituated ritual activities as a strategy for the purpose of maintaining *order* and *harmony* in both sacred and secular worlds. These worlds intersect in the house. Everyone, including children, plays a role in maintaining that order (Brown 1991:69–82; Child and Child 1992; O'Bryan 1956; Opler 1946; Yue and Yue 1986). Çatalhöyük's consistent plastering practices and figurine constructions are hallmarks of habituated activities in a traditional society.

Children learn that spirits, ancestors, and other mythical or supernatural entities must be respected and will be content and cooperative as long as religio-cultural rules are observed; these inspire conformity, a sense of responsibility, and begin the process of cultural bonding between the child and household but also the wider community of which they are a member.

Children are taught the meaning of rituals and how they must be done by giving the child an appropriate role in order to participate (Markstrom 2008:46–122). Healing ceremonies conducted in the home, for instance, are designed to restore mental or physical order that has been lost (Bunzel 1992; Child and Child 1992; Epes and Cousins 2001; Parsons 1996; Schaafsma 2000; Turner 1969; Van Gennep 1960). Healers attempt to identify the source of imbalance in a sick person's life by first looking in the home. Thus, it can be said, children learn very early that the home is a micro universe to the larger world and that they must care for it as one would care for a family member. They come to understand that their well-being and that of the entire community is interdependent.

Conclusion

Differentiated spaces within the houses based upon floor demarcations (ridges, partitions, and curbs), wall paintings, faunal installations, and other architectural features suggest imbued meanings to the inhabitants at Çatalhöyük. Household behaviors were likely structured and framed in tradition and repetitious acts, in some ways becoming unconscious performances that could be characterized by the concept of *habitus* (Bourdieu 1977). Current discussions about household rituals in the scholarship of Çatalhöyük do not specifically address children's roles in these ritualized and habitualized behaviors (Asouti 2005; Hodder 2006; Hodder and Cessford 2004; Last 1996, 2005).

I argue that socialization and traditional teaching would have been strongest at the household level for egalitarian and preliterate communities; children would have been the focus of these efforts. Çatalhöyük's intramural burials suggest a strong connection to the past, to kinship or lineage, and that the house itself was a collection of traditional knowledge and memories (Baxter 2005; Child and Child 1993; Hodder 2006; Hodder and Cessford 2004; Keith 2005). I propose that children were living symbols of ancestral continuity and that their participation in the ritual life of the house would have been seen as a necessity.

I propose that figurine fragments in plastered surfaces were not inadvertent. Unlike fill material, mortar, and mud brick constructions taken from available resource areas around the settlement and then remolded, these fragments were left visibly obvious on platform, wall, and floor surfaces in the plastering process in an otherwise meticulously cleaned house. They would not have been overlooked. Inhabitants were obsessively conscientious about removing debris from their houses, and the inclusion of figurine pieces at literally the last stage of completing this responsibility would have been untenable.

The fragments themselves indicate purposeful selection; the majority of them appear to be miniature horns from cattle figurines. When one considers these fragments within the context of bull symbolism in wall paintings, plastered bucrania installations, or the hidden inclusion of cattle scapula or horn cores purposely placed inside walls, this would seem to indicate a ritual correlation that is hard to ignore.

It is impossible to determine definitively the meaning of miniature figurine horns on plastered platforms, walls, and other surfaces in the house. However, I would offer the possibility that *mimicry* of adult ritual symbolism is present. Children learning sacred significances of the bull may have been encouraged to gather "horns" from figurines as safe symbolic scatter deposits in the plaster. In this way the significance of the bull and its parts, visible and hidden on the walls, would have been reinforced at the level of children's participation in a habituated ritual household event. Such a possibility would be consistent with ethnographic examples of mimicry as a learning tool among traditional peoples.

In general, figurines are not found within Çatalhöyük's houses except on rare occasions as purposeful deposits. The general absence of figurines within houses and, most pointedly, their complete absence from intramural children's burials suggests a social construct that generally prohibited them from indoor spaces in a secular way (Meskell et al. 2008; Meskell and Nakamura 2005:161–188; 2006:226–240). For this reason, Çatalhöyük's figurines as "toys" have been contested. The argument against them as toys or as part of children's material culture per se, is largely predicated on the belief that one should expect to find "toys" in homes or that they should be among children's grave goods; because they are not, *ergo* their purpose must not be related to children. This is inherently a Western notion.

In many indigenous cultures, children's toys may have restrictions placed upon them because they are often perceived as simultaneously playthings as well as objects of *agency* with spiritual lives of their own, capable of doing harm under certain conditions. For example, Eskimos and other Bering Strait peoples' traditions prohibited children from bringing their dolls inside the house at night or to sleep with because it was believed that dolls had the ability to become animate at night. In southwestern regions of Alaska, dolls were considered a seasonal plaything (summer specific—perhaps based in part upon availability of materials) and were relegated to the outdoors. The belief was that, as a seasonal object, a doll brought inside the house or kept during the winter would bring bad luck upon the entire village (Fair 1982). As a seasonal being, created with materials attainable only in summer, a doll entity might not want to be "kept" in an environment that was not "natural" for it and retaliate.

One certainly would not expect to place an object imbued with a spirit or agency in a grave. Objects such as these enjoy both sacred and secular designations simultaneously, and depend largely upon context to derive meaning, as opposed to a Western notion that a child's "toy" is nothing more.

Ideas about dolls and children's association with them are contextually defined. If a figurine in prehistory was also thought capable of animation, for instance, or embodied concepts of seasonality, which precluded appropriateness indoors, one would neither expect to find them in houses nor in children's burials, except perhaps, in rare exceptions as household ritual deposits, as has been seen at Çatalhöyük.

The debate over whether figurines were "wish vehicles," teaching aids, children's toys, or cult objects is unlikely to be settled in the near future. I argue that by placing figurines in one category or another and making them mutually exclusive, we preclude the multivocal meanings with which figurines and related creations are often imbued in traditional societies.

Ethnographic and historic accounts of children's behavior demonstrate that children usually fashion playthings out of readily available materials, which are often expendable after short periods of use, and that these playthings fulfill an important role in the socialization process on several levels (Baxter 2005:41–50; Daiken 1965:13–20; Lee 1999; Sutton-Smith 1986:26–27). The reconfiguration of plaything to sacred object is not an alien concept in many indigenous cultures, because sacred and secular often overlap or are indistinguishable from one another in daily life.

REFERENCES CITED

Andrews, P., T. Molleson, and B. Boz 2005 The Human Burials at Çatalhöyük. In *Inhabiting Çatalhöyük, Reports from the 1995–99 Seasons*, edited by I. Hodder, pp. 261–278. Çatalhöyük Research Project, Vol. 4, McDonald Institute for Archaeological Research, Cambridge.

Asouti, E. 2005 Group Identity and the Politics of Dwelling at Neolithic Çatalhöyük. In *Çatalhöyük Perspectives: Reports from the 1995–99 Seasons*, edited by I. Hodder, pp. 75–92. Çatalhöyük Research Project, Vol. 6, McDonald Institute for Archaeological Research, Cambridge.

Baxter, J. E. 2005 *The Archaeology of Childhood*. Altamira Press, Walnut Creek, California.

Bell, C. 1992 *Ritual Theory, Ritual Practice*. Oxford University Press, Oxford.

Bourdieu, P. 1977 *Outline of a Theory of Practice*. Cambridge University Press, Cambridge.

Brown, J. E. 1991 *The Spiritual Legacy of the American Indian*. Crossroad Publishing, New York.

Brown, J. E., and E. Cousins 2001 *Teaching Spirits: Understanding Native American Religious Traditions*. Oxford University Press, Oxford and New York.

Brown, L. 2000 From Discard to Divination: Demarcating the Sacred through the Collection and Curation of Discarded Objects. *Latin American Antiquity* 11(4):319–333.

Bunzel, R. L. 1992 *Zuni Ceremonialism*. University of New Mexico Press, Albuquerque.

Cessford, C. 2007 Level Pre-XII.E-A and Levels XII and XI, Spaces 181, 199 and 198. In *Excavating Çatalhöyük: South, North, and KOPAL Area Reports from the 1995–99 Seasons*, edited by I. Hodder, pp. 59–101. Çatalhöyük Research Project, Vol. 3, McDonald Institute for Archaeological Research, Cambridge.

Child, A. B., and I. L. Child 1993 *Religion and Magic in the Life of Traditional Peoples*. Prentice-Hall, Englewood Cliffs, New Jersey.

Cook, A. 1987 The Middle Horizon Ceramic Offering from Conchopata. *Ñawpa Pacha* 22–23(1984–1985):49–90.

Crown, P. L. 2002 Learning and Teaching in the Prehispanic American Southwest. In *Children in the Prehistoric Puebloan Southwest*, edited by K. A. Kamp, pp. 108–124, University of Utah Press, Salt Lake City.

Daiken, L. 1965 *Children's Toys through Ages*. Spring Books, London.

Deal, M. 1985 Household Pottery Disposal in the Maya Highlands: An Ethnoarchaeological Interpretation. *Journal of Anthropological Archaeology* 4:243–291.

Fair, S. 1982 *Eskimo dolls*. Exhibit catalog, edited by S. Jones. Alaska State Council on the Arts, Anchorage.

Goldberg, M. Y. 1999 Spatial and Behavioral Negotiation in Classical Athenian City Houses. In *The Archaeology of Household Activities*, edited by P. M. Allison, pp. 142–161. Routledge, New York.

Hamilton, N. 2005 The Figurines. In *Changing Materialities at Çatalhöyük: Reports from the 1995–99 Seasons*, edited by I. Hodder, pp. 187–214. Çatalhöyük Research Project Vol. 5, McDonald Institute for Archaeological Research, Cambridge.

Halperin, C. T. 2001 *Ritual Cave Use by the Ancient Maya: An Investigation of Jolja' Cave in Chiapas, Mexico*. Research Report to the National Speleological Society, Huntsville.

Halperin, C. T, S. Garza, K. M. Prufer, and J. E. Brady 2003 Caves and Ancient Maya Ritual Use of Jute. *Latin American Antiquity* 14(2):207–219.

Hendon, J. 1999 Having and Holding: Storage, Memory, Knowledge, and Social Relations. *American Anthropologist* 102(1):42–53.

Hodder, I. 2005 Women and Men at Çatalhöyük. *Scientific American* 15(1):34–41.

Hodder, I. 2006 *The Leopard's Tale: Revealing the Mysteries of Çatalhöyük*. Thames and Hudson, London.

Hodder, I., and C. Cessford 2004 Daily Practice and Social Memory at Çatalhöyük. *American Antiquity* 1(69):17–40.

Kamp, K. A. 2002 Working for a Living: Childhood in the Prehistoric Southwestern Pueblos. In *Children in the Prehistoric Puebloan Southwest*, edited by K. A. Kamp, pp. 71–89. University of Utah Press, Salt Lake City.

Keith, K. 2005 Childhood Learning and the Distribution of Knowledge in Foraging Societies. In *Children in Action: Perspectives on the Archaeology of Childhood*, edited by J. E. Baxter. Archaeological Papers of the American Anthropological Association 15.

Last, J. 1996 A design for life: Interpreting the art of Çatalhöyük. *Journal of Material Culture* 3(3):355–378.

Last, J. 2005 Art. In *Çatalhöyük Perspectives: Reports from the 1995–99 Seasons*, edited by Ian Hodder, pp. 197–208. Çatalhöyük Research Project, Vol. 6. McDonald Institute for Archaeological Research, Cambridge.

Lawrence, S. 1999 Towards a Feminist Archaeology of Households: Gender and Household Structure on the Australian Goldfields. In *The Archaeology of Household Activities*, edited by P. M. Allison, pp. 121–141. Routledge, New York.

Lee, M. C. (editor) 1999 *Not Just a Pretty Face: Dolls and Human Figurines in Alaska Native Cultures*. University of Alaska Museum, Fairbanks.

Markstrom, C. A. 2008 *Empowerment of North American Indian Girls: Ritual Expressions at Puberty*. University of Nebraska Press, Lincoln.

Matthews, W. 2005 Micromorphological and Microstratigraphic Traces of Uses and Concepts of Space. In *Inhabiting Çatalhöyük, Reports from the 1995–99 Seasons*, edited by I. Hodder, pp. 335–398. Çatalhöyük Research Project, Vol. 4, McDonald Institute for Archaeological Research, Cambridge.

Matthews, W., C. French, T. Lawrence, and D. Cutler 1996 Multiple Surfaces: The Micromorphology. In *On the Surface: Çatalhöyük 1993–95*, edited by I. Hodder, pp. 301–342. McDonald Institute Monographs. Oxbow Books, Oxford.

McAnany, P. A. 2000 *Living with the Ancestors: Kinship and Kingship in Ancient Maya Society.* University of Texas Press, Austin.

Mellaart, J. 1967 *Catal Höyük: A Neolithic Town in Anatolia.* Thames and Hudson, London.

Mellaart, J. 1998 Catal Höyük: The 1960s Seasons. In *Ancient Anatolia: Fifty Years' Work by The British Institute of Archaeology at Ankara*, edited by R. Matthews, pp. 35–41. British Institute of Archaeology at Ankara.

Metcalf, P., and R. Huntington 1991 *Celebrations of Death: The Anthropology of Mortuary Ritual.* 2nd edition. Cambridge University Press, New York.

Meskell, L., and C. Nakamura 2005 Figurines. In Çatalhöyük 2005 Archive Report, pp. 161–188. Electronic document, http://www.catalhoyuk.com/downloads/Archive_Report_2005.pdf; accessed July 13, 2013.

Meskell, L., and C. Nakamura 2006 Figurines. In Çatalhöyük 2006 Archive Report, pp. 226–240. Electronic document, http://www.catalhoyuk.com/downloads/Archive_Report_2006.pdf; accessed July 13, 2013.

Meskell, L., C. Nakamura, R. King, and S. Farid 2008 Figured Lifeworlds and Depositional Practices at Çatalhöyük. *Cambridge Archaeological Journal* 18(2):139–161.

Molleson, T., and P. Andrews 1996 Çatalhöyük 1996 Archive Report. Electronic document, http://www.catalhoyuk.com/archive_reports/1996/index.html; accessed July 13, 2013.

O'Bryan, A. 1956 *The Diné: Origin Myths of the Navaho Indians.* Smithsonian Institution Bureau of American Ethnology Bulletin 16. Smithsonian Institution, Washington, D.C.

Opler, M. E. 1946 *Childhood and Youth in Jicarilla Apache Society.* Southwest Museum, Los Angeles.

Parsons, E. C. 1996 *Pueblo Indian Religion.* University of Nebraska Press, Lincoln.

Pendergast, D. 1969 *The Prehistory of Actun Balam, British Honduras.* Art and Archaeology Occasional Papers 16. Royal Ontario Museum, Toronto.

Rainey, F. G. 1947 The Whale Hunters of Tigara. *Anthropological Papers of the AMNH* 41(2):231–283. New York.

Russell, N., and L. Martin 2005 Çatalhöyük Mammal Remains. In *Inhabiting Çatalhöyük, Reports from the 1995–99 Seasons*, edited by Ian Hodder, pp. 33–98. Çatalhöyük Research Project, Vol. 4. McDonald Institute for Archaeological Research, Cambridge.

Russell, N., and S. Meece 2005 Animal Representations and Animal Remains at Çatalhöyük. In *Çatalhöyük Perspectives: Reports from the 1995–99 Seasons*, edited by Ian Hodder, pp. 209–230. Çatalhöyük Research Project, Vol. 6. McDonald Institute for Archaeological Research, Cambridge.

Schaafsma, P. 2000 *Kachinas in the Pueblo World.* University of Utah Press, Salt Lake City.

Schiffer, M. 1987 *Formation Processes of the Archaeological Record.* University of Utah Press, Salt Lake City.

Schmandt-Besserat, D. 1997 Animal Symbols at 'Ain Ghazal. *Expedition* 39(1):48–58.

Scott, E. 1999 *Archaeology of Infancy and Infant Death.* British Archaeology Reports #819, Oxford.

Stearns, P. N. 2006 *Childhood in World History.* Routledge, New York.

Sutton-Smith, B. 1986 *Toys as Culture.* Gardner Press, New York.

Turner, V. 1969 *The Ritual Process.* Aldine, Chicago.

Van Gennep, A. 1960 *The Rites of Passage.* University of Chicago Press, Chicago.

Verhoeven, M. 2002a Transformations of Society: The Changing Role of Ritual and Symbolism in the PPNB and the PN in the Levant, Syria and South-east Anatolia. *Paleorient* 28(1):5–14.

Verhoeven, M. 2002b Ritual and Ideology in the Pre-Pottery Neolithic B of the Levant and Southeast Anatolia. *Cambridge Archaeological Journal* 12(2):233–258.

Verhoeven, M. 2002c Ritual and its Investigation in Prehistory. In *Magic Practices and Ritual in the Near Eastern Neolithic*, edited by H. Georg, K. Gebel, B. D. Hermansen, and C. H. Jensen, pp. 5–40. Studies in Early Near Eastern Production, Subsistence, and Environment, Vol. 8. Ex Oriente, Berlin.

Verhoeven, M. 2004 Beyond Boundaries: Nature, Culture and a Holistic Approach to Domestication in the Levant. *Journal of World Prehistory* 18(3):179–282.

Walker, W. H. 1995 Ceremonial Trash? In *Expanding Archaeology*, edited by J. M. Skibo, W. Walker, and A. Nielsen, pp. 67–79. University of Utah Press, Salt Lake City.

Yue, C., and D. Yue 1986 *The Pueblo*. Houghton Mifflin, Boston.

Zehren, E. 2006 [1962] *The Crescent and the Bull: A Survey of Archaeology In the Near East*. Translated by J. Cleugh. Kessinger, Whitefish, Montana.

Chapter Twelve

The Ends and Means of Childhood

Mourning Children in Early Greece

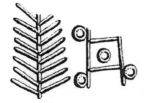

Susan Langdon

Abstract *The archaeology of childhood in early cultures has for obvious reasons been dominated by mortuary studies. Small bones and child-specific grave goods make their burials detectable and rich in potential social and political information. Rarely has the child's perspective been considered. As death was a common fact of life, children were themselves often among the mourners. Their involvement in funerary rituals would have been a necessary part of their socialization into the values, religious beliefs, and customs of family and community. While this childhood experience leaves few archaeological traces, two categories of material from Early Iron Age Athens provide evidence for children as mourners: a distinctive class of decorated ceramic grave markers, and the presence in graves of miniature vessels that can be connected with children. By investigating various modes of representation and seeing children as partners in the rituals of mourning, we can better understand a culture's social and political patterns.*

The archaeology of children and childhood in prehistoric and proto-literate cultures to date has been dominated by mortuary studies, and for obvious reasons. Small bones and child-specific grave goods make their burials readily detectable, and the information to be derived from the data is full of social and political potential. In many early cultures, moreover, graves are the only places where children are indisputably visible. Investigations of child burials are usually situated in the perspective of the family and community, and look for mortality data, signs of gender or status in the grave assemblage, or political meaning in the location of child burials relative to public cemeteries and habitation areas (Scott 1999). There is another dimension of childhood experience that has rarely been considered. Death and its commemoration were inescapable features of life in past societies, and children were themselves often among the mourners. Their involvement in funerary rituals would have been a necessary part of their socialization into the values, religious beliefs, and customs of their family and community. Participation in private and public rituals required learning properly gendered behavior and acceptable demonstrations of grief. A funeral offered an opportunity to explain and reinforce family histories and begin a process of memorializing the deceased, placing him or her into the ancestral lineage. The presence of children at a funeral was palpable assurance of generational continuity.

While the archaeological evidence of this childhood experience is ordinarily non-existent, two categories of material from Early Iron Age Athens, Greece, provide rich evidence for children as mourners: a distinctive class of decorated pottery that was used to mark graves and the presence in graves of miniature vessels that can be connected with children. If the material considered here is specific to Early Iron Age Athens (1000–700 B.C.), the issues involved in investigating early Greek children extend to other archaeological cultures with few or no written texts, sparse or poorly preserved material remains, archaeological evidence skewed to the ritual contexts of sanctuaries and cemeteries, and underexplored settlements. In a time of high birth rate and lower life expectancy, we can assume both a generally younger population and a higher value accorded to children (Baxter 2005; Lucy 2005). The experience of childhood as a time of dependency and free play would likely have been brief, with the gendering process beginning early. These assumptions urge us to consider the dominant cultural discourse through the lens of child agency and reception. Making children more visible also requires avoiding an essentializing view of childhood; a child's life experience, like that of any adult, was shaped in important ways by his or her class, gender, and ethnicity. The most archaeologically visible children will undoubtedly be those who were accorded more material investment because of their family's prominent status (Morris 1987). While it is always more difficult to access the representations and realities of nonelite children, some cultural norms were no doubt shared at all social levels. The experiences of children in mourning the loss of family members and friends will have been differently affected by class status. The iconographic tradition on elite grave markers, newly instituted around 760 B.C., includes children in funerary gatherings. This underexplored visual resource of approximately 60 known monuments illustrates the importance of children in family identity as well as perceptions of children's behavior. While these images reflect adult perspectives and intentions, we can approach a child's experience of loss through offerings in child graves that might have been left by siblings or young friends of the deceased.

CHILDREN AS MOURNERS

After several nearly picture-less centuries, the figural arts were revived in Athens around 760 B.C. for elite funerals and grave markers, adding a permanent visual record to the most crucial of social crises: the deaths of prominent community members, whose demise not only kindled family grief but could stir rivalries and power shifts. The creation of figured funerary vases used as markers of adult burials addressed both aspects of loss through a formulaic scene: the *prothesis,* or lying in state of the deceased man or woman surrounded by mourners (Figure 12.1). The vessel forms used above ground continued a long-traditional gender symbolism of kraters for men and belly-handled amphorae for women. It is important to note that most graves of the period throughout Greece have left no visible marking system. Some had stones, others might have had wooden stakes or planks, but none is preserved. Only a select few for a couple of decades in Athens carried a monumental krater or towering amphora. On men's kraters, which could exceed 1.5 meters in height, the mourning scenes may be accompanied by a heroic land or ship battle, a muster of chariot-borne warriors, or the *ekphora,* the ritual transport of the corpse by mourners to the cemetery. Except for one amphora with an *ekphora,* women's vases carry only the *prothesis.* Figures tend to be clearly gendered in appearance and

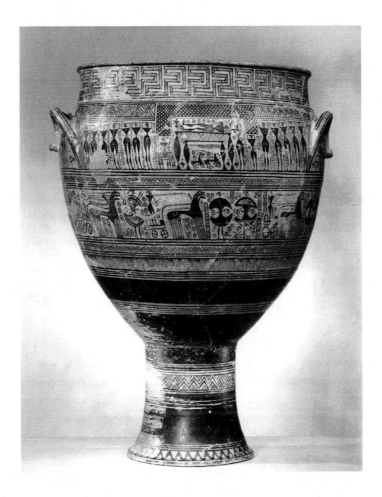

FIGURE 12.1 Attic Late Geometric krater with prothesis and chariot file. The Metropolitan Museum of Art, Rogers Fund, 1914 (14.130.14). Image © The Metropolitan Museum of Art.

behavior. Mourning females hold both hands to their heads and stand or sit beside the bier; they may touch the head of the deceased as well. By contrast, men raise one hand to the head in a formal salute and stand at a distance from the corpse, usually beyond the female mourners, where they display proper masculine emotional control and avoid the pollution of death (Ahlberg 1971; Rombos 1988; Shapiro 1991; van Wees 1998b).

While the presence of mourning warriors projects a clear message of status, group cohesion, and peaceful continuity, the mixed group of mourners also memorializes the kin-group by alluding to personal grief and family continuity. Children in these formulaic scenes have been noted, though little discussed, as small figures sitting on women's laps and standing among the adults. This neglect is partly due to the problematic conventions of Geometric style: since elements of a scene, including its figures, might be scale-adjusted for compositional reasons, how can we know when small figures in a mourning group represent children? In her authoritative analysis of *prothesis* scenes, Gudrun Ahlberg questioned whether reduced figures might be children (1971:97–101). Assuming that spatial layout overruled other factors, she first eliminated figures whose small size was constrained by framing elements, then sought variations in physical appearance or signs of dependence on larger figures (e.g., hand-holding). She concluded that few figures could be classed as children. To her thinking, no undersized figure who touches or tends the body could be a child because only adults would have "ritual concern" with a corpse (1971:134). Small figures who climb on top of the couch and even onto the corpse are seen as adults shrunk to fit the space or meant as standing behind the bier. Despite the logic of her approach, Ahlberg's underlying assumption that all actors are adults unless proven otherwise makes all but the most conspicuous child invisible.

There may be times and cultures where public memorialization of the dead would reasonably involve only adult mourners. As an era when new hierarchies and social institutions were forming, however, Early Iron Age Greece seems an unlikely place. From this perspective, Attic Geometric funeral scenes require fresh examination through a child-centered lens. Focusing on the smaller figures reveals unsuspected variety among these scenes, created through particularizing details inserted into a formulaic scheme. For this reason no two vessels are alike. This is exactly what we might expect for the first generation of Athenian grave markers, whose monumentality and limited distribution suggest they were made for a handful of elite families (Snodgrass 1987:149–150). These vessels were likely commissioned at the time of a death. As will be more fully explored below, the variety in the ages, gender, and number of mourners among these monuments suggests painters planned their scenes around figures of the requisite ages and roles for the families of the deceased. Before examining the small figures in Attic scenes, this approach can be tested by analyzing an unusually detailed funerary scene painted by a Boeotian artist who drew heavily on Attic models.

A Late Geometric hydria from Thebes presents a woman lying in *prothesis* surrounded by 18 mourners whose varied hair, clothing, placement, and behavior represent a group of mixed ages and genders (Figure 12.2; Ruckert 1976:Plate 15). Adults have long, full hair, while children are generally dressed as small adults with short spiky hair. Proximity to a corpse is determined by gender hierarchy. The body is tended by grown

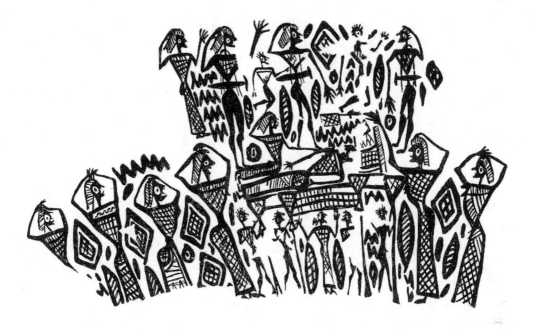

FIGURE 12.2 Prothesis scene from Boeotian hydria. Louvre A 575 (CA 639).

women and children while older males mourn at a distance. A young girl (with adult hair but no breasts) has climbed onto the couch and grasps the arm of the deceased. Standing among the women, four small boys and a girl touch the legs and underside of the bier. Above, two men are shown with full hair and with swords hanging from baldrics. A third figure has a sword but short hair, suggesting he is younger. Among the men are two small, swordless boys who dance, presumably to a funeral dirge. This remarkably detailed image suggests two broad observations. First, children are distinguished from adults by physique (lack of breasts, smaller stature), behavior (emotional conduct), and attributes (short hair, lack of swords). Second, specific activities are allocated by age and gender, with boys and adolescent males joining the men, while younger children of both sexes remain with the women to participate in their own way.

This model allows us to interpret many more of the small figures in Attic scenes as children while still acknowledging the constraints of Geometric style. That is, some small figures may indeed be reduced only for compositional requirements. Yet the adult-child dichotomy that yielded few children can be replaced by a model of multiple child stages differentiated by appearance and activity as suggested by the Theban hydria. Children can be classed in the following categories: held as lap infants, standing on top of the bier and/or corpse, touching the legs or underside of the bier, as "older" children (described below) standing with the men or women directly beside the bier, and standing with men or women at some distance from the bier. The decoration of these grave markers is typically plotted symmetrically around the focal scene of the *prothesis* or *ekphora* in which the deceased is immediately surrounded by what appears to be the family unit:

the most varied figures will be here, while lines of identical mourners frame the central element. Occasional small figures serve as generic space fillers, but these are not set within the family scene.

The results of this new analysis are dramatic. Already in the first generation of Geometric funerary scenes, children appear everywhere. They are present in 14 to 16 of the 29 Late Geometric I (LG I) funerary scenes collected by Ahlberg (1971) and augmented by Rombos (1988), and listed here in the appendix. Of the remaining 13 scenes, 10 are too fragmentary to determine; only two, possibly three seem clearly to exclude children. In other words, nearly 90 percent of the known LGI grave markers include recognizable subadults, from infant to adolescent, as a regular part of the funerary proceedings.

A closer look reveals further details of the pattern. The presence of a subadult girl crouched on the bier on the Theban hydria supports our reading of small figures as children in five similar Attic scenes. An unusually emotional scene on a krater fragment in Athens shows a woman mourning beside the deceased, a man reaching toward the latter from the foot of the couch, and a child straddling the corpse (Figure 12.3). Similarly, a belly-handled amphora in Brussels features six mourners arranged around the bier and a small figure sitting on the corpse (Ahlberg 1971:Figure 21b). A dramatic moment is invoked on a krater where a woman (mother?) holds a small child out over a corpse (Figure 12.4). On a giant krater in the Metropolitan Museum of Art, New York, a deceased warrior of heroic scale lies on the bier, while mourning women sit below and men arrive bearing strings of fish, fowl, and rabbits for a funeral feast (Figure 12.5; Ahlberg 1971:Figure 22; Boardman 1966). Two small figures are on the couch: one sits at the feet of the corpse, while the other stands and reaches over its helmeted head to the mouth as if feeding it, perhaps a fish like the tiny one by the legs of the child (Boardman 1966, Plate IIa). It is a rare glimpse of funerary rituals that may have included not only feeding the living but symbolic nourishment of the deceased. On another well-known krater in New York, the extensive crowd of mourners includes a baby seated

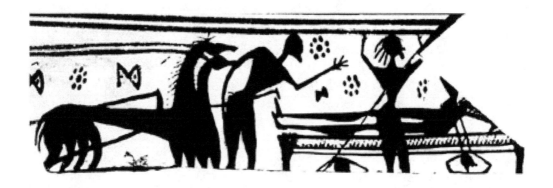

FIGURE 12.3 Part of funerary scene on fragmentary Attic Late Geometric krater, Athens NM 806 (after Archaiologikon Deltion 28:Plate 128). Drawing by author.

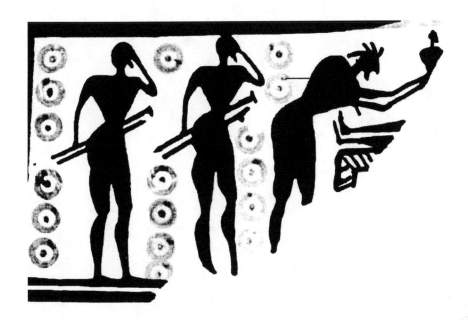

FIGURE 12.4 Krater fragment with child held over corpse (after Archaiologikon Deltion 28:Plate 127b). Drawing by author.

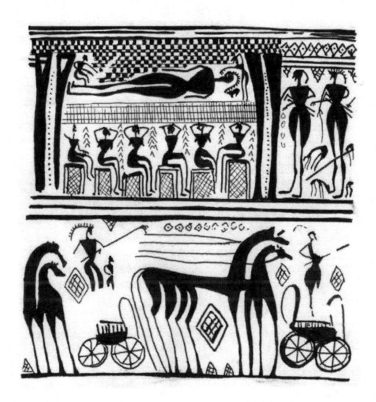

FIGURE 12.5 Detail of Attic Late Geometric krater with children on bier. The Metropolitan Museum of Art, Rogers Fund, 1914 (14.130.15). Drawing by author.

on a woman's lap and two youngsters holding hands at the corpse's feet as they gaze at his heroic form—surely the deceased's immediate family (Ahlberg 1971:Figure 25). Like the Boeotian *prothesis,* these scenes acknowledge the strongly emotional responses of those too young to understand the nature of death.

Having recognized the shorthaired boy with a sword on the Theban hydria as adolescent or older, we can find at least five and as many as seven similar figures on the Attic vessels. Ahlberg assumed these to be men because of their swords, and indeed they usually stand with the men, as opposed to the women-and-children groups. Around the extensive *prothesis* on a krater in the Louvre (Appendix 6), small bareheaded male figures standing under the chariot horses wear a single sword at their waists, in contrast to the helmeted adult warriors around them who wear two blades (Ahlberg 1971:Figure 4a-d). On a Late Geometric neck-handled amphora in Karlsruhe, the deceased lies between two groups of adult mourners, men with helmets and swords standing to the left, women to the right. At the head of each line, touching the bed or bier cloth, is a smaller figure: on the left a bareheaded youth with sword, on the right a girl unrobed like the women behind her (Figure 12.6; same scheme on an amphora in Oxford, Appendix 37). The

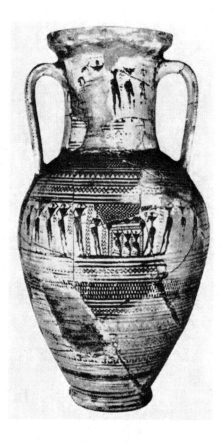

FIGURE 12.6 Attic Late Geometric amphora with funerary scene. Karlsruhe, Badisches Landesmuseum B 2674.

ekphora on a krater in Athens segregates the mourners by gender, with females to the left of the cart and sword-wearing males to the right. In an upper panel, next to the bier, a boy with a sword holds the hand of the warrior beside him (Appendix 5).

The inclusion of swords as an attribute suggests that this was the premier symbol of manhood acquired in adolescence, perhaps more because of its symbolic than practical status. From the tenth to early eighth centuries B.C., Greece shared in the widespread European phenomenon of weapons burials. Comparison with the European evidence suggests these individuals were buried not as warriors per se (swords are sometimes found with adolescent boys or physically infirm men), but simply in their customary peacetime dress with swords and spears but not armor. The emphasis on offensive rather than defensive dress characterizes the deceased (and the living) as a man of action and potential force (Sofaer Derevenski 2000:6–7; Van Wees 1998a; Whitley 2002). This is equally characteristic of Geometric art, where the sword is basic equipment, routinely shown even in peaceable scenes of funerals and horse training. In this light, the Late Geometric krater scenes add rising male heirs to the elite warrior kit of weapons, horses, and chariots that idealize the deceased. A similar notion seems clear in the chariot frieze below the mourning scene on the Attic krater, where one vehicle carries a small figure along with the warrior-charioteer (Figure 12.5; for detail, see Boardman 1966:Plate IIIa). Directly aligned with the bier, this chariot links the child to the deceased, perhaps a son now old enough to join the men. He might well be the older sibling of the other children above, whose age or gender allows him to join the parade to the cemetery. Although he has no sword, the message is the same assurance of continuity of family and cohort.

By the second generation (LGII) children appear less frequently in the *prothesis*, most likely due to changes in the use of grave pottery. The large grave marker vessels fall from favor except in provincial Attica (including krater Figure 12.4), to be replaced by smaller vessels that are briefly displayed during the funeral and then interred with the deceased. Athenian *prothesis* scenes now appear on these much smaller amphorae and pitchers, carrying reduced picture zones with fewer and more formulaic mourners. Children are present in five to seven of 29 LGII *prothesis* scenes, including three products of provincial Attic workshops that still adhere to the LGI conventions (Appendix 30, 57, 58). Eight scenes are too fragmentary to judge; 14 definitely lack children. As in LGI, children continue to touch the legs or the underside of the funeral couch, and less often simply stand beside it. That the decline in children in the latest Geometric funerary scenes reflects changes within pottery traditions rather than funerary custom is seen in the increased presence of children in the newly elaborated *prothesis* images of the seventh and sixth centuries (Boardman 1955; Shapiro 1991).

Mourning scenes offer not a snapshot of the bereaved but a schema of proper ritual procedure and behavior in the interest of restoring social order and delivering the deceased to the realm of death (Sourvinou-Inwood 1983). In this important task everyone has a role appropriate to his or her nature and status: young children caress and perhaps symbolically feed the dead, while older children dance (in the Boeotian scene) and touch the bier. Their regular proximity to the corpse suggests that either the young were naturally protected from pollution, or more likely that the concept had not yet developed in Greece. Still older adolescents or preadults resemble smaller versions of the adults beside whom they stand. Girls learn to care for the corpse. Youths with swords (or daggers) join the men at a safe distance from the corpse. They mourn like men, with a single hand raised in grief or salute. The emotional displays of the young and their need for contact with the deceased are presented as a natural part of these idealizing images. This perception continued into the seventh century as seen in a terracotta *ekphora* model from Vari (Kurtz and Boardman 1971:78; Oakley 2003:Figure 6). A shroud-covered bier stands on a wagon surrounded by four adult mourners and a horseman. On top of the shroud, a small child lies sprawled on his back, reaching upward. A bird beside him may represent the departing soul (Vermeule 1979:18).

The chronological pattern reveals yet more. The great LGI grave markers were sites of remembrance and belonging, their imagery providing a strong statement of familial attachment. Children shown seated on the bier or touching the corpse are the very picture of Philippe Ariès's "Tamed Death," a situation in which death is familiar and unfeared (Johnston 1999:30–31, 96; Sourvinou-Inwood 1995). This accords with the representation of death in Homeric epic around this time. Given proper burial rites, the heroic and nonheroic dead are equally out of reach of the living. Death is sudden and absolute, and affects the grief of the survivors in its own way, but not through fear of the corpse or the departed ghost. Fear of anonymity and oblivion is a natural correlative of this view, and a strong motivation for both Homeric heroes and eighth-century grave marking. If prominent families could publicly proclaim status, prosperity, and divine favor through mourning imagery, it may not be too much to imagine that scenes were individualized to depict specific family groupings, schematic portraits. The variety of ages, gender, and number of mourners in the centered *prothesis* panels suggests that painters planned their commissioned scenes to draw attention to the number and gender of the rising generation in families of the deceased. Framing and filling elements, including additional mourners, would have been added after a scene was properly set. The innovative LGI scenes embody socially constructed emotions in their gendered formulas for adult mourners. Among them the children's more random and overt responses to the corpse appear startlingly natural, underscoring the "emotional basis of group identity" (Tarlow 1997:106). No less culturally constructed, the representation of children's emotions effectively expressed both the force of family grief and the legacy of the deceased. While Greek funerary symbolism lacked overt references to fertility, the presence of children helped knit the fact of death into the fabric of life. Visually capturing the "cycle of life" at the time of a death is a persistent human impulse (e.g., Metcalf and Huntington 1991:Figure 7).

CHILDREN AND MINIATURE GRAVE POTTERY

It is important to bear in mind that what burials give us is burial practices (Lucy 2005), yet assemblages can sometimes offer a view of social perspectives and expectations. Children might be conceptualized through grave goods as the infants, toddlers, or children of their parents' experience, or as once-future adults and members of a kin or social group. The difference, which likely correlates with age of the deceased and identity of the buriers, could lead to quite different patterns in burial style and furnishing. One way to address this is by comparing children's assemblages with those of adults. The availability of more than 600 published graves from Early Iron Age Attica provides a way to distinguish separate stages of childhood and the differential treatment of boys and girls (Langdon 2008; Strömberg 1993; Whitley 1991).

Throughout these centuries (1000–700 B.C.) most graves, both child and adult, were sparsely furnished with only a couple of simple vessels. Those with more numerous and varied grave goods look relatively lavish and assure us that status is a strong determinant of visibility as social individuals. Just as in the ritual scenes, age distinctions suggest broad burial categories of infant, toddler, and older children merging into adolescents. Infants from birth to about one year of age had spouted feeders and miniature vessels for eating and drinking; toddlers (aged one to three or four years) additionally received small terracotta toys such as rattles and wheeled animals (Oakley 2003:176–177). Older children, from around age eight or 10 through adolescent, begin to receive certain items that have often been called toys, but whose unworn and fragile nature suggests are more likely gender-specific symbols or ritual goods (Langdon 2008, chapter 3). At least the first two categories seem to reflect a direct experience of the tiny person (sometimes including even a used toy), so one can theorize that immediate families, especially women, were in charge of burying the very young.

Archaeologists often accept without closer examination miniature vessels as appropriate grave goods for children. These diminutive objects are seen to represent toys and child-scale versions of items through which children can be socialized into gender-appropriate tasks and behaviors (Baxter 2005:46–50). Going beyond these anthropologically well-attested categories takes us into interpretations of intentionality that are difficult to demonstrate archaeologically. Nevertheless, there are certain instances when the small vessels in a child's grave appear to have been made by a child's hands, and in such cases may represent the gifts of child mourners or perhaps the handiwork of the deceased. Criteria for identifying child-produced pottery have been much discussed (Bagwell 2002; Kamp 2001; Crown 2001 and 2002) and recently applied to Greek pottery (Langdon 2014). Briefly, the work of young potters and painters can be distinguished from that of adult learners through nonstandard forming techniques and traits that reveal immature motor and cognitive development, such as unintentional asymmetry, small-scale pots with thick and uneven walls, poor understanding of motif concepts, painstaking but inept brushwork, and problems with planning and spacing. Obviously, these signs will be less apparent if an adult teacher were closely monitoring and correcting mistakes. One of the many difficulties in seeking the products of children in the archaeological record is the likelihood that they will have been incompletely published or entirely neglected in publications when only a representative sample of pottery from a site is published. A promising context is children's graves containing miniature vessels. An example from the Athenian Agora is a Late Geometric pithos burial (D16:3) of a two-month-old infant

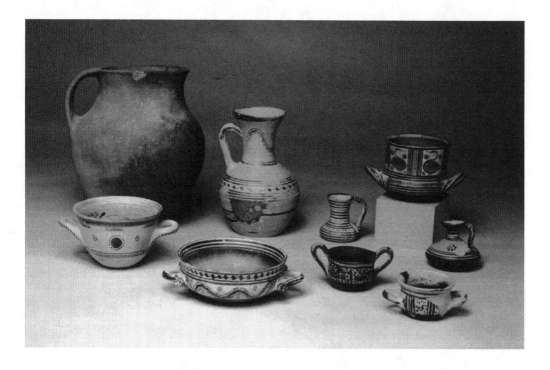

FIGURE 12.7 Infant burial assemblage from the Athenian Agora, D 16:3 (courtesy of the Trustees of the American School of Classical Studies at Athens).

(Figure 12.7; Thompson 1950:330–331). Among the fine grave pottery are three cups with figural panels: a beautiful high-rimmed skyphos with plump birds and two much poorer versions of the same idea. The published commentary in the Agora volume is revealing: "The miniature skyphos 368 in the same deposit with 319 shows that the finest and the worst painting was done at the same time" (Brann 1962:72). The small bird-panel skyphos is based on a very common type of vessel. The even humbler little kantharos, with sloppy lines, poorly smoothed surface, and awkward figures of birds and perhaps boats, was not mentioned or given a catalog entry in the final Agora volume. Dismissive language serves as a useful indicator to the researcher of potential child work meriting further investigation. In this case, the extremely young age of the recipient makes it likely that the miniature kantharos and perhaps the skyphos were gifts from the hands of older siblings or young family friends.

The Kerameikos cemetery has a high correlation between miniature cups that appear to have been produced by young workers and their deposition in child burials. Excavations for the Athens subway uncovered several child graves in the vicinity of the Kerameikos station. One of these graves contained a small cup painted with a unique scene of two ships, each populated with a crudely outlined but cheerful crew (Parlama and Stampolidis 2001:286). The boats are backward, the number of rowers does not match with oars, the rays are shaky and drippy, and the cup was unusually painted resting upside down on its rim as if for maximum stability. While it is not entirely clear how to interpret the presence of possibly child-produced pottery in children's graves, it is significant that the Athenian Agora and the Kerameikos burials are located in potters' quarters where potters' families likely resided. Some apprentice pots might have been the deceased child's own handiwork, and in other cases might have been gifts by potters' children. A further stage of this study would compare child graves at other sites to see how often the presence of a potters' quarter is a factor in the presence of child-produced works in graves.

CONCLUSION

There is a long way to go before scholarship grants children more than a passive, symbolic role in ancient societies. The demographic factor of large subadult populations in antiquity demands that we begin from theoretical perspectives attuned to finding children throughout the archaeological record. This study uses two different material categories to explore the potential for approaching children, not just as passive recipients of culture but as agents in the creation of new social and political structures. The inclusion of children in funerary scenes on grave markers turns out to be more extensive than previously thought, showing that the young were much more integral to the markers' messages of status, group cohesion, and continuity. Even in the relatively limited syntax of Geometric style, the care artists took to signify age groups and roles in the proceedings makes the children not just sentimental ambiance but partners in the appropriate discharge of funerary ritual. Identifying the ceramic offerings of child learners documents a new aspect of their emotional life as well as their participation in the economic life of the community. To a great extent a new society is built at the household level, where child rearing adjusts traditional norms and values to the new institutions and authority structure of the community. By investigating cultural categories that reveal children as partners in this effort, we can more fully understand social change in early Greece. If the *means* of childhood was using material culture to mold girls and boys to properly gendered maturity, its *ends* can be seen in the foundation of new communities.

APPENDIX

Late Geometric *prothesis* and *ekphora* scenes noting absence and presence of children. Small figures with no child-linked physical or behavioral characteristics are not included. "Fragmentary" indicates that major portions of the main scene are missing. References are to Ahlberg 1971 and Rombos 1988.

LATE GEOMETRIC I

1.   Krater. NY, Metropolitan Museum 34.11.2. Child on bier. (Ahlberg cat. 1)
2.   Amphora. Athens NM 804. Child touching bier. (Ahlberg cat. 2)
3.   Amphora. Athens, NM 803. Child touching bier. (Ahlberg cat. 53)

4. Amphora. Sèvres, Musée National de Céramique. Two children stand below bier, two touch bier at sides. (Ahlberg cat. 3)
5. Krater. Athens, NM 990. Child with sword touching bier. (Ahlberg cat. 54)
6. Krater. Paris, Louvre A 517. Child with sword under horses. (Ahlberg cat. 4)
7. Krater. Paris, Louvre A 522. Fragmentary. (Ahlberg cat. 5)
8. Krater. Halle, Robertinum 58/58 A 1–2. Fragmentary. (Ahlberg cat. 6)
9. Krater. Athens NM 802. Child on lap. (Ahlberg cat. 7)
10. Krater. Athens, Piraeus Street. Child stands beside shroud, three children touch bier, one stands beneath. (Ahlberg cat. 8)
11. Krater. Amsterdam, Allard Pierson Museum 2015. Fragmentary. (Ahlberg cat. 9)
12. Krater. Paris, Louvre CA 3391. Fragmentary. (Ahlberg cat. 10)
13. Krater. Paris, Louvre A 545. Child stands under bier. (Ahlberg cat. 11)
14. Krater. Athens NM. Fragmentary. (Ahlberg cat. 12)
15. Krater. Paris, Louvre A 547. Fragmentary. (Ahlberg cat. 13)
16. Krater. Sydney, Nicholson Museum 46.41. Possible child under horse. (Ahlberg cat. 14)
17. Krater. Paris, Louvre A 541. Fragmentary, possible child under horse. (Ahlberg cat. 15)
18. Krater. Paris, Louvre A 552. One child touches bier outside, possibly others below. (Ahlberg cat. 16)
19. Amphora. Athens, Agora Museum P 10664. Fragmentary. (Ahlberg cat. 17)
20. Krater. Athens NM 812. Small figures alternate with larger, no clear indications of age. (Ahlberg cat. 18)
21. Krater. Athens NM 4310. Child seated on corpse. (Ahlberg cat. 19)
22 Krater. Athens NM 806. Fragmentary; *prothesis* scene missing. (Ahlberg cat. 20)
23. Krater. Athens, Third Ephoria. Child held in arms. (Rombos cat. 75)
24. Amphora. Brussels, Musées royaux d'Art et d'Histoire A 1506. Child seated on corpse. (Ahlberg cat. 21)
25. Pitcher. Dresden, Stattl. Kunstsamm. ZV 1635. No apparent children. (Ahlberg cat. 23)
26. Amphora. Athens NM 18062. No children. (Ahlberg cat. 24)
27. Krater. NY, Metropolitan Museum 14.130.14. One child on lap, two on bier. (Ahlberg cat. 25)
28. Krater. Athens, Kerameikos Museum Fragmentary. (Ahlberg cat. 26)
29. Amphora. Athens, Kriezi Street. Incompletely illustrated. (Ahlberg text Figure 3)

Late Geometric II

30. Krater. NY, Metropolitan Museum 14.130.15. Two children on bier, child in chariot. (Ahlberg cat. 22)
31. Krater. Florence, Museo Archeologico 86.415.85/86. Fragmentary. (Ahlberg cat. 27)
32. Krater. Uppsala University 137. Fragmentary. (Ahlberg cat. 28)

33. Amphora. Copenhagen, Ny Carlsberg Glyptothek 2680. No children. (Ahlberg cat. 29)

34. Krater. Thorikos TC 65.666. Fragmentary. (Ahlberg cat. 30)

35. Amphora. Berlin, Staatl. Mus. 1963.13. No children. (Ahlberg cat. 31)

36. Amphora. Karlsruhe, Badisches Landesmuseum B2674. Two children touching bier, one with sword. (Ahlberg cat. 32)

37. Amphora. Oxford, Ashmolean Museum 1916.55. Two children touching bier, one with sword. (Ahlberg cat. 33)

38. Pitcher. Athens NM 18474. Fragmentary. (Ahlberg cat. 34)

39. Amphora. Myrrhinous, Brauron Museum. No children. (Ahlberg cat. 35)

40. Amphora. Houston, Museum of Fine Arts. No children. (Rombos cat. 147)

41. Amphora. Cleveland, Museum of Art 1927.27.6. Two possible children touching bier. (Ahlberg cat. 36)

42. Amphora. Baltimore, Walters Art Gallery 48.2231. One possible child touching bier. (Ahlberg cat. 37)

43. Amphora. Athens, private collection. No children. (Ahlberg cat. 38)

44. Amphora. Athens, Agora P4990. Poorly preserved, no clear children. (Ahlberg cat. 39)

45. Amphora. Athens, Stathatou collection 222. No children. (Ahlberg cat. 40)

46. Amphora. Essen, Folkwang Mus. K 969. No children. (Ahlberg cat. 41)

47. Amphora. Athens, Kerameikos Mus. 1371. No children. (Ahlberg cat. 42)

48. Amphora. Kerameikos Museum 5643. No children. (Rombos cat. 172)

49. Amphora. Hamburg, Museum für Kunst und Gewerbe 1966.89. No children. (Ahlberg cat. 43)

50. Amphora. Athens, Vlastos collection. Fragmentary. (Ahlberg cat. 44)

51. Pitcher. London, British Museum 1912.5.22.1. No children. (Ahlberg cat. 45)

52. Amphora. Athens, Benaki Museum 7675. No children. (Ahlberg cat. 46)

53. Oinochoe. Paris, Louvre CA 3283. No children. (Ahlberg cat. 47)

54. Amphora. London market. No children. (Ahlberg cat. 48)

55. Sherd. Athens NM 283. Fragmentary. (Ahlberg cat. 49)

56. Sherd. Athens, Acropolis Museum 255. Fragmentary. (Ahlberg cat. 50)

57. Krater. Merenda 6–IX–61. Child held in arms. (Rombos cat. 315)

58. Krater. Merenda, Brauron Museum. Child standing by bier. (Rombos cat. 388)

REFERENCES CITED

Ahlberg, G. 1971 *Prothesis and Ekphora in Greek Geometric Art*. Studies in Mediterranean Archaeology 32. Paul Åström, Göteborg.

Bagwell, E. A. 2002 Ceramic Form and Skill: Attempting to Identify Child Producers at Pecos Pueblo, New Mexico. In *Children in the Prehistoric Puebloan Southwest*, edited by K. A. Kamp, pp. 90–107. University of Utah Press, Salt Lake City.

Baxter, J. E. 2005 *The Archaeology of Childhood: Children, Gender, and Material Culture*. Altamira Press, Walnut Creek, California.

Boardman, J. 1955 Painted Funerary Plaques and Some Comments on *Prothesis*. *Annual of the British School at Athens* 50:51–66.

Boardman, J. 1966 Attic Geometric Vase Scenes, Old and New. *Journal of Hellenic Studies* 86: 1–5.

Brann, E. 1962 *Late Geometric and Protoattic Pottery*. Agora Vol. 8. American School of Classical Studies, Princeton.

Crown, P. 2001 Learning to Make Pottery in the Prehispanic American Southwest. *Journal of Anthropological Research* 57:451–469.

Crown, P. 2002 Learning and Teaching in the Prehispanic American Southwest. In *Children in the Prehistoric Puebloan Southwest*, edited by K. A. Kamp, pp. 108–24. University of Utah Press, Salt Lake City.

Johnston, S. I. 1999 *Restless Dead: Encounters Between the Living and the Dead in Ancient Greece*. University of California Press, Berkeley and Los Angeles.

Kamp, K. A. 2001 Prehistoric Children Working and Playing. A Southwestern Case Study in Learning Ceramics. *Journal of Anthropological Research* 57:427–450.

Kurtz, D. C., and J. Boardman 1971 *Greek Burial Customs*. Cornell University Press, Ithaca.

Langdon, S. 2008 *Art and Identity in Dark Age Greece, 1100–700 BCE*. Cambridge University Press, New York and London.

Langdon, S. 2013 Children and Material Culture in Early Greece. In *The Oxford Handbook of Childhood and Education in the Classical World*, edited by T. Parkin and J. Evans-Grubbs. Oxford University Press, Oxford.

Lucy, S. 2005 The Archaeology of Age. In *The Archaeology of Identity: Approaches to Gender, Age, Status, Ethnicity, and Religion*, edited by M. Díaz-Andreu, S. Lucy, S. Babic, and D. N. Edwards, pp. 43–66. Routledge, London.

Metcalf, P., and R. Huntington 1991 *Celebrations of Death: The Anthropology of Mortuary Ritual*. 2nd edition. Cambridge University Press, Cambridge.

Morris, I. 1987 *Burial and Ancient Society: The Rise of the Greek City-State*. Cambridge University Press, New York and London.

Oakley, J. 2003 Death and the Child. In *Coming of Age in Ancient Greece: Images of Childhood from the Classical Past*, edited by J. Neils and J. Oakley, pp. 163–194. Yale University Press, New Haven and London.

Parlama, L., and N. Stampolidis 2001 *Athens: The City Beneath the City: Antiquities from the Metropolitan Railway Excavations*. Greek Ministry of Culture, Athens.

Rombos, T. 1988 *The Iconography of Attic Late Geometric II Pottery*. Studies in Mediterranean Archaeology-PB 68. Paul Åström, Jonsered.

Ruckert, A. 1976 *Frühe Keramik Böotiens*. Antike Kunst Beiheft 10. Franke, Bern.

Scott, E. 1999 *Archaeology of Infancy and Infant Death*. Archaeopress, Oxford.

Shapiro, H. A. 1991 The Iconography of Mourning in Athenian Art. *American Journal of Archaeology* 95:629–656.

Snodgrass, A. M. 1987 *An Archaeology of Greece: The Present State and Future Scope of a Discipline*. University of California Press, Berkeley.

Sofaer Derevenski, J. 2000 Material Culture Shock: Confronting Expectations in the Material Culture of Children. In *Children and Material Culture*, edited by J. Sofaer Derevenski, pp. 3–16. Routledge, London and New York.

Sourvinou-Inwood, C. 1983 A Trauma in Flux: Death in the Eighth Century and After. In *The Greek Renaissance of the Eighth Century B.C.: Tradition and Innovation*, edited by R. Hägg, pp. 33–48. *SkrAth* 4, 30. Stockholm.

Sourvinou-Inwood, C. 1995 *"Reading" Greek Death to the End of the Classical Period.* Oxford University Press, Oxford.

Strömberg, A. 1993 *Male or Female? A Methodological Study of Grave Gifts as Sex Indicators in Iron Age Burials in Athens.* SIMA-PB 123. Paul Åström, Jonsered.

Tarlow, S. 1997 An Archaeology of Remembering: Death, Bereavement, and the First World War. *Cambridge Archaeological Journal* 7:105–121.

Thompson, H. 1950 Excavations in the Athenian Agora: 1949. *Hesperia* 19:313–337.

van Wees, H. 1998a Greeks Bearing Arms: The State, the Leisure Class, and the Display of Weapons in Archaic Greece. In *Archaic Greece: New Approaches and New Evidence*, edited by N. Fisher and Hans van Wees, pp. 333–378. Duckworth, London.

van Wees, H. 1998b A Brief History of Tears: Gender Differentiation in Archaic Greece. In *When Men Were Men: Masculinity, Power, and Identity in Classical Antiquity*, edited by L. Foxhall and J. Salmon, pp. 10–53. Routledge, London and New York.

Vermeule, E. 1979 *Aspects of Death in Early Greek Art and Poetry.* University of California Press, Berkeley.

Whitley, J. 1991 *Style and Society in Dark Age Greece: The Changing Face of a Pre--Literate Society.* Cambridge University Press, Cambridge.

Whitley, J. 2002 Objects with Attitude: Biographical Facts and Fallacies in the Study of Late Bronze Age and Early Iron Age Warrior Graves. *Cambridge Archaeological Journal* 12:217–232.

CHAPTER THIRTEEN

The Children's Cemetery of Lugnano in Teverina, Umbria

Hierarchy, Magic, and Malaria

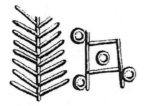

David Soren

Abstract *Throughout classical antiquity infant cemeteries existed to provide a means of disposing of unwanted children or dealing with victims of disease. It is therefore important, when archaeologists excavate a children's cemetery (or any cemetery), to consider whether the cemetery is normal or abnormal in order to understand why the children were buried as they were. A normal cemetery contains bodies placed one at a time or occasionally in paired groups when, perhaps, stillborn twins die. Such a cemetery grows horizontally (the more typical way most cemeteries expand) as more bodies are interred. But an abnormal cemetery may contain features that are unexpected. These include vertical depositions or placing of bodies in groups one above the other. These cemeteries may take advantage of abandoned areas, filling up pits and disposing of infants in a rapid manner. In order to investigate such cemeteries certain criteria should be developed and certain questions asked. When these questions are asked and answered they can help to determine if the cemetery is normal or abnormal and can also help to identify why the burials were made. These conclusions were developed during the excavation of Italy's largest known infant cemetery, found in 1988 in Lugnano in Teverina, Italy, which has become a type site for forensic and parasitological studies resulting in the extraction of the oldest DNA evidence for an epidemic of Plasmodium falciparum malaria known from an archaeological site.*

In 1999 the results of the University of Arizona excavations at Poggio Gramignano, near Lugnano in Teverina (Umbria), Italy, were published (Soren and Soren 1999). This gently rolling hill was the site of one of the largest Roman villas in Umbria, constructed circa 15 B.C. in the Augustan period and intended to take advantage of abundant farmland and a magnificent view of the Tiber River (Figures 13.1, 13.2, and 13.3 on page 238). The villa featured uniquely innovative architecture, which included using roof tiles broken up as if they were building bricks (i.e., proto-bricks), done at a time before actual bricks had come into use in the Roman empire. It also featured a *triclinium* or dining area with columns lining three sides, three barrel vaulted walkways, and a central pyramidal-shaped ceiling with a flattened apex (Figure 13.4 on page 239; Soren and Aylward 1994; Soren and Borghetti 1992; Soren and Soren 1992).

This architectural experiment proved to be too dynamic, however, because the villa was not founded on solid bedrock and its shifting substructure and overly top-heavy concrete ceiling vaulting caused the villa to crack and collapse within a century after it was constructed. Eventually, by the third century A.D., with depressed economic times having set in, it was impossible to maintain the sizable villa even in a dilapidated state, and the structure became a ruin.

In the mid-fifth century A.D. the part of the villa on the hillside facing the Tiber, which originally had been used as storage magazines and kitchen and service areas, was reused as an infant cemetery (Pimpolari 2006; Soren 2002; Soren, Fenton, and Birkby 1995). The vaulted ceilings and roofs of this part of the villa were by now missing and the villa was unusable except as a squatter habitation. This was evidenced by circular areas of burning, indicating campfires directly on the floor of a beautiful mosaic.

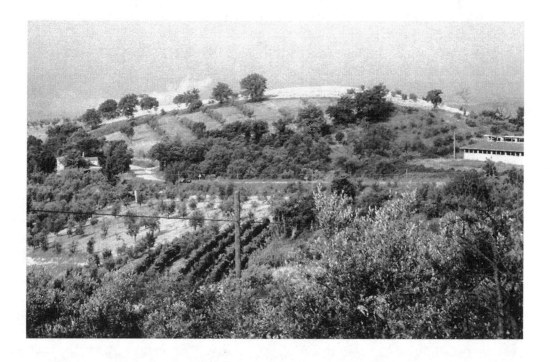

FIGURE 13.1 View over the hilltop of Poggio Gramignano in the area of Lugnano in Teverina, Umbria, Italy (photo by Noelle Soren).

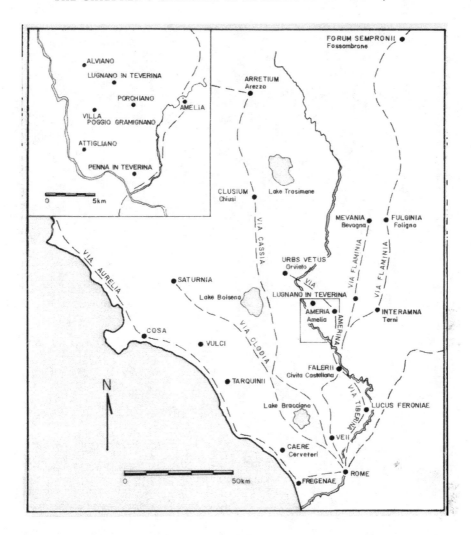

FIGURE 13.2 Map showing the location of the villa near Lugnano in Teverina (map by Jose Olivas, Reality Bytes).

To make the infant cemetery, five rooms were pressed into service during an emergency which saw 47 infants and 13 young dogs buried (Figures 13.5 on page 239 and 13.6 on page 240). Twenty-two of the infant burials were premature births and most of the other burials were neonates. The American excavation of the cemetery was halted when the permit to excavate expired, but most of the cemetery had been excavated, leaving approximately 10 square meters remaining to dig. The question then turned to what happened to the infants of Lugnano.

In order to answer this question it was necessary to effect a detailed excavation of the cemetery and analyze the results. When human remains first began to appear during the excavations in 1989 a specific methodology was developed to dig the area using the concept of Formation Processes developed by anthropologist Michael Schiffer (Schiffer

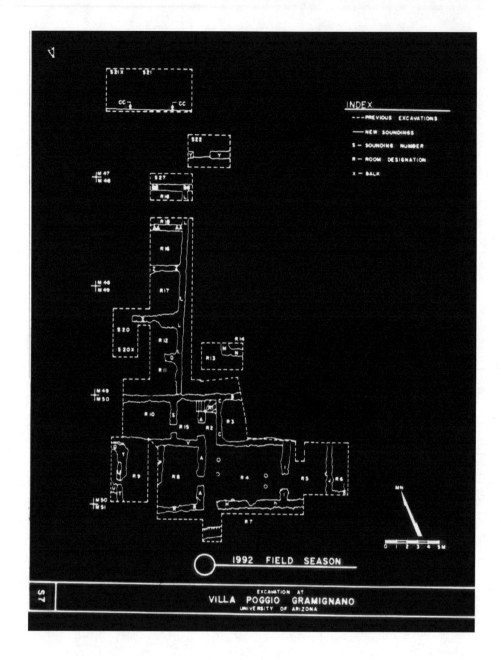

FIGURE 13.3 Plan of the villa of Lugnano in Teverina (Jose Olivas, Reality Bytes).

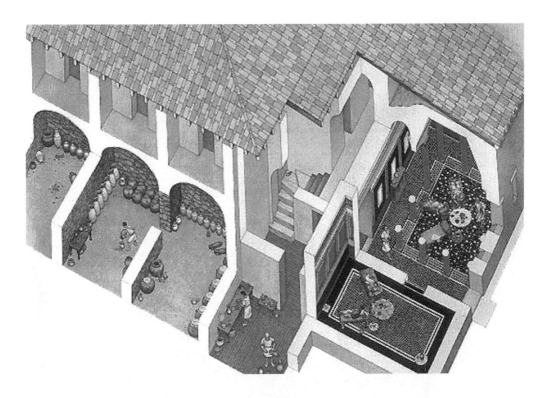

FIGURE 13.4 Reconstruction of the main triclinium and secondary triclinium at right with service quarters and stairs to second floor at left (David Vandenberg).

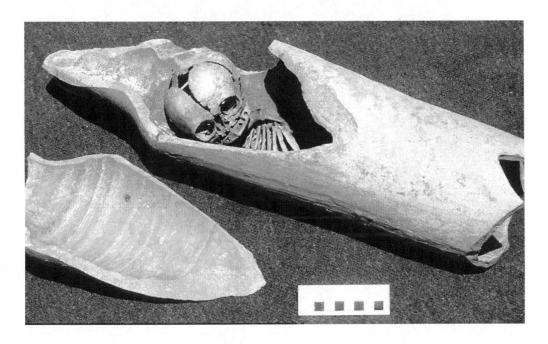

FIGURE 13.5 Neonate burial IB1 in African spatheion amphora, as reconstructed by Walter Birkby (Photo by Noelle Soren).

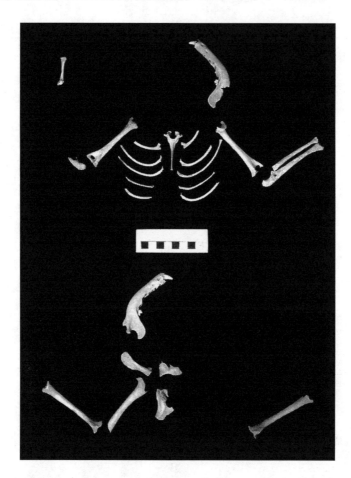

FIGURE 13.6 Skeletal remains of an immature dog aged five to six months found severed in half with each half separately buried within the infant cemetery (Photo by Noelle Soren).

1987). Instead of excavating by loci or individual layers, it was decided to dig down in approximately 10 cm passes, changing basket numbers with each pass. Whenever even slight changes in the soil composition or color were noted, a new locus or layer was declared. In this manner, using micro-stratigraphy, it was possible to be sure of what finds were found at what levels and any subtle changes in the makeup of the fill within the cemetery could be noted, allowing a final analysis of the area to determine how it was created.

It became clear very quickly that the cemetery was filled with loosely compacted earth, much of it burned. The soil appeared to be put in either at one time or, more likely, over a very short period of time over the former storage rooms and kitchen of the destroyed Roman villa. The soil was not uniform but was not at all tamped down or "metaled" into a floor surface at any point and it raised the level of the rooms approximately three meters. There were many small pockets or lenses of different-colored earth throughout, much of it with traces of ash. The highest part of the fill contained a higher percentage of ash. Burials were found throughout the fill, both of infants and canines and all but one of the canines were between five and six months in age. Furthermore, there were abundant scattered potsherds throughout, several of which were found in the bottom layers of the fill and which joined to potsherds in the top layers. There were some earlier potsherd scraps dating back to the time of the original construction of the villa and suggesting that the fill had been brought in from a location where it had been used as a previous fill but mixed in with it was a significant quantity of pottery, which suggested a date around the middle of the fifth century A.D.

To date, 45 infants were discovered in these rooms. It was also decided to excavate the still-remaining piles of backfill from the previous excavations of Daniela Monacchi in the earlier 1980s and even to sift the soil, since these excavations focused on Room 10, the kitchen area of the villa, as well as the corridor leading to the former triclinium (number 4). This laborious work yielded the scattered remains of two more partially complete infants, probably from Room 10, and this raised the total to 47. Since a small area was left unexcavated in Rooms 11 and 12 when the excavation permit was not renewed, there probably are more infant burials waiting to be unearthed, but exactly how many is difficult to estimate because of the manner in which they were sometimes single and sometimes clustered. Only the sex of female burial 36 was determined by specialists.

The reason that so much time was taken excavating the cemetery was that this did not parallel any other ancient cemetery that the excavators had ever encountered. Instead of being placed in a horizontally emphasized grouping, the human interments began with a single burial at the very bottom of the cemetery and as the cemetery progressed with its fill toward the top, paired burials were found. At or near the top, burials of up to seven infants at once were noted. If the cemetery was installed over a very brief period of time, as the evidence suggested, then the burials were placed in a gradually escalating fashion from the bottom to the top.

Each of the burials, human and canine, was analyzed by forensic anthropologists Walter Birkby and Charles Fenton. Twenty-two of the infants were premature and likely aborted fetuses, eighteen were newborns, and the others were up to six months in age, with the exception of one two to three-year-old child. Six different types of burial were encountered: simple inhumation, burial under or within reused roof cover-tiles from the destroyed villa, interment with a gabled triangle of pan tiles, burial inside a crudely made little "house" built up of tiles, or burial within an amphora (transport jar) either in a nearly complete or fragmentary state. All of the burials were simple and there were few finds to suggest wealth.

Also of interest was the hierarchic dispersal of the burials. With a few exceptions, the eldest infants were placed in the three northernmost rooms and were afforded the most elaborate burials. Neonates and the premature or aborted fetuses were generally restricted to the simplest inhumations in the two southernmost rooms. A striking feature of the burials in the southern rooms was that the fill in this area contained a considerable amount of debris, particularly refuse from the villa in the form of roof tiles, pottery fragments, and ash. The dump continued south of the burials into Room 9. This suggested that in general (but with a few exceptions) the younger children were buried most perfunctorily, almost to be considered scattered amid a dump of fill and debris from the decaying ruin of the villa. In general, the older the child, the more care was provided in terms of burial. However, it appeared that some younger children could be given more attention, making an exception to the rule. This would make sense in that families might be less attached to an aborted fetus but more attached to a child the longer it lived with the family and yet some families would be equally devastated no matter what age their child. Since infant death was much more common than it is in developed countries today, the view of infant death differed from our own, especially in a rural area of the later Roman empire (Hope 2009).

Although the cemetery showed evidence of considerable poverty in the types of tombs, there were nonetheless offerings present, and particular attention was placed on documenting them and attempting to interpret their meaning from the context in which they were found. Among the neonates and premature burials were finds that one might expect in a normal cemetery, but there were also objects that suggested that magic was being employed in conjunction with the burials. Magic rituals and the fear of ghosts and unexplained events were not uncommon in a rural community such as this, which was facing some sort of major crisis that was causing an increasing number of deaths in a short period of time (Ogden 2009). Something needed to be done to try to protect the community and deliver it from whatever was affecting it. As the excavation progressed and the unusual finds in the cemetery proliferated, it was determined that the burials had resulted from an epidemic of some kind, although the precise nature of it remained to be determined pending further examination of the evidence.

Some of the responses of this mid-fifth-century A.D. rural community to the as yet undetermined epidemic included the burial of 12 puppies all less than six months in age (Figure 13.6) and one dog aged ca. 14 months. These animals were analyzed by Michael MacKinnon of the Department of Anthropology of the University of Winnipeg who showed that the slaughtered puppies were generally buried with the younger children (MacKinnon 1999:542–543). One dog skeleton was found severed in two and buried in two parts while others showed evidence of having their mandibles ripped away by force. MacKinnon concluded that the dogs were used in "some religious ritual or sacrifice" in which "some puppies appear to have been dismembered or beheaded." The magic healing power of sacrificed puppies was well established in the ancient Mediterranean world long before late antiquity, even among the Hittites and ancient Greeks (Soren 1999a:621).

Other finds placed on the infants that suggested the use of magic included one raven's talon (on Infant Burial 3) and the skeleton of a small toad (IB33). The talon might be interpreted as a chthonic symbol or talisman against evil. The raven and the crow, with their sinister beaks and gleaming eyes, were particularly associated with evil, death, and destruction, with the raven being used often as an apotropaic (Virgil, *Ecl.* IX.15). The raven was particularly associated with underground pits, wells, and graves because of its chthonic connections:

[The raven formed] a line of communication between the living and the dead, the earth and the underworld of powers. Ravens and crows, with their black plumage and their habit of feeding off of dead things, were clearly seen as messengers from the Otherworld. (Green 1992:126)

Toads and frogs have been associated with magic and sorcery since remote antiquity due to the fact that they were considered repugnant to touch and view and because their breath was considered poisonous (Summers 1992). Roman frog part amulets were particularly popular as talismans with curative powers (Pliny *N.H.*XXII.74) and toad entrails were used in magic rites such as prognostication (Juvenal III.44–45). A primitive bone doll was also found and, although such an offering may be perceived as normal in a child's grave (Shumka 1999), this doll had no arms or legs (Figures 13.7 and 13.8) and as such may have been intended as a human substitute or *effigies* such as was done in tombs at Pompeii for freeborn men and women (Jongman 1991:296).

In Room 17, generally reserved for older infants, was found the oldest child, two to three years of age. The child had been laid out simply but had stones placed over the hands and a heavy tile over the feet, suggesting that the female had been deliberately

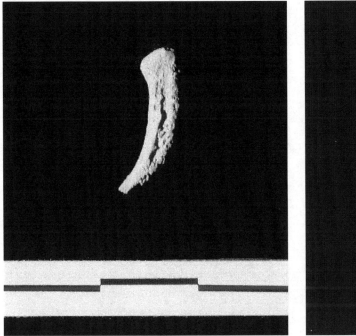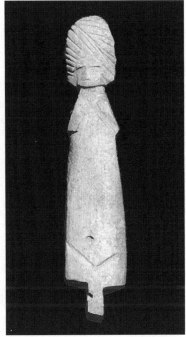

FIGURE 13.7 (left) Raven talon found inside the amphora and on the skeleton of IB 3 (Photo by Noelle Soren).

FIGURE 13.8 (right) Bone doll found within the infant cemetery (Photo by Noelle Soren).

weighed down so as not to be able to rise from the grave and harm the living (Figure 13.9). There were also two bronze cauldrons, one inside the other, with one containing ash. Palynologist Karen Adams observed that several tombs contained seeds of *Lonicera caprifolia* or honeysuckle, which was known to Pliny the Elder as *periclymenon*, Honeysuckle blooms in later July or August, giving a possible clue as to the time of year of the epidemic.

The mid-fifth century A.D. was a time when the late Roman empire had been officially Christianized, but of course in many areas, including rural Umbria, old values died hard and nothing in the infant cemetery of Poggio Gramignano reflected Christian burial practices. Instead, it reflected what Eleanor Scott has termed a "revitalization movement" (Scott 1991), a going back to the practices of female witches (*sagae*) of earlier times such as were invoked by Virgil and Horace. In fact, the parallels between the

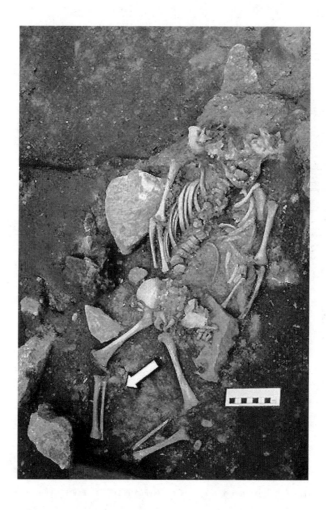

FIGURE 13.9 Infant burial 36 weighted down with stones over the hands and a large tile over the feet (Photo by Noelle Soren).

cemetery finds at Poggio Gramignano and the evidence found in the poetry of Virgil and Horace are remarkably striking.

Virgil in *Eclogue* 9.15 mentions graveyards, ravens, toads, and dolls. Horace in *Satire* 1.8 offers a comic description of two witches, Canidia and Sagana, whose practices were nonetheless already well known to his readers. In the dark of the night, they tear apart a black lamb in a cemetery and pour its blood into a trench in order to attract the attention of available human souls. Wax and wooden dolls are used in the invocation of daimonic gods such as Hecate and Tisiphone while hellish dogs and snakes roam freely among the tombs. Blazing fires are set at the graveyard and the white excrement of ravens is also offered. The witches in the graveyard are seeking to gain control of the souls of the dead, and human bones are used in their spells and potions to vex living humans. This account offers striking parallels to the remains found at the Lugnano excavations.

In *Epode* 5. 43–46 Horace has Sagana and Canidia joined by two other witches. One of them is Folia of Arminium, now the town of Rimini in Umbria, who is a powerful witch who employs eggs, birds, hideous toads, and jawbones from a starving bitch. These elements are used to invoke Hecate/Diana. In *Epode* 17, Horace refers to wax dolls used to influence Hecate. While the precise rituals do not exactly match the mysterious goings on at the Poggio Gramignano site in the area of Lugnano, there are enough parallels to suggest most strongly that magic rituals and even witchcraft were employed there to expiate a suddenly arriving terror such as an epidemic from the community. Such practices would have received a boost in popularity when, after the epidemic ran its seasonal course, the community appeared to have been saved!

If the honeysuckle found in the cemetery was placed there when honeysuckle was in bloom, this could have had significance for the inclusion of the slaughtered canines in the cemetery. The presence of the puppies during the "dog days" (*dies caniculares*) of summer, might be related to the rising and setting with the sun of the dog star Sirius between July 3 and 11, a time noted for fevers and heatstroke when people could be *astrobletoi* or starstruck (Soren 1999a:628). An epidemic arriving at this time could have been ascribed to the dog days of the summertime.

Once all of the evidence for the cemetery was assembled, it was time to ask experts what happened to the infants of Lugnano in Teverina. Infectious disease specialist and professor of medicine Eskild Pedersen of the University of Arizona and malariologists Mario Coluzzi and Lorenza Merzagora of the Istituto di Parassitologia, University of Rome, La Sapienza were consulted and they offered a range of possible diseases and epidemics, but the only one of their suggestions that fit the archaeological scenario was *Plasmodium falciparum* malaria (Merzagora 1996). Simply put, this disease is spread by mosquitoes drawing out parasite-tainted blood from one human and depositing the parasites into another human. The parasite invades the liver eight to 12 days later. Arizona State Museum forensic anthropologists Walter Birkby and Todd Fenton were apprised of the suggestions made by the other specialists.

The cemetery presented a clear pattern. It contained aborted fetuses, neonates, and a few older children. A few children died at first and then the epidemic escalated, killing up to seven at a time. This occurred over a very short period of time, perhaps weeks or a month but not much longer, and the bodies were interred quickly. The large number of aborted fetuses and neonates was particularly important in interpreting the site since maternal malaria in the last week of pregnancy is particularly associated with neonatal mortality. Also, the town of Orte, very near to Lugnano and on the Tiber, was a center for flooding and standing water in antiquity (particularly in the fifth century A.D. when ports and commerce were being disrupted) and malarial outbreaks are well documented even into the nineteenth century (Romer 1999). Circumstantial evidence suggested that Lugnano was a prime candidate for an ancient summertime malaria epidemic (Soren 1993).

When the preliminary results of the excavation were published and became the subject of a *Learning Channel* television special called *A Roman Plague*, produced by Peter Young and *Archaeology Magazine* in 1991, criticism poured in regarding the identification of the epidemic as malaria. An attempt was made to have the bones of the infants analyzed to see if traces of *Plasmodium falciparum* malaria might be found through a process of DNA extraction that was just being perfected at the time in a variety of institutions. Phone calls to the Centers for Disease Control and Prevention in Atlanta and the National Institutes of Health in Bethesda were greeted with derision or disinterest. Then professor of anthropology Marshall Becker of West Chester State University stated on *The Learning Channel* program: "The evidence for malaria (at Lugnano) is in effect nonexistent."

However, Robert Sallares, research fellow in the Institute of Science and Technology and the Department of Biomolecular Sciences at the University of Manchester, tested and confirmed the malaria hypothesis by extracting the oldest evidence of *Plasmodium falciparum* malaria known (although recent studies by Hawass et al. 2010 have provided evidence for malaria in the mummy of King Tutankhamun). The genome sequence for *Plasmodium falciparum,* consisting of the entire sequence of DNA molecules found within a single parasite, was only worked out in 2002 (Humphries 2010). Sallares removed DNA from the two- to three-year-old child (Burial 36) in two separate extractions. The fact that this extraction could be done from such an old skeleton was evidence of a massive infection of the infant and proved that the disease was a major factor at Lugnano.

Sallares's discovery also provided insight into what happened to the infants of Lugnano (Sallares 2002:67; Sallares, Bouwman, and Anderung 2004). A summertime epidemic had swept through the area, probably due to unseasonably warm temperatures, leaving the community, which was not normally subject to this form of malaria, devastated and desperate to find a solution to expiate the terrifying symptoms they were experiencing: excruciating headaches, nausea, paroxysms, chills, tertian fevers, vomiting, severe gastric pain, enlarged spleen, physical weakness, an emaciated and gaunt appearance, and death. Pregnant mothers suffered aborted fetuses and experienced toxemia or blood poisoning. The disease had likely spread from Africa by trade to Rome's harbor Ostia, because much of the finer pottery of the fifth century came from North Africa including tableware and the very amphorae in which the infants of Lugnano were buried. The malaria epidemic then continued along the Tiber during a warm summer period, perhaps promoted also by flooding in the Lugnano to Orte area (Merzagora 1996).

The Romans never understood what malaria really was, so when an epidemic struck they couldn't stop it and witchcraft was employed because it was more hopeful than doing nothing and watching people panic and die horrible moaning deaths. The apotropaics employed, such as raven's talon and toad, would be appropriate and the use of honeysuckle in Roman times, an unusual offering in a tomb, was a remedy employed for 30 days dissolved in white wine to cure splenomegaly, or enlarged spleen, one of the symptoms of *Plasmodium falciparum* malaria (Pliny *N.H.* XXVII.XCIV.120; Soren 1999b:518).

Since the event occurred at or just after the middle of the fifth century A.D., one might expect that the community would have made a Christian response, but the evidence showed otherwise. The members of the community had to make critical decisions about where and how to bury the dead. The ruined villa, useless for habitation, was a perfect location and, apparently, it was not near the town of the living, which has not yet been located. A special hierarchy was observed for infants because at this time in the late Roman world, the infant mortality rate was so high (some estimates suggesting 30 to 40 percent) even under normal conditions that aborted fetuses or stillborn neonates were virtually discarded (Golden 1988:155; Soren 1999b:482).

In the ruined villa at Poggio Gramignano the youngest infants and fetuses were placed in several rooms along with trash from the tidying up of the villa for the cemetery installation, but in other rooms farther to the southwest, away from the trash, older children were buried along with a few other neonates, suggesting two things. First, the older children tended to be buried in rooms away from the younger ones and were more respected. Second, a few of the younger ones were possibly also respected. That the people of the village were poor is shown by the types of burials.

No adults were found, because at this time adults would be buried in a separate cemetery which has not yet been located but which may lie near the bottom of the southwest slope of the hilltop where farmers plowing their fields have turned up roof tiles that may have been reused for tombs. The Roman tradition was not to pay attention to the death of an aborted fetus or an unwanted diseased neonate, but it is clear that some Romans could not help mourning the death of a child at birth (Bradley 1991:28–29). The Christian tradition, which was gaining sway by the fifth century A.D., argued that all infants should be baptized and respected (Cyprian *Ad Fidum* 2–3). Hence, some infant burials were treated as discards and some were buried with more tender care. But all of the slightly older children were given some sort of attention at burial.

The fear of the epidemic is reflected in the special practices revealed in some of the burials. It is probable that *sagae* or *magi* were summoned; these were individuals in the community believed to have the ability to use supernatural means to achieve a desired effect versus evil forces. At Poggio Gramignano this meant a number of measures had to be taken. First, the affected children needed to be buried in isolation from the rest of the community, not only because this was still the normal way infants who died before their time were buried but also because it was necessary to remove their ability to pollute the living (Horace *Epod.* 5.92; Johnston 1990:144–145; Plutarch, *De genio Socratis* 22; Sallares, Bouman, and Anderung 2004; Tertullian, *De Anima* 57; Virgil, *Aen.* VI.426).

A particular hierarchy was observed whereby the children who never lived were generally treated as nonhuman discards and separated from actual proper burials of older children. Magical spells or incantations would have accompanied the burials and these would have been augmented by the sacrifice of animals traditionally associated with the dead and the underworld and with the power to heal. It is likely that local gods or spirits (*daimones*) might be prayed to as well in hopes of their halting the disease contaminating the community and offerings made in the bronze cauldrons found stacked together with ash inside of them.

The excavations of Lugnano are important for the insight they give into how an Umbrian rural community of the middle fifth century responded to a terrifying epidemic and how they viewed and treated their dead children in this time of sorrow and urgency. Even though this community was devastated, it does not prove that all of Italy fell victim to malaria epidemics. For malaria to thrive, conditions must be very specific. Times of drought may even contribute to drying up of waterways, leaving standing water pools along the Tiber. Intense summer heat may also have fueled the epidemic. Slaves and field workers in low-lying areas would have suffered most from such an epidemic while those on higher ground would be more protected from the mosquitoes. This may be the reason that Lugnano in Teverina was founded on the top of a hill. Fluctuations in temperature or extended periods of heat also would have affected the occurrence of malaria. Thus, malaria would have struck intermittently and only in the summer months and it would tend to harm those of the poor who experienced extended exposure to the mosquitoes.

Lugnano is only one excavation site. More comparative data is needed. Archaeologists excavating other cemeteries may wish to answer the following questions when excavating a cemetery site:

1. What is the stratigraphy of the cemetery and, if it is an infant cemetery, does it have a horizontal or a vertical emphasis in the depositions of the infants? In other words, are the bodies dispersed vertically over a short period of time or are they buried horizontally in the manner of a typical cemetery?

2. Is there evidence of mass burials and if so how are the bodies grouped? If there is a vertical emphasis to the cemetery, do the burials increase in frequency over time? In short, is the diachronic span, if it exists at all, extremely short or long?

3. Is the material culture found consistent with one period of time or with a lapse of time, and what is the nature of the burial goods?

4. What is the palynological evidence and what are its social and temporal implications? For example, is honeysuckle present? Can the time of year or season of deposition be determined?

5. What conditions or pathology do the preserved bones display?

6. What animal bones are present and where and how are they placed?

7. Is there evidence of ritual or magic in the tomb or tomb area?

8. How does the known history of the area support the archaeological finds?

9. Are there parallels for the evidence found in the cemetery at other sites?

10. Is there evidence of an ancient disease or epidemic?

11. Based on the above, what conclusions may be reached about the nature of the cemetery? Is it a typical or abnormal cemetery?

In order to attempt to answer these questions and to formulate new ones using modern scientific techniques, Jonathan Weiland, currently a doctoral student at Stanford, is using Bio-Archaeology to attempt to put together a map of areas that may have been affected in later Roman antiquity by malaria in hopes of examining archeological sites within this zone that suggest the presence of the disease. He hopes to examine skeletal material from ongoing or recently completed excavations in Italy for which data may be readily available, including grave sites at San Donato and Vivio (Urbino area), Lucus Feroniae (near Capena in Lazio), and Vallerano (Viterbo area), as well as other sites in Umbria close to Lugnano in Teverina, such as Alviano (Weiland 2011). Only by micro-stratigraphy and laboratory analysis of ancient burial sites can we hope to have enough data to formulate more definitive conclusions about the diseases and responses to them of the ancient Romans. Soon it may be possible to learn even more about what happened to the unfortunate infants of Lugnano.

REFERENCES CITED

Bradley, K. 1991 *Discovering the Roman Family.* Oxford University Press, Oxford.

Carroll, M., and J. Rempel (editors) 2011 *Living Through the Dead: Burial and Commemoration in the Classical World (Studies in Funerary Archaeology).* Oxbow, Oxford.

Golden, M. 1988 Did the Ancients Care When Their Children Died? *Greece and Rome* 35(2):152–163.

Green, M. 1992 *Animals in Celtic Life and Myth.* Routledge, London.

Hawass, Z., Y. Z. Gad, S. Ismail, R. Khairat, D. Fathalla, N. Hasan, A. Ahmed, H. Elleithy, M. Ball, F. Gaballah, S. Wasef, M. Fateen, H. Amer, P. Gostner, A. Selim, A. Zink, and C. M. Pusch 2010 Ancestry and Pathology in King Tutankhamun's Family. *Journal of the American Medical Association* 303(7):638–647.

Hope, V. M. 2010 *Roman Death: The Dying and the Dead in Ancient Rome.* Continuum, London.

Humphries, Courtney 2010 An Evolving Foe: Applying Genomic Tools to the Fight Against Malaria. *Harvard Magazine* (March/April):42–47, 75.

Johnston, S. I. 1990 *Hecate Soteira: A Study of Hekate's Roles in the Chaldean Oracles and Related Literature* (Homage Series). Oxford University Press, Oxford.

Jongman, W. 1991 *The Economy and Society of Pompeii.* John Benjamins, Amsterdam.

MacKinnon, M. 1999 Animal bones. In *Roman Villa and a Late Roman Infant Cemetery*, edited by D. Soren and N. Soren, pp. 533–594. L'Erma di Bretschneider, Rome.

Merzagora, L. 1996 *L'altra battaglia di Cassino Contro la malaria a cinquant'anni dall'epidemia della Valle dei Liri 1946–1996*. Società Italiana di Parassitologia, Gaeta.

Millett, M., J. Pearce, and M. Struck (editors) 2013 *Burial, Society, and Context in the Roman World*. Oxbow, Oxford.

Morris, I. 1992 *Death-Ritual and Social Structure in Classical Antiquity (Key Themes in Ancient History)*. Cambridge University Press, Cambridge.

Ogden, D. 2009 *Magic, Witchcraft and Ghosts in the Greco-Roman World: A Sourcebook*. Oxford University Press, Oxford.

Pimpolari, T. 2006 *Villa romana di Poggio Gramignano, cimitero di bambini a Lugnano in Teverina*. Leader Plus, Terni.

Romer, F. 1999 Famine, Pestilence, and Brigandage in Italy in the Fifth Century AD. In *Roman Villa and a Late Roman Infant Cemetery*, edited by D. Soren and N. Soren, pp. 465–475. L'Erma di Bretschneider, Rome.

Sallares, R. 2002 *Malaria and Rome: A History of Malaria in Ancient Italy*. Oxford University Press, Oxford.

Sallares, R., A. Bouwman, and C. Anderung 2004 The Spread of Malaria to Southern Europe in Antiquity: New Approaches to Old Problems. *Medical History* 48(3):311–328.

Schiffer, M. B. 1987 *Formation Processes of the Archaeological Record*. University of New Mexico Press, Albuquerque.

Scott, E. 1991 Animal and Infant Burials in Romano-British Villas: a Revitalization Movement? In *Sacred and Profane: Proceedings of a Conference on Archaeology, Ritual, and Religion. Oxford, 1989*, edited by P. Garwood, D. Jennings, R. Skeates and J. Toms, pp. 115–121. Oxford University Committee for Archaeology, Oxford.

Scott, E. 1999 *The Archaeology of Infancy and Infant Death*. British Archaeological Reports International Series 819.

Shumka, L. 1999 A Bone Doll from the Infant Cemetery at Poggio Gramignano. In *Roman Villa and a Late Roman Infant Cemetery*, edited by D. Soren and N. Soren. L'Erma di Bretschneider, Rome.

Soren, D. 1993 Can Archaeologists Excavate Evidence of Malaria? *World Archaeology* 35(2):193–209.

Soren, D. 1995 Morte tra le rovine. *Storia* 10(94):36–41.

Soren, D. 1999a Hecate and the Infant Cemetery at Poggio Gramignano. In *Roman Villa and a Late Roman Infant Cemetery*, edited by D. Soren and N. Soren, pp. 619–631. L'Erma di Bretschneider, Rome.

Soren, D. 1999b The Infant Cemetery at Poggio Gramignano: Description and Analysis. In *Roman Villa and a Late Roman Infant Cemetery*, edited by D. Soren and N. Soren, pp. 477–527. L'Erma di Bretschneider, Rome.

Soren, D., and W. Aylward 1994 Dazzling Spaces. *Archaeology* July/August:24–28.

Soren, D., and G. Borghetti 1992 Villa a Lugnano. *Archeo* 12(2):18–19.

Soren, D., and N. Soren 1992 The Life and Death of an Italian Villa. *The Italian Journal* 6(2–3):52–57.

Soren, D., and N. Soren (editors) 1999 *Roman Villa and a Late Roman Infant Cemetery*. L'Erma di Bretschneider, Rome.

Summers, M. 1992 *The History of Witchcraft and Demonology*. Citadel, Secaucus.

Weiland, J. 2011 Malaria in Etruria, *Etruscan Studies* 14(1):97–106.

CHAPTER FOURTEEN

The Age of Consent

Children and Sexuality in Ancient Greece and Rome

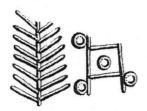

Jeannine Diddle Uzzi

Abstract *In this chapter I demonstrate that the non-Roman child from the Clementia Sarcophagus reflects and reinforces the power dynamic between Roman and non-Roman in which the Roman subject uses the non-Roman object not only for the purposes of Empire but also for sexual enjoyment. Since the publication of Craig Williams's Roman Homosexuality, it has been impossible to ignore the likelihood that pederasty was practiced at Rome. This chapter interrogates the concepts of sexuality and the age of consent, to which any notion of childhood is inextricably linked, in the hope that a frank conversation about the relationship among childhood, ethnicity, and sexuality at Rome can unfold.*

In November 2009, at the Arachne Conference in Göteborg, Sweden, I showed an image of a captive, non-Roman child from the so-called Clementia Sarcophagus (Figure 14.1 on page 252) and asked whether that image might have been an object of sexual interest for the Roman viewer. My question sparked heated debate, with some members of the audience insisting that such an interpretation was impossible, ridiculous, and informed by what they characterized as the sexual depravity of the modern world. Indeed, it is troubling for the modern mind to consider a child's body, rife with its potential for growth and change and so often held innocent and inviolable, an object of sexual interest. The funerary context of the Clementia Sarcophagus might also seem a deterrent to such an interpretation; however, there is ample evidence, both literary and visual, compelling us to consider the child on the Clementia Sarcophagus an object of erotic interest for the Roman viewer.

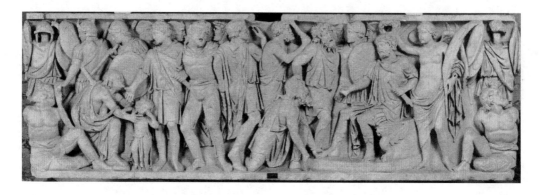

FIGURE 14.1 Clementia Sarcophagus (DAI 93/VAT.13, after Uzzi 2005).

In this chapter, I demonstrate that the Clementia child and children from similar Roman reliefs reflect and reinforce the power dynamic between Roman and non-Roman in which the Roman subject uses the non-Roman object not only for the purposes of empire but also for sexual enjoyment. Far from being shielded from the erotic gaze, images such as the Clementia child invite that gaze in a number of ways. To imagine that the erotic relationship between Rome and her conquests runs both ways, that the Romans both imagine their captives desiring Roman imperialism and at the same time gaze at non-Romans as erotic objects is not at all radical. Since the advent of postcolonialism, theorists have recognized the sexual politics of the colonial narrative. Said, for instance, while denying that the sexual politics of imperialism were "the province of his analysis" in *Orientalism*, at the same time took as given "not only [the] fecundity but [the] sexual promise (and threat)" of the Orient in the colonial narrative (1979:188). Joseph Boone has argued that Said's analysis of colonialist erotics is limited by his assumption of a heteroerotic framework and has attempted to broaden our understanding of the narrative of colonialism to include homoerotic elements (Boone 2001:90). I extend Boone's analysis to children.

Research on homoeroticism and pederasty in classical Athens blazed the trail for classicists interested in exploring the sexuality of children and the age of consent. Since the publication of Craig Williams's *Roman Homosexuality*, it has been impossible to ignore the likelihood that there was also a tradition (or at least a practice) of pederasty in Rome; however, research on Roman pederasty has been sporadic, and, as Paolo Asso notes in his treatment of Statius's *Silvae* 2.1, Latinists seem to avoid the topic of pederasty for reasons he ascribes to cultural perspective: "In previous interpretations of Statius' poem, scholars have focused on the fostering frame at the expense of the homoerotic dimension. Why leave the homoerotic man-boy rapport out of the frame? One obvious deterrent is that Glaucias was a 12 year old boy when he died and, therefore, from certain modern perspectives, Atedius Melior is a child molester. However, the sexual joys of boy-toys were far from uncommon in ancient Greece and Rome" (Asso 2010:664).

Asso is only partially correct: Amy Richlin's *The Garden of Priapus: Sexuality and Aggression in Roman Humor* entered these waters in 1983, and she was not alone. Since the publication of Kenneth Dover's groundbreaking *Greek Homosexuality*, Jonathan Walters, Marilyn Skinner, and others have joined the inquiry, including Niall McKeown, who concludes in his brief treatment of Martial that when the poet expresses interest in pretty young slave children, "[n]othing in our evidence allows us to assume that Martial's general tastes belong to some kind of deviant social sub-group within Rome" (2007:61). In fact, he notes that "[t]here were, apparently, no *legal* restrictions on Martial and his audience moving from poetic fantasy to reality, so long as the object of their desires was a slave" (McKeown 2007:61). Nevertheless, resistance to the idea of Roman pederasty lingers. Perhaps Roman pederastic practice has been easier to ignore than Greek because it is less obvious in the Roman visual record than in the Greek; perhaps this difference in the visual record has led modern viewers to surmise that pederasty was less normative for the Romans than it was in fifth-century B.C. Athens; perhaps the modern inheritance of Roman culture—especially law—and the eventual conversion of the Romans to Christianity has made us in the modern era less willing to confront aspects of Roman practice we find disturbing or distasteful. Whatever the case, instead of opening a wider field of discussion around children and sexuality, scholarly focus on classical Athenian pederasty has drawn our attention in such a way that it has become the exception to what seems an otherwise unspoken rule that children were not generally considered objects of sexual interest in the ancient world. Putting aside direct refutations of the denial of Roman pederasty that come not only from Latin poetry[1] but also from Arretine Ware, erotic frescoes, and, most elegantly, the Warren Cup, this chapter seeks to deepen our understanding of Roman sexuality and the age of consent through the interrogation of images of non-Roman children in Roman imperial relief.

Like all primary sources, the Clementia Sarcophagus benefits from the careful consideration not only of the images it contains but also its contemporary contexts—visual, funerary, and literary—as well as the precedents for it and potential influences on it. The Clementia Sarcophagus presents a non-Roman child among sexualized non-Roman adults: the child appears alongside captives, many of whom are displayed for the viewer in a way that emphasizes their position as political and sexual objects: three non-Roman men in the scene are bare-chested and frontal, displayed as what Shapiro might call "pinup boys" (1992:72). The standing figure closest to the child opens his mouth and tilts his head back as a Roman magistrate points a dagger at his genitals, which are emphasized in outline by his garments. The captives who flank the scene are used almost decoratively, their bodies like erotic bookends, mirror images of one another with hands bound behind them, opening their torsos for the viewer. The drapery of the submissive figure before the general slides from his shoulder, exposing his chest. While the kneeling woman at left may be the child's nurse, she functions in the scene as a mother figure, and her drapery also slips, exposing her breasts (see esp. Bonfante 1997:184–88). The child himself is frontal, and his body is revealed as much as concealed by his garments. The erotic nature of this scene is reinforced by the side panel of the sarcophagus where we see a non-Roman mother and child captive on a cart. That child touches the tip of a Roman soldier's spear in a suggestive gesture.

Statius's *Silvae* 2.1, which predates the Clementia Sarcophagus by 60–70 years, offers telling literary context for the relief. In his careful and convincing treatment, Paolo

Asso acknowledges the poem's homoerotic, pederastic narrative in which Statius's patron Melior mourns his foster son and beloved Glaucias, *puer delicatus,* dead at age 12. Of such *delicati,* Rawson notes that "[p]retty little boy or girl slaves were . . . welcome in adults' company as pets and adornments. These were *delicia/deliciae* (or associated terms), "delights" or "little darlings." The line between indulgent affection and sexual exploitation must have been blurred" (Rawson 2003:261; see also Richlin 1983:32–44 on pederasty and the erotic appeal of youth). Glaucias was not a slave, but he was a former slave, Melior's *libertus.* In the poem, Statius employs the homoerotic pairs Hercules and Hylas and Apollo and Hyacinthus as mythological parallels for Melior and Glaucias, and there is even a tradition in which Hercules is figured as the foster parent of Hylas.[2] Whatever the historical relationship between Melior and Glaucias, within the narrative of *Silvae* 2.1, the 12-year-old Glaucias is clearly an object of sexual interest for Melior.

The poem, a *consolatio* written for Melior on the occasion of Glaucias's death, is similar to the Clementia sarcophagus in two noteworthy ways. First, both poem and relief are funerary, and both exhibit an erotic subtext. Second, and even more important for our purposes, is the difference in status between the elite sexual actor, Melior, and the object of his erotic gaze: the social status of Glaucias as *alumnus libertus* (foster child and former slave) is similar to that of the child on the Clementia Sarcophagus, who, himself of servile status as a non-Roman captive, draws the gaze of the elite Romans wealthy enough to purchase such a work of art. As Natalie Kampen notes, "[t]he famous beloved boys—such as Domitian's favorite, the eunuch slave Earinus or Hadrian's Antinoos—are always of much lower status than the lover" (2009:65).[3]

While parallels between the Clementia Sarcophagus and *Silvae* 2.1 may be compelling, literary parallels for ancient works of art can be difficult to sustain. As tempting as it is to read the Clementia child as something of a Glaucias figure, at least 60 years separate the poetic text from the sarcophagus, and no clear causal link exists between them. Before we go any farther, therefore, we ought to consider methodology. How can we identify a work of art as erotic? If a work of art does not depict the sex act itself, that is, if it is not sexually explicit, pornographic,[4] how can we read its sexual content? To say that pornography is erotic is a tautology, but what of images such as those found on the Clementia Sarcophagus? Is it possible to unearth an erotic gaze for an image that is not pornographic? When we consider an art object, how can we locate the desire of the subject in the object viewed?

Where female images are concerned, and especially if we assume a male viewer, which we must do if we wish to reflect the patriarchies that were Greece and Rome, it is culturally normative both for us and the ancients to identify a heteroerotic object for the male gaze.[5] Whatever other sexual practices Greek and Roman men undertook—and there were certainly many—they were expected to enter into marriages and engage in sexual intercourse for the production of children. In an excellent chapter on sculpted female figures in Greek art, Robin Osborne uses Praxiteles's Aphrodite of Knidos to demonstrate how, using only the object itself, one can indeed locate the erotic gaze of the viewer. He writes, "Both ancient and modern commentators agree that Aphrodite is engaged in the private activity of bathing, but that the gesture of the right hand acknowledges that a viewer has intruded . . ." (1994:83). Aphrodite's gesture allows modern readers not only to assume a viewer but to assume something specific about that viewer: he is interested in the very thing Aphrodite tries to hide, and therefore her gesture is not only revealing but also emphatic. In this particular case, our assumptions about the erotic gaze of the ancient viewer are confirmed by the literary record, which preserves multiple erotic homages to this very sculpture, one of which claims to be an epigram of Plato.[6]

Consider likewise images of captive women from the Column of Marcus Aurelius (Figure 14.2). Of such images, Dillon remarks, "loose hair perhaps signals sexual violation, since the dress of one of these women also slips down on her arm, revealing a bare shoulder" (2006:249). Dillon claims that "drapery that slips off the shoulder, sometimes exposing the breasts, signifies physical vulnerability and sexual availability. . . . Rape is probably also implied in scenes in which women are grabbed by the hair. Bare shoulders, beautifully flowing drapery, and long, loose hair give many of these figures an erotic charge" (2006:258). We may believe that a bare breast would have elicited an erotic response in a male viewer, and we may know that the exposure of the shoulder bore erotic connotations in the ancient world, but Dillon's analysis goes so far as to suggest that the implication of rape in these scenes would have been appealing to the Roman viewer. While we might not make the same intellectual leap, there is a solid tradition in classical mythology wherein rape has an affinity with love and marriage. Images such as the Meidias Painter's rape of the Leucippidae (Sutton Figure 1.12) and stories like the rape of Persephone or the Sabine women in Livy (1.9) illustrate the conflation of marriage and rape in Greek and Roman texts (e.g., Souvrinou-Inwood, Lefkowitz, and Richlin

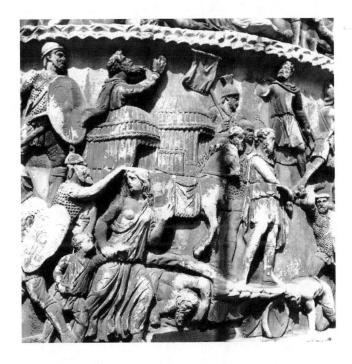

FIGURE 14.2 Column of Marcus Aurelius, Scene XX (DAI 43.84, after Uzzi 2005).

1992). Of Rome in particular, Marilyn Skinner writes, "Sex and violence . . . [were] linked . . . in . . . Roman mentality. . . . In a culture where sex was so unashamedly on display, where violence was accepted as routine, and where bodily penetration was synonymous with domination, brutality may have been erotically stimulating" (2005:197, 208).

Beth Cohen's thoughtful study of female breast baring in classical art concludes that in depictions of the rape of Leda, for example, accidental breast baring can be read as a "positive erotic symbol" for a woman who is unexpectedly raped by a god (1997:70). Similarly, of Greek art, Larissa Bonfante writes that "women appear with bared breasts in moments of great danger, to indicate their weakness and vulnerability" (1997:175). Of Roman images, Bonfante links "the barbarian captive, with one breast uncovered . . . to earlier representations of vulnerability of slaves and prisoners, and the primitive, uncivilized aspect of barbarians and other wild creatures" (1997:184). That is, while the bare breast is certainly associated with fertility, female beauty, and erotic desire, these associations must be understood alongside the "earliest and broadest context" in which the female breast is bared: scenes of rape or scenes in which violence is perpetrated against women (Cohen 1997:79). Thus, we find that erotic images of women intended for a heterosexual gaze, in addition to baring the breasts and other parts of the female body, may also conflate the sexual with the violent.[7] In fact, in scene 97 of the Column of Marcus Aurelius, a woman is stabbed in the breast. Might this image be comparable to stories in Ovid where, as Amy Richlin has suggested, the author uses mutilation of the female body to stand in for the act of rape he does not depict explicitly (1992:64)?

What of the male object? Again, Greek tradition is fundamental to our understanding of Roman imagery. Broadly speaking, there are two kinds of homoerotic imagery in Greek vase painting, depictions of the mortal male couple, *erastes* and *eromenos,* and illustrations of myths with homoerotic content, the abduction of Ganymede by Zeus, for instance. There are striking differences between depictions of human couples and depictions of mythological couples; a great deal of tenderness and restraint is shown between mortal couples, both in Greek and Roman depictions.[8] Often these images include eye contact or loving gestures between lover and beloved (Figure 14.3). In depictions of homoerotic abductions of humans by gods, in contrast, artists seem particularly interested in the body of the love object, who is often shown in frontal or three-quarter view and splayed out for the viewer (Figure 14.4). In addition, divine-human homoerotic scenes clearly present the force of the abduction, with rape often implied, especially if we can identify the myth behind the image. The hand on wrist gesture is typical, whereas in images of mortal couples, that gesture is absent.

The difference in status between divine subject and mortal object in homoerotic scenes parallels that between mortal male subject and female object in heteroerotic images. As a result, it is possible that the implied violence of homoerotic scenes added to their appeal, as appears to have happened in the heteroerotic scenes treated by Cohen and Dillon. While our concern here is not Greek and Roman pornography, the violence of heteroerotic scenes with prostitutes in Greek vase painting are often quite violent, with women bent over, beaten, and generally abused (see Shapiro 1992:64; Shapiro 1992:Figure 3.6). As Shapiro notes, however, homoerotic Greek art, even when rape is implied, prefers the depiction of pursuit to the depiction of rape per se; we can count on one

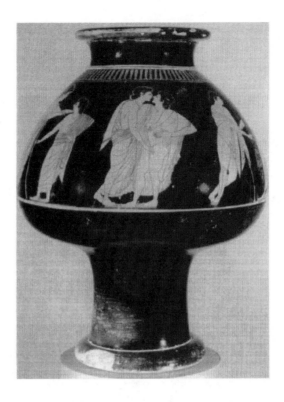

FIGURE 14.3 Homoerotic couples, red figure cup exterior (after Sutton 1992:Figure 1.4) (from his chapter in Amy Richlin's book *Pornography and Representation*).

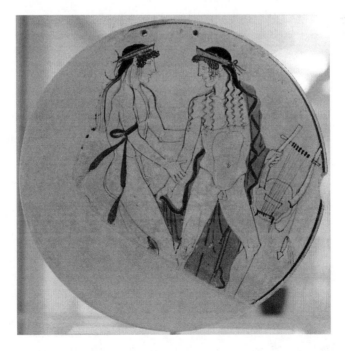

FIGURE 14.4 Eros with youth, Athenian white-ground bobbin (Metropolitan Museum of Art 28.167. Fletcher Fund 1928).

hand the number of possible scenes of forcible homoerotic intercourse that survive from all of Greek vase painting.[9]

The Barberini Faun (Pollitt 1986:Figure 146), sleeping and splayed out vulnerably, is posed something like the beloved in a homoerotic rape scene, and the Faun's arm-over-head gesture is considered by John Clarke (after Sichtermann) to be an erotic invitation, perhaps the male equivalent of drapery slipping from the shoulder of a woman.[10] Early occurrences of the gesture indicate sleep, innocence, and vulnerability more clearly perhaps than sexual availability; however, as Clarke notes, in light of such representations of Endymion and Ariadne, "a sexual interpretation is convincing, since the gesture occurs in conjunction with the motif of baring the body" (1998:68). Clarke's analysis of a silver cup from the House of Menander at Pompeii, which contains a sexually explicit scene, this time of heteroeroticism (1998:Figure 23), concludes that the man's gesture, "with right arm crooked over his head," signals a "readiness for love"—indeed a "less innocent sexual readiness"—that would have been clear to the Roman viewer following from artistic precedents both Greek and Roman, hetero- and homoerotic (Clarke 1998:68).[11] And Christopher Hallett finds that in Roman culture, the "association of near nakedness with surrender and punishment is . . . apparent in [an] early Roman custom: the repudiation of a treaty by handing over to the enemy the Roman commander who had agreed to it—*nudus*, with his hands tied behind his back" (2005: 64), a posture that opens the upper body to vulnerability and view like the hand-over-head gesture. Hallett notes that this denuding of soldiers symbolized their "total helplessness" and surrender (2005:64).

Thus, we find that nonpornographic images can exhibit something of a visual language for the artistic representation of erotic objects. Erotic images of women tend to show hair unbound and bodies partially divested of drapery. The upper shoulder and breast are often revealed. The depiction of a private moment, such as Aphrodite's bath, may disrupt the viewer's expectation for a public art object, and this may indicate that object's performance of an erotic function. The gestures and postures of objectified women may draw attention to body parts likely to have been particularly compelling for the viewer. Erotic images of men show the male body at least partially nude and often in three-quarter or frontal (or sometimes dorsal) view and splayed out for the viewer. In depictions of pursuit, the arms of the erotic object spread out, opening the chest to view. The hand-over-head gesture, which perhaps originally indicated vulnerability or helplessness, can also indicate sexual availability or readiness. These postures, characterized by the opening of the arms, chest, neck, and upper body, offer the object to the erotic gaze. Recall, for example, how one of the bare-chested non-Roman men on the Clementia Sarcophagus tilts his head in such a way as to reveal his neck: this posture participates in the language of sexual availability. Women and men alike appear in distress or as victims of violence, and the violence of such scenes may have enhanced their erotic appeal for the intended viewer. Finally, there is often a status differential in which the lover (the subject or viewer) is of higher status than the beloved (the object or the viewed).

With this language in hand, we can turn back to images of children. For children as recipients of the erotic gaze there is one clear, thoroughly vetted ancient precedent: the *erastes-eromenos* relationship is well attested not only in literary sources but also on archaic and classical black and red figure pottery such as this late archaic cup by the Brygos Painter (Figure 14.5). While widespread acknowledgment of the *erastes-eromenos* relationship in many ways revolutionized the field of classics and the study of children, specifically, it is far from our only evidence that children performed sexual functions in the fabric of Greek and Roman society. We have considered briefly Statius's *Silvae* 2.1 and the figure of the *delicatus/a* at Rome. Statius is by no means unique among Roman poets in his presentation of a youthful figure as an object of erotic interest. Catullus, Horace, Ovid, and Propertius all write poems of this nature. Catullus 48 and 99, for instance, express the speaker's erotic desire for the boy Juventius, and Horace's speaker in Epode 11 characterizes himself as burning for soft boys and girls (*mollibus in pueris aut puellis urere*).

In both Greece and Rome, girls were married at or about the time of menarche. Xenophon's *Oeconomicus* reports that Isocrates married a girl not yet fifteen years of age (7.5). Of hysteria in women, the Hippocratic corpus claims that "virgins who do not take a husband at the appropriate time for marriage experience [hysterical] visions more frequently, especially at the time of their first monthly period" (Hippocrates *On Virgins* VIII:466–470; translation from Lefkowitz and Fant 1992:Passage 349, p. 242), implying that the healthiest age of marriage for girls is at the very onset of menstruation. In Sophocles's *Women of Trachis*, Deianeira's speech poignantly imagines two distinct (although perhaps unequal) halves of a woman's life, girlhood and marriage, in which marriage defines the end of girlhood per se: "For a young life grows just so in its own place, and the heat of the sun-god and rain and winds do not strike it, but it uplifts its untroubled life in pleasure until she is called a wife instead of a girl. . ." (Sophocles 141–152; Lefkowitz and Fant 1992:Passage 31, p. 12). Note here the absence of a concept of youth as a transitional period; in this speech a girl is transformed directly into a wife with the singular act of marriage.

Roman marriage is treated similarly, with girls usually marrying between the ages of 12 and 16, but it is clear that menarche was not necessarily a precondition for marriage

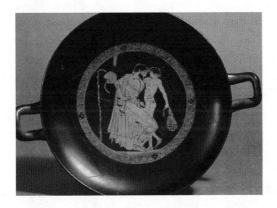

FIGURE 14.5 Homoerotic Cup Tondo, Brygos Painter (Boardman Red Figure Archaic 260, Oxford Ashmolean Museum 1967.304, from Vulci, Beazley's ARV 378, 137). After Johns 1982:Figure X.

(Hopkins 1965:309–310). Susan Treggiari's monograph reports some measure of scholarly agreement that a girl's minimum age for valid marriage was 12 years, although legal texts also assume that a girl of 12 years is *viripotens* ("ready for a husband" or "capable of taking a man") (Justinian *Institutes* 1.10); that is, textual evidence suggests that 12 is the symbolic age of sexual maturity for girls rather than a marker for the actual beginning of menarche proper (Treggiari 1991:39). Funerary epigraphs from Rome indicate that while men begin to be commemorated by wives (rather than fathers and mothers) around the age of 25, women begin to be commemorated by husbands at the age of 15 (Treggiari 1991:399–400), and it was not unusual for girls to be betrothed to men before puberty; in fact, Dio reports that Augustus, "to stop men engaging themselves to very young girls in order to claim the privileges granted to husbands and fiancés in his new law on marriage, tightened up the law disallowing engagements which did not result in marriage within two years" (Treggiari 1991:41; Dio 54.16.7).

From Dio's account we can deduce that prior to this legislative "tightening" it had been legal and apparently socially acceptable for men to engage themselves to girls who were not yet 10 years of age. Postclassical jurists set the minimum age for betrothal at seven years (*Digest* of Justinian 23.1.14), but there is evidence of much earlier betrothal, especially within the imperial family, with Vipsania Agrippina, for instance, betrothed to Tiberius at just one year of age (Treggiari 1991:153–154). Of course, betrothal is no necessary indication of sexual activity or interest, and betrothal within the imperial family had everything to do with politics and very little to do with erotic desire. For those outside the imperial family, marriage served two primary purposes: the creation of alliances between families (men) and the production of legal heirs who could inherit the property of the male line and care for their aging parents. In such a climate, girls were currency, a medium of exchange for the maintenance of patriarchy; however, understanding that the production of heirs necessarily requires sexual reproduction, the fact that girls could be betrothed before puberty and married around the age of twelve to men often twice their age or older indicates that men were able to consider very young girls objects of normative sexual interest.

Moreover, Roman authors report that in times of war or civil unrest, the Romans feared the sexual violation of their children, providing reasonable evidence that Roman soldiers might likewise have considered enemy children objects of sexual interest. Cicero claims that if Clodius had not been restrained, for example, "that man would never have held back from your children and wives his own unbridled lust" (Cic. *Mil.*76). In his speeches against Verres, accused, among other things, of seducing the daughter of Philodamus in Lampsacus, Cicero imagines the misfortune of those who were not able to keep their wives and children *integras* ("intact," "uncorrupted," or even "free") because of the *petulantia* ("wantonness" or "impudence") of Verres (Cic.*Verr.*1.14). In retelling the story of the Bacchanalian scandal, Livy wonders whether men who themselves had been shamed could defend the "chastity[12] of [their] wives and children" (Livy 39.15.14).[13] These examples do not address children in their own right but rather present "wives and children" as a combined unit of concern, supporting Dillon's claim that women and children can be read as synecdoche for an entire community; however, these few examples are sufficient to demonstrate that the sexual violation of children was imagined as a real possibility by the Romans, that the threat of this violation was even imagined to come from within their own community, and that as a result, Roman soldiers probably considered enemy children sexually available. Although they predate the Clementia Sarcophagus by many years, the fears expressed by Cicero and Livy provide a frame of reference for the non-Roman child on the sarcophagus, whose status as prisoner of war parallels that of the victims imagined above: the Clementia child found himself on the wrong side of Roman political conflict.

While legal and literary sources provide important context from which to work, our primary concern here is visual evidence. Michel Foucault wrote that "[t]he Greeks of the classical period *said* less than they *showed*" (1982:27; this claim may not strike the casual reader as odd, but it has always struck my ancient Greek students as remarkable!). Twenty years later, David Halperin used Foucault's claim to inform his thinking about the difference between, on the one hand, what people do and, on the other hand, how they talk about it. In *How to Do the History of Homosexuality*, Halperin cautions his reader not to move too quickly from the world of words to the world of deeds, recognizing a fundamental disconnect between discourse and social practice. If Foucault and Halperin are correct, it follows that when it comes to sexuality, what the ancients showed in the art they produced is just as important, and perhaps even more so, than what comes down to us in the literary, epigraphic, and legal records.

With all this in mind, let us consider a few of the visual predecessors of the Clementia Sarcophagus. Roman relief is the product of a rich visual tradition that not only informed and inspired Roman artists but provided them precedent and context for their work. By dint of its repetition, classicists and historians have made famous Horace's lines, "[C]aptive Greece seized its savage captor and brought culture to the rustic Latins" (*Epistles* 2.1.156–7),[14] and with good reason: while Greece indeed lost political hegemony to Rome, Greek art, literature, and philosophy captivated the attention and imagination of the Romans, and Roman artists in some cases spent entire careers copying Greek works of art. In his consideration of Greek influence on Roman sexual practices, Williams concludes the following:

> In view of the fact that pederasty formed an important part of Greek traditions, it is a reasonable enough supposition that among the results of Greek influence was an increase in the acceptance and practice among Roman aristocrats of romantic relationships with freeborn youth. Indeed, whereas Catullus, writing in the 60s and 50s B.C., assumed the persona of a man in love with the freeborn youth Juventius, less than a century earlier a certain Valerius Valentinus had been condemned by public opinion for having written a poem on his relationships with a freeborn boy and a freeborn girl . . . the work of such other Roman love poets as Horace, Tibullus, Propertius, and Ovid reflects a cultural environment in which men might openly express desire for both boys and girls. (Williams 1999:64–65)

Williams's conclusions can certainly be extended to the world of art, and it will serve us well to consider the Clementia child and his contemporaries not only in the context of *erastes-eromenos* images but also in the context of Greek and Roman child images that expose children's bodies in culturally significant or problematic ways, thereby offering those bodies as notable items of display.

The first of these is the *arrhephoros* ("symbol carrier") from the Parthenon frieze; second is the Dove Girl funerary stele from Paros, along with two *stelai* similar to it; the final precedents are Roman, from the Augustan Ara Pacis and Tiberian Boscoreale Cup. John Younger's analysis of the *arrhephoros* child (Figure 14.6) from the central frieze of the east side of the Parthenon takes up the sexuality of the controversial young figure who assists an older, bearded man with what is probably Athena's new *peplos*. While the specifics of the procession depicted on the frieze are a matter of ongoing debate, it is certainly an official civic procession associated with the cult of the goddess Athena. Scholarly disagreement over this child, one of the most prominent figures on the frieze of the Parthenon, arguably the most important piece of public architecture in fifth-century B.C. Athens, stems from two questions: (1) What is the gender of the child? and (2) Why are the child's buttocks exposed? Using comparative evidence from other portions of the frieze, Younger argues convincingly that the child is male. The child's costume, with *himation* draped in such a way as to reveal his body beneath, is not so easily explained. As Younger notes, it was not uncommon for boys to appear nude in public, nor was

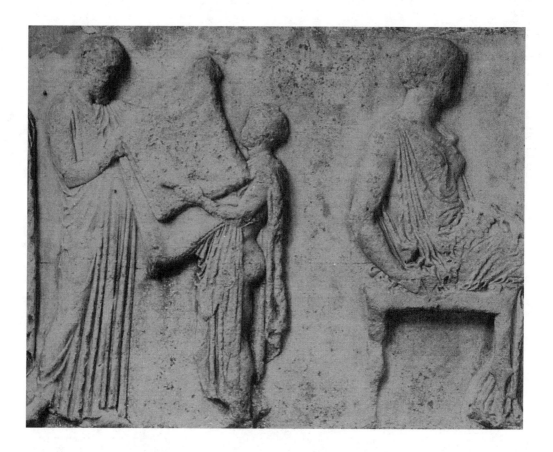

FIGURE 14.6 *Arrhephoros*, Parthenon East frieze block V, peplos-folding scene (after Younger 1997:19).

it common for boys to wear *chitons* beneath their *himations* as girls did; however, the artist in this case seems to have taken special care to expose the child's buttocks as the focal point of the frieze. Viewed within the context of the Athenian *erastes-eromenos* relationship, it is impossible not to see this pair, an older bearded man with a partially nude boy, as homoerotic.

Most important for our purposes is Younger's compelling observation that the boy from the east frieze has "a sexuality long before his puberty" (1997:138). The relationship between *erastes* and *eromenos*, like most normative sexual relationships in archaic and classical Athens, and, as we have seen, in Rome as well, was essentially imbalanced: "While faithful and abiding love was certainly possible, more often than not the homoerotic relationship lasted only as long as the younger partner, the *eromenos,* stayed young. . . . The sexual element was certainly a component but while the older *erastes* could actively pursue and take pleasure, the younger *eromenos* was expected to maintain both his emotional and physical distance" (Younger 1997:130). That is, the sexually mature partner in the relationship was expected to act in a sexually mature way, taking pleasure as he pleased, while the immature partner was expected to behave in an almost presexual way, resisting but not altogether refusing the sexual advances of the older man. The *eromenos* seems to play an important sexual role in society before he is mature enough to understand, embrace, or perhaps even experience his own sexuality. One wonders if this combination of resistance and capitulation could possibly have amounted to consent on the part of the boy: after all, as we have seen, the element of pursuit in Athenian vase painting is itself erotic, not to mention the threat of violence implied thereby. The question of consent may seem moot in a relationship characterized by such uneven power dynamics: while the *eromenos* will eventually grow up to become the political equal of his *erastes,* the power differential between a sexual adult and a pubescent or prepubescent child is clear. On the other hand, the Athenian law of *hubris,* the term for coerced homo- or heterosexual relations, applied to children as powerfully as it did to adults and probably provided some means of regulating the *erastes-eromenos* relationship (Cohen 1993:15).[15]

In his analysis of the Parthenon child, Younger uses for comparison the so-called Dove Girl (Figure 14.7 on page 264), now in the Metropolitan Museum of Art, from a funerary *stele* from the island of Paros. The girl appears in profile like the Parthenon boy, and her buttocks are likewise exposed. As Younger notes, the exposure of this child's buttocks is particularly strange because girls did not normally appear nude in public. Girls wore *chitons* beneath their *himations,* but this girl wears an open-sided *peplos* that reveals her young form beneath (Younger 1997:122). A stele from Chalkidike[16] presents a similarly exposed female child. A third example, the Giustiniani *stele,* now in Berlin, shows a similar female figure whose short, Ionic *himation* covers her buttocks but whose type seems to have served as a model for the Dove Girl. According to Younger, "the sculptor of 'Doves' started with drapery like that of 'Giustiniani' but cut out a window, as it were, to 'expose' the buttocks of the girl with the doves. The act was deliberate, though the reasons remain obscure" (Younger 1997:142, footnote 25).

These images of exposed female children are every bit as intriguing as the Parthenon boy, and the reasons for their exposure may not be as altogether obscure as Younger

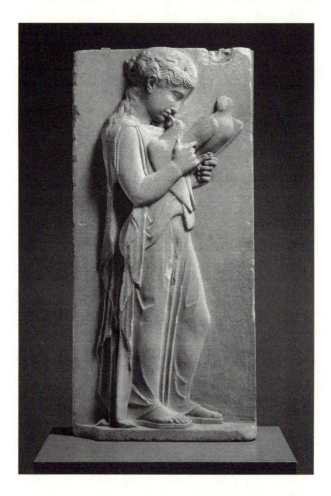

FIGURE 14.7 Dove Girl, Metropolitan Museum of Art, N.Y. (after Younger 1997).

thinks. While images of female children cannot be read within the specific context of the *erastes-eromenos* relationship per se, Julie Laskaris believes they should be read alongside it. At the 2003 meeting of the American Philological Association, Laskaris presented her initial work on children and sexuality, finding that "an important factor in Greek marriage of the classical period was sexual attraction to barely pubescent or early adolescent girls that is parallel to the attraction to boys of the same age. . . . [A]n erotics centered on the (apparent) asexuality of the childish or immature body," Laskaris claims, "was a powerful motive for marrying very young girls," and she concludes that "the pederastic ethos was not, in short, limited to same sex relationships" (Laskaris 2003).[17] If Laskaris is correct, we ought to consider the possibility that the Dove Girl, the Chalkidike *stele,* and probably the Giustiniani *stele* are images intended at least in part for the erotic gaze. A comparison of these *stelai* with other mid-fifth-century B.C. depictions illustrates how unusual they are: on the Parthenon, for instance, maidens are thoroughly and modestly draped. Considering the tender age of girls at betrothal and marriage it seems reasonable, and perhaps even necessary, to imagine that like Athenian boys, girls may also have had, as Younger terms it, sexuality before puberty. If the funerary context of the *stelai* troubles us, we ought to consider the ample evidence for the conflation of marriage and death in classical Greek art and literature, which often figures girls who die before marriage as brides of Hades (for an exhaustive list of examples, see Keuls 1985:129–152; Lefkowitz 1993; Loraux 1991; and Rehm 1994). The age of Greek girls at marriage, along with the tendency of Greek culture not only to sexualize the presexual but also to ascribe bridal qualities to a girl who died before marriage, suggests that we might reasonably reconstruct an erotic gaze for the girls on these *stelai*.

The processional frieze from the enclosure wall of the Ara Pacis depicts an official procession similar in its ceremonial, civic, and religious functions to that of the Parthenon frieze. Included in the procession are Roman children in traditionally modest Roman dress as well as two children whose bodies are revealed to the viewer. In contrast to the Parthenon boy and the Dove Girl, however, who were ethnically Greek and therefore cultural insiders, these children are dressed as non-Romans. The older boy from the south side of the frieze wears a tight diadem as well as a torque and a short tunic that slips from his shoulder like the drapery of captive women on the Column of Marcus Aurelius (Figure 14.8). His shoes are eastern, with long laces and tongues pulled up over their fronts. The younger child on the north frieze also wears a torque and a tunic that

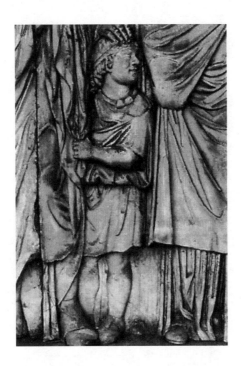

FIGURE 14.8 Ara Pacis, South Frieze Child (after Uzzi 2005).

exposes his chest and is too short to cover his buttocks (Figure 14.9). The curly, unbound hair of both children on the Ara Pacis calls to mind the hair of captive women from the Column of Marcus Aurelius. The costumes of these two children contrast markedly with the garb of the six Roman children in the processional friezes, all of whom wear full *togas* and have close-cropped or tightly bound hair.[18]

Paul Zanker identifies the younger Ara Pacis child as Lucius Caesar dressed as a "little Trojan" to remind viewers of Aeneas (1988:217); Charles Brian Rose identifies the older child from the south frieze as the son of Queen Dynamis of Bosporus (1997:57), while Erika Simon calls them simply Eastern royalty (1967:18). Corollaries for the younger Ara Pacis child are found on the Tiberian Boscoreale cup, which depicts the submission of a group of non-Romans before the emperor Augustus. Offered by their fathers (or father figures) as symbols of submission are two small children, both with exposed buttocks. In his monograph *The Roman Nude*, Christopher Hallett says the following of nudity at Rome:

> From the Roman perspective, to be stripped and exposed to public view was something that was inflicted on condemned criminals or on slaves being displayed for purchase. Accordingly in Roman society the first and most obvious connotation with public nudity was with punishment and humiliation. But even in the case of criminals and slaves, persons morally beyond

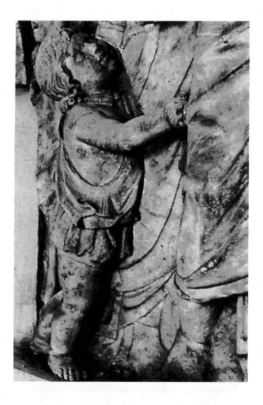

FIGURE 14.9 Ara Pacis, North Frieze Child (after Uzzi 2005).

the pale, Roman feelings of modesty were so strong that . . . those described in our ancient sources as "stripped" (*nudus*) will mostly have retained an undergarment which at least kept their sexual organs covered. (2005:61)

These children may represent the children of non-Roman rulers friendly to Rome; they may stand for captives from significant non-Roman families who were incorporated in some way into the imperial family; they may simply call to mind prisoners of war, displayed for the Roman public as in a triumph to symbolize the subjugation of their ethnic group (see Uzzi 2005:chapter 9 for a more complete analysis and interpretation of the non-Roman children on this frieze). Whatever the historical fact implied by the reliefs, these children are first and foremost artistic constructions, and, as such, their bodies are exposed in a way that echoes C. Hallett's description of the criminal and the servile, status groups associated with *infames,* those without bodily integrity under Roman law (Edwards 1997). In fact, in addition to other visual roles these boys perform—sons of foreign kings loyal to Rome, non-Roman captives, trophies of war, slaves of the imperial family, even "little Trojans," if we trust Zanker—we might consider adding *delicati* to the list.

Furthermore, the Ara Pacis and Boscoreale cup are informed by a literary tradition in which military and sexual conquest are conflated: Roman imperialism is presented as sexually desirable and captivity to the Romans as erotically charged. Consider Livy's presentation of the rape of the Sabine women, in which women whom the Romans seize by force eventually capitulate, accepting the Roman arguments that (1) "often, out of injury, gratitude soon arises," and (2) "the [Romans'] act of rape was excused by their desire and love [for the Sabine women]."[19] The following excerpt from Catullus's Poem 11 employs sex as a metaphor for territorial expansion, with the Roman male literally penetrating (*penetrabit*) a foreign space, exposing the connection between sexuality and imperialism:

> Furius and Aurelius, friends of mine—
> whether Catullus is on the outskirts
> invading Indians on Aurora's echoing shore
> or penetrating Persians or soft Arabs,
> Scythians or Parthian sharp-shooters,
> crossing seas tinged by the gaping Nile or the high Alps,
> taking it all in Caesar's wake,
> the Gallic Rhine or the terrible Brits on the final frontier,
> ready to master anything,
> following the will of the sky—

Catullus's poem clearly imagines the penetration of the non-Roman male ("soft Arab") by the Roman male ("Catullus"), and Craig Williams provides exhaustive literary evidence for male homoeroticism in the Roman world, but the homoerotic aspect of Roman imperialism has yet to enter the scholarly discourse in earnest. Instead, scholarly consensus has allowed that "territorial conquest is figured as rape of the (female) land" (Dillon 2006:262; here, Dillon follows Bahrani's analysis). As a result, few doubt that captive women were objects of sexual interest for the Roman viewer:

> Because they lack clear public roles and have no real place in Roman state art . . . women with children can serve as a synecdoche for the entire community, for a people and their future. . . . In the imperialist narrative imaged on the column [of Marcus Aurelius], a decisive and comprehensive Roman victory could only be visualized through the insertion of women into the narrative. Female bodies have long functioned in Roman imperial art as symbols both of Rome's stability and its imperial domination. Bodies of women provide a particularly expressive and supple medium with which to write the visual language of Roman victory. (Dillon 2006:262–263)

The children in these scenes have been almost entirely absent from the discussion. Even Dillon, who takes particular interest in some of the images with which I am concerned, pairs children with women, addressing the non-Roman family and the non-Roman community writ large rather than children in their own right. These children, like their male and female adult counterparts, served an erotic function for the Roman viewer.

As we have seen, the Clementia child is surrounded by sexualized non-Roman figures, figures who exhibit the types of gestures, postures, and bodily display explored in this chapter and who thereby signal their performance of erotic functions. In the context of such a sexualized kin group, the child himself becomes an erotic figure: in fact, the position of his arms can now be read in light of the erotic hand-over-head gesture discussed above. The image of Victoria at the far right of the scene, which resembles Venus or Aphrodite more than any other sculptural precedent, stands as a reminder that Roman imperial culture conflates conquest and desire. Rachel Kousser has argued effectively that the "Aphrodite-like qualities [of Victoria from the Column of Marcus Aurelius] intimate the desirable aspects of Roman imperialism" (Kousser 2006:220), the "seductions of civilization," as Kousser calls it (Woolf 1998:67–68). In addition to its demonstration of the desirability of Roman conquest, a narrative in which the conquered desires the conquerer, Victoria's sensual qualities, in conjunction with the sexualization of non-Roman figures in Roman imperial relief, show the state of captivity to the Romans—the state of being a non-Roman prisoner of war—to be essentially erotic.[21] These images demonstrate what Rome wants, and what Rome wants is the non-Roman body.

A sarcophagus from the Uffizi contemporary with the Clementia Sarcophagus includes a scene in which a non-Roman woman and child submit to a victorious Roman general. As we might expect, the woman's garment slides from her shoulder, and in this case the child is fully nude and shown from behind. Unlike the Clementia sarcophagus, whose side panel directly reinforces the narrative of the main panel, the Uffizi sarcophagus also depicts a *dextrarum iunctio* (marriage) with baby Hymen holding the marriage torch along with another nude child in a scene of bathing on the side panel. The bathing scene is clearly to be associated with the *dextrarum iunctio,* where the child stands for the first fruits of legal Roman marriage. The contrast between these reliefs highlights the difference in status between the two children, one a future citizen, the other a prisoner of war: perhaps the Uffizi sarcophagus displays with unusual clarity the ambivalent nature of the body of the child in imperial art and culture and the importance of status in defining the role of the child in the social fabric. A sarcophagus nearly identical to the Uffizi in every way can be found in Mantua at the Palazzo Ducale (Kleiner 1992:Figure 271); while the child in this case is clothed, his buttocks are emphasized rather than hidden by his trousers (for additional contemporary parallels see Brilliant 1963:154–161).

CONCLUSION

The visual record from Greece and Rome has preserved for us images of children that have perplexed classicists and art historians alike, the Parthenon *arrhephoros* and the non-Roman children from the Ara Pacis among them. If we consider these images within the context of Athenian pederasty, normative marriage to barely pubescent girls, a tradition of poetics in which young boys and girls were regular objects of erotic interest, the essential inequity of most ancient sexual relationships, and the conflation of sexual and military conquest, we find that the *erastes-eromenos* relationship is far from the exception to any rule. Far from being shielded from the erotic gaze, both male and female children seem often to have been objects of sexual interest for the adult viewer, and even images of children without explicit sexual content in this context can be seen to function as erotic objects. Literary and visual evidence compiled in this chapter demonstrates the exploitation of inequities of age (*erastes-eromenos*), gender (normative marriage), power (divine-human), ethnicity (Roman–non-Roman), and social status (freeborn-slave/freedperson) in ancient sexual relations. Therefore, while it might disturb us to imagine that children participated in this practical world of sex, playing a sexual role in society and sometimes having a sexuality before puberty, knowing what we do about the worlds of ancient Greece and Rome, perhaps it ought not surprise us.

NOTES

1. See especially Martial 9.6.4–7 and 9.8.3–4, which document the preparation of infants for the sex trade.
2. Ap. Rh. *Arg.* 1.1211. See Asso 2010:683, footnote 65.
3. See Kampen 2009:156, footnote 4 for an extensive treatment of evidence re: Earinus and Antinoos.
4. I appreciate Shapiro's analysis of the term *pornography,* which means literally in Greek "drawings of prostitutes" but which was not used in English until the nineteenth century as a term for erotic Roman paintings discovered at Pompeii (1992:53). As Shapiro says, "erotic scenes on Greek vases . . . illustrate perfectly the literal, etymological meaning of pornography" (1992:54) in that they show encounters between Athenian men and prostitutes; however, I will use the term *pornography* to refer to works of art that are explicitly erotic, many of which depict the sex act itself.
5. It is possible, and to my mind likely, that female viewers also found Praxitiles's Aphrodite erotically appealing; unfortunately, the literary and archaeological records preserve little in the way of evidence for female homoeroticism in ancient Greece or Rome. Sappho's

poetry is, of course, the most well-known evidence for female homoeroticism in ancient Greece, but classicists have shown how problematic it can be to read Sappho within a modern concept of homosexuality. See, for example, chapter 1 of duBois or Lombardo's introduction to his translation of Sappho. There is one extant red-figure Attic attributed to Apollodorus that may depict female homoeroticism, although it has also been identified as a depiction of two prostitutes (*ARV* 1565.1), and there is a smattering of literary evidence for female homoeroticism from texts such as Aristophanes's speech in Plato's *Symposium*. For an overview of Greek and Roman evidence, see Rabinowitz and Auanger. For analysis of Roman literary evidence, see Hallett 1997.

6.   "Paphian Kytherieia came through the waves to Knidos/Wanting to see her own image./ She gazed all round in an open space and/Said: Where did Praxiteles see me naked?/ Praxiteles did not see what he should not, but/The iron carved such a Paphian goddess as Ares desired!" Translated here by Page 1976.

7.   See also archaic and classical Attic pottery, on which heterosexual encounters with female prostitutes are often quite violent, as in a red-figure cup by the Brygos Painter circa 480 B.C. (Johns 1982:Figure 93; Sutton 1992).

8.   I must give credit here to Alan Shapiro for his thoughtful (1992) analysis of Greek homo-erotic vase paintings.

9.   One such rare scene may be found on an Athenian red figure cup fragment circa 480 B.C. (MFA, Boston 13.94. *ARV2* 1570, 30 (Shapiro 1992:Figure 3.6).

10.   Zahra Newby's (2002) work on Roman art follows the analysis of Sichtermann and Clarke where this gesture is concerned.

11.   For an exhaustive list of examples of the history of this particular gesture of erotic avail-ability, see Clarke's analysis of the Warren Cup, especially 1998:61–72.

12.   I render the Latin *pudicitia* here as "chastity."

13.   I am in debt to Craig Williams for compiling these examples together in his third chapter on the Roman concept of *struprum*.

14.   *Graecia capta ferum victorem cepit et artis/intulit agresti Latio.*

15.   One ought to note that it is not unusual in Athenian vase painting for the beloved, the *eromenos,* to take a certain amount of pleasure in the encounter. In some cases the *eromenos* is visibly aroused; in other instances, as in Figure 2, the *eromenos* pulls the *erastes* to him, perhaps not taking an active role but certainly not resisting either.

16.   *Archaeological Reports* 28:Figure 74. On the Dove Girl and Giustiniani *stele* see Ridgway 1970:Figures 66 and 67.

17.   Laskaris relies heavily on Henderson's analysis of Attic comedy in which he finds among the Greeks a "preference . . . for sexual objects which are sexually incompletely identified, not fully developed, and combine the physical characteristics of both sexes—women or girls who have trim, firm bodies with neat features (small breasts and hips like unripe fruit, and a minimum of pubic hair), and young, undeveloped boys who display the 'feminine' mental qualities of shyness, coyness, modesty, and the need for instruction and assistance from older men. There is a constantly expressed preference for more or less ambiguously defined sexual characteristics, a preference reflecting well-known features of pubertal sexu-ality" (1991:207).

18.   One Roman child in the processional frieze wears a belted tunic and is best read as a *camillus,* an acolyte of sorts.

19.   Livy, *Ab Urbe Condita (From the Founding of the City* or *Early History of Rome)* 1.9.15 and 1.9.16.

20. A contemporary sarcophagus from Via Collatina (Uzzi 2005:Figure 58) appears similar to the Clementia Sarcophagus in composition. At left we see a group of captive non-Romans with a non-Roman child at center. The child is nude but for a cape that flies out behind him, emphasizing his position as he strides forward; he is also frontal and splayed out. The woman behind the child, probably his mother, has unbound hair and drapery sliding from her shoulder, and the child's father, seated with hands bound behind his chest, is bare-chested and nearly frontal. Decorative male figures like the captive bookends from the Clementia Sarcophagus pepper the lid of the Via Collatina Sarcophagus, and a single bound, nude male figure appears at right. Finally, two additional male captives, one standing bare-chested near the child and the other submitting at right, have hands bound behind their backs. While many of the elements of the Via Collatina Sarcophagus echo elements of the Clementia Sarcophagus, and while I have considered it a parallel for the Clementia Sarcophagus, the apparent identification of this as a Neoptolemus scene problematizes it for the purposes of this study, which attempts to reconstruct not mythological narrative but a historical Roman gaze. Another contemporary sarcophagus from the Los Angeles County Museum of Art offers a similar scene, but the child is too poorly preserved to say anything specific about his or her role in the scene (Uzzi 2005:Figure 41).

21. While Kousser is concerned specifically with the presentation of Victoria on the Column of Marcus Aurelius, the Clementia Sarcophagus and other reliefs approximately contemporary with the column portray Victoria similarly.

REFERENCES CITED

Asso, P. 2010 Queer Consolation: Melior's Dead Boy in Statius' Silvae 2.1. *American Journal of Philology* 131:663–697.

Bahrani, Z. 2001 *Women of Babylon: Gender and Representation in Mesopotamia.* Routledge, New York.

Bonfante, L. 1997 Nursing Mothers in Classical Art. In *Naked Truths*, edited by A. O. Koloski-Ostrow and C. L. Lyons, pp. 174–196. Routledge, London.

Boone, J. 2001 Vacation Cruises; or, the Homoerotics of Orientalism. In *Post-Colonial, Queer*, edited by J. C. Hawley, pp. 89–107. State University of New York Press, Albany.

Brilliant, R. 1963 *Gesture and Rank in Roman Art.* Connecticut Academy of Arts and Sciences, New Haven.

Clarke, J. R. 1998 *Looking at Lovemaking: Constructions of Sexuality in Roman Art, 100 B.C.–A.D. 250.* University of California Press, Berkeley.

Cohen, B. 1997 Divesting the Female Breast of Clothes in Classical Sculpture. In *Naked Truths*, edited by A. O. Koloski-Ostrow and C. L. Lyons, pp. 66–92. Routledge, London.

Cohen, D. 1993 Consent and Sexual Relations in Classical Athens. In *Consent and Coercion to Sex and Marriage in Ancient and Medieval Societies*, edited by A. E. Laiou, pp. 1–16. Dumbarton Oaks Research Library and Collection, Washington, D.C.

Dillon, S. 2006 Women on the Columns of Trajan and Marcus Aurelius and the Visual Language of Roman Victory In *Representations of War in Ancient Rome*, edited by S. Dillon and K. E. Welch, pp. 244–271. Cambridge University Press, Cambridge.

duBois, P. 1995 *Sappho Is Burning.* University of Chicago Press, Chicago.

Edwards, C. 1997 Unspeakable Professions: Prostitution and Performance in Ancient Rome. In *Roman Sexualities*, edited by J. Hallett and M. Skinner, pp. 66–95. Princeton University Press, Princeton.

Foucault, M. 1982 Des caresses d'hommes considérées comme un art. *Libération* 1:27.

Hallett, C. 2005 *The Roman Nude: Heroic Portrait Statuary 200 BC–AD 300*. Oxford University Press.

Hallett, J. 1997 Female Homoeroticism and the Denial of Roman Reality in Latin Literature. In *Roman Sexualities*, edited by J. Hallett and M. Skinner, pp. 255–273. Princeton University Press, Princeton.

Halperin, D. 2002 *How to Do the History of Homosexuality*. University of Chicago Press, Chicago.

Henderson, J. 1991 *The Maculate Muse: Obscene Language in Attic Comedy*. Oxford University Press, New York.

Hopkins, M. K. 1965 The Age of Roman Girls at Marriage. *Population Studies* 18(3):309–327.

Johns, C. 1982 *Sex or Symbol? Erotic Images of Greece and Rome*. Routledge, New York.

Kampen, N. B. 2009 *Family Fictions in Roman Art*. Cambridge University Press, New York.

Keuls, E. 1985 *The Reign of the Phallus*. University of California Press, Berkeley.

Kleiner, D. 1992 *Roman Sculpture*. Yale University Press, New Haven.

Kousser, R. 2006 Conquest and Desire: Roman *Victoria* in Public and Provincial Sculpture. In *Representations of War in Ancient Rome*, edited by S. Dillon and K. E. Welch, pp. 218–243. Cambridge University Press, Cambridge.

Laskaris, Julie 2003 The Erotics of the "Asexual": The Paederastic Ideal in Greek Marriage. American Philological Association Abstracts. Electronic document, http://apaclassics.org/images/uploads/documents/abstracts/Laskaris.pdf; accessed July 15, 2013.

Lefkowitz, M. 1993 Seduction and Rape in Greek Myth. In *Consent and Coercion to Sex and Marriage in Ancient and Medieval Societies*, edited by A. E. Laiou, pp. 17–38. Dumbarton Oaks, Washington, D.C.

Lefkowitz, M., and M. Fant 1992 *Women's Life in Greece and Rome: A Sourcebook in Translation*. The Johns Hopkins University Press, Baltimore.

Lombardo, S. 2002 *Sappho: Poems and Fragments*. Hackett, Indianapolis.

Loraux, N. 1991 *Tragic Ways of Killing a Woman*. Harvard University Press, Cambridge.

McKeown, N. 2007 Had They No Shame? Martial, Statius, and Roman Sexual Attitudes toward Slave Children. In *Children, Childhood, and Society*, edited by S. Crawford and G. Shepherd, pp. 57–61. Archaeopress (British Archaeological Reports), Oxford.

Newby, Z. 2002 Reading Programs in Greco-Roman Art: Reflections on the Spada Reliefs. In *The Roman Gaze. Vision, Power, and the Body*, edited by D. Frederick, pp. 110–148. Johns Hopkins University Press, Baltimore.

Osborne, R. 1994 Looking On—Greek Style. Does the Sculpted Girl Speak to Women too? In *Classical Greece: Ancient Histories and Modern Archaeologies*, edited by I. Morris, pp. 81–96. Cambridge University Press, Cambridge.

Pollitt, J. J. 1986 *Art in the Hellenistic Age*. Cambridge University Press, New York.

Rabinowitz, N., and L. Auanger 2002 *Among Women: From the Homosocial to the Homoerotic in the Ancient World*. University of Texas Press, Austin.

Rawson, B. 2003 *Children and Childhood in Roman Italy*. Oxford University Press, Oxford.

Rehm, R. 1994 *Marriage to Death: The Conflation of Wedding and Funeral Rituals in Greek Tragedy*. Princeton University Press, Princeton.

Richlin, A. 1983 *The Garden of Priapus: Sexuality and Aggression in Roman Humor*. Oxford University Press, Oxford.

Richlin, A. 1992 Reading Ovid's Rapes. In *Pornography and Representation in Greece and Rome*, edited by A. Richlin, pp. 158–179. Oxford University Press, Oxford.

Ridgway, B. S. 1970 *The Severe Style in Classical Sculpture*. Princeton University Press, Princeton.

Rose, C. B. 1997 *Dynastic Commemoration and Imperial Portraiture in the Julio-Claudian Period*. Cambridge University Press, New York.

Said, E. W. 1979 *Orientalism*. Vintage Books.

Shapiro, H. A. 1992 Eros in Love: Pederasty and Pornography in Greece In *Pornography and Representation in Greece and Rome*, edited by A. Richlin, pp. 53–72. Oxford University Press, Oxford.

Skinner, M. 2005 *Sexuality in Greek and Roman Culture*. Blackwell, Malden, Massachusetts.

Simon, E. 1967 *Ara Pacis Augustae*. Verlag Ernst Wasmuth, Tübingen.

Souvrinou-Inwood, C. 1987 A Series of Erotic Pursuits: Images and Meanings. *Journal of Hellenic Studies* 107:131–153.

Stewart, A. 1992 *Greek Sculpture: An Exploration*. Yale University Press, New Haven.

Sutton, R. F., Jr. 1992 Pornography and Persuasion on Attic Pottery. In *Pornography and Representation in Greece and Rome*, edited by Amy Richlin, pp. 3–35. Oxford University Press, Oxford.

Treggiari, S. 1991 *Roman Marriage:* Iusti Coniuges *from the Time of Cicero to the Time of Ulpian*. Oxford University Press, Oxford.

Uzzi, J. D. 2005 *Children in the Visual Arts of Imperial Rome*. Cambridge University Press, New York.

Williams, C. A. 1999 *Roman Homosexuality: Ideologies of Masculinity in Classical Antiquity*. Oxford University Press, Oxford.

Woolf, G. 1998 *Becoming Roman: The Origins of Provincial Civilization in Gaul*. Cambridge University Press, Cambridge.

Younger, J. 1997 Gender and Sexuality on the Parthenon Frieze. In *Naked Truths*, edited by A. O. Koloski-Ostrow and C. L. Lyons, pp. 120–153. Routledge, London.

Zanker, P. 1988 *The Power of Images in the Age of Augustus*. University of Michigan, Ann Arbor.

Chapter Fifteen

"A Place for Everything and Everything in Its Place"

The Cultural Context of Late Victorian Toys

Kyle Somerville

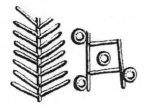

Abstract   *The Victorian period (1837–1901) saw the mass production of thousands of toys, dolls, and games designed and made specifically for children. However, in many ways these amusements say more about adult conceptions of childhood and children than they do about the children for whom they were ostensibly made. This paper explores the origins and nature of late Victorian conceptions of children and childhood, and how the material culture reflects Victorian cultural values, using both documentary evidence and examples of toys from the collection at the Margaret Woodbury Strong Museum of Play in Rochester, New York.*

For most historical archaeologists, toys, or what remains of them, are common finds on historical sites. Fragments of a bisque doll's head, a stray marble here or there, perhaps even a soldier figurine, make up most of the playthings found on nineteenth- and twentieth-century sites. And yet, these objects require us to ask a further question: Where are the rest of the toys? After all, even the game of marbles requires more than one marble to play. This question of "where" can be answered, at least partially, by entering almost any antique shop, where countless old train sets, dolls of every shape and form, board games, and mechanical toys rest on shelves or in neat little boxes.

In the strictest archaeological sense, these toys often lack the controlled provenience and contextual information of those fragmentary artifacts pulled out of the ground. While this is indeed disappointing, an examination of the cultural and social contexts in which these objects were manufactured and used can help make sense of these objects that no longer have a provenience, and can further inform upon the past lives of children and adult conceptions of what childhood was and what it should be. This chapter focuses on Victorian toys, those manufactured between roughly 1837 and 1901, and those toys, such as board games, ornate dolls, tin and steel trains and carts, mechanical banks and automatons that are rarely, if ever, found in traditional archaeological contexts.

This chapter considers what the existence of these "contextless" toys says about middle-class Victorian conceptions of children, childhood, and play, the place of these conceptions in Victorian society, and where these conceptions come from and how might toys embody them. Here, the term *child* as a distinct social being is defined according to middle-class Victorian notions of childhood, that is to say from birth to approximately early twenties, and which does not socioeconomically participate in the family unit (Calvert 1992). However, the toys under consideration here are those that were considered appropriate for children at the older end of that scale, from approximately seven to 12 years of age. All of the objects on which the remarks in this chapter draw come from the extensive collection of toys and playthings in the possession of the Margaret Woodbury Strong Museum of Play in Rochester, New York.

Because the material objects discussed below were generally only affordable by those with a disposable income, we might expect toy manufacturers to design products that reflect middle-class cultural values, thereby reinforcing them while also making money off them. As the historian Doris Wilkinson (1974:100) observes:

> Play objects are not merely items for fun, but function directly and indirectly to maintain existing beliefs and behavioral systems. They are not material trivialities. . . . Both games and toys provide a looking-glass reflection of the larger society; and one cannot offer a meaningful commentary on these cultural artifacts without evaluating them in the broader network of the systems in which they were constructed and in which they were played with.

A BRIEF OVERVIEW OF VICTORIAN CULTURE

Victorian America is generally defined by a number of different "cultural motifs" (Howe 1977). First, the Victorian period is virtually synonymous with industrial capitalism, and although the social relations between and among its classic upper, bourgeois, and proletariat delineations are the source of much archaeological research, Victorian Americans were much less class conscious than their British counterparts. That said, the most deeply held Victorian cultural values were middle-class in nature and practice. Therefore, the toys described in this paper would presumably appeal to middle-class people.

As a mosaic of social and technological changes, the Industrial Revolution introduced faster modes of transport such as steam-powered railways, and transatlantic shipping and communication such as the telegraph brought Europeans into much closer contact with other cultures, particular those of East Asia and Africa, than in previous decades, leading to an increased self-awareness of American/European culture, disseminated by the fledgling practice of anthropology and ethnographic publications. Travel, too, as a pastime of the middle class would also enhance this cultural self-consciousness, and would strongly influence middle-class perceptions about the world and its peoples, particularly with regard to nationalistic attitudes (Howe 1977). Education quickly gained in importance, and featured the establishment of numerous public schools and, in particular, kindergartens for teaching very young children (Schlereth 1991). The increase of education fueled the mass production of reading materials of all types, especially books of advice on a number of topics from health and maintenance of the home to, significantly, child rearing (Calvert 1992, Schlereth 1991).

In one sense, the Victorian period was a time of great contradiction, as society was uneasily caught between the technological wonders of the Machine Age and the social changes and problems of industrialization and urbanization. The rapid pace of these social issues thusly led to a near obsession with order: order within the universe, within society, and finally within the individual. The individual was an important component of Victorian society because it was the individual who embodied the central Victorian cultural values of hard work, morality, sexual repression, improvement of self, conscientiousness, compulsivity, and competitiveness (Howe 1977). An ordered individual would to lead to an ordered society, and ultimately, to an ordered world. These cultural values were reflected by a new materialism, in which material goods became a physical manifestation of these values within the individual (Cross 2004:32). Vices and flaws such as drunkenness and laziness were considered the result of personal failings on the part of the individual but, with discipline and will, an individual could redeem himself or herself. This sort of "moral urgency" was linked to a strong emphasis on didactic persuasion instead of physical coercion as a means of social control, resulting in a now familiar myriad of institutions such as the penitentiary, the Christian mission, and the public school (Howe 1977:20). In short, Victorian didacticism was meant to produce "a person who would no longer need reminding of his duties, who would have internalized a powerful sense of obligation and could then be safely left to his own volitions" (Howe 1977:24).

The Foundations of Victorian Conceptions of Children and Childhood

In this light, toys therefore can also be considered another form of Victorian didacticism, and an attempt to instill order within the individual at a young age. Underlying these sociocultural dimensions was an implicit tension between rationality, exemplified by the wonders of industry, and emotionalism, the very real and perceivable problems brought along by modernization. This tension, in part, accounts for the sentimentalization of childhood and desire to protect children from vice, and hence a strong emphasis on the moral individual.

Childhood, in the modern sense and usage, emerged during the Victorian period and was at least partially related to demography. Beginning in 1800, a precipitous decline in national birthrates occurred, as the average number of children born to one woman at the beginning of the century was just over seven children, falling to about five by mid-century and just over three and a half by 1900 (Cross 2004:27). Despite this decline, children still made up 22 percent of the United States' population (Calvert 1992:221). Fewer children within families led to parents having more time and resources for their children, subsequently leading to strong delineation between children and adults (Chudacoff 2007:69–70).

Victorian notions of childhood innocence built on earlier seventeenth- and eighteenth-century ideas of childhood as a time of susceptibility to influence, both good and evil. Under this view, childhood was synonymous with innocence, and therefore childhood had a particular sense of sacredness, which was corrupted by adult intervention or simply life experience. Childhood was seen as the antithesis of the modern world, full of stress and anxiety and the boredom of work. Children, on the other hand, were wondrously innocent, and "gave delight and assurance to the anxious adult, fearful of the future and alienated from the past" (Cross 2004:27). Children were thusly reified, prized simply because they were children (Cook 2004).

This view of children as pure and innocent coexisted uneasily with the notion that, as humans, children were also susceptible to evil and corruption from within themselves. As the great disseminator of manners and social grace Thomas Hill opined in 1873:

> It is painful to contemplate how many bright, beautiful children come into this world of sunshine, to sink into habits that will shadow their after-years. In all the great cities, there are large numbers of women who have been unfortunate and have left all hope behind. There were periods in their childhood when, in their girlish dreams, the world seemed all beautiful and bright. . . . In the haunts of vice and in the prisons there tens of thousands of men to-day that stood, at one time in their childhood, where the road divides . . . at the diverging point, a kind, judicious, and wise teacher might have directed them into the better way. (Hill 1967[1873]:120)

Parenting, thusly, became a struggle to foster the good within the child while controlling the potential for evil. It was this inherent duality, combined with the strong imperative to raise children to become good, moral, and ultimately ordered citizens that defined the Victorian conception of childhood, and what made childhood and children so interesting, and thus special, to American society (Calvert 1992:104).

Victorian childhood, however, was not a uniform construct but instead included a number of different stages. Very young children, from newborns to young toddlers, were considered asexual. Between the ages of three and seven, children of both sexes were dressed in clothes that combined masculine and feminine elements. This practice blurred the sexual division between boy and girl, and asserted that gender differences were irrelevant to young children while simultaneously reinforcing the notion of childhood as a stage separate and distinct from adulthood (Calvert 1992:103). Yet, this androgynous image of children was acceptable to Victorian parents so long as the "nature and destiny of each sex seemed unalterable and secure . . . and . . . that any child would be able to fill its proper place in society" (Calvert 1992:110). Therefore, gender-specific toys were the means by which parents encouraged socially correct behavior for boys and girls.

The analysis of Victorian children and their toys is therefore intimately bound up in the study of Victorian gender roles. One fundamental social change caused by industrialization was the introduction of the factory system, in which labor and its means of production are removed from individual homes into a centralized location. In turn, the home moved from a unit of production into a unit of consumption. The movement of production outside the home created a separation between the formerly connected home and workplace into the public and domestic spheres with their own prescriptions of gender roles. Men were expected to provide for their families, while women were expected to shape the home into "a temple of hearth watched over by the Household Gods" (Ruskin 1865:161); a refuge from the noise and toil of the workplace. The ideal Victorian home could only exist with the ideal Victorian woman who, in contrast to the virtues of aggression and competitiveness in the productive masculine public sphere, embodied the virtues of gentleness and compassion in the nonproductive, feminine domestic sphere, which included children (Cook 2004:31). As the keepers of the home, women were responsible for instilling in their children these values so that they might grow up to be good, moral, and productive citizens.

The different roles of gender thusly extended into notions of acceptable toys and kinds of play for boys and girls. As opposed to boyhood which was considered "unfettered and self-invested," girlhood was for "encouraging girls to view themselves as social conscious beings in constant negotiation with the expectations that surrounded them," in essence to prepare them for motherhood (Dawson 2003:63–64). Indeed, during the Victorian period, " 'boys will be boys,' had no feminine counterpart" (Calvert 1992:113). Toys thus were disciplining mechanisms to engage the child's body into his or her appropriate place within Victorian society. Bodily gestures were facilitated both by the toy itself and the material of which it was made, and children learned how to handle miniature versions of adult objects in culturally appropriate manners (Sofaer, this volume).

Consequently, boys had access to a greater number and variety of toys than girls, such as mechanical banks, train sets, and automatons, which were often made of robust materials such as metal or wood. Girls' toys, on the other hand, were often delicate, made of paper or wax, which encouraged careful handling during play. Boys' play developed courage, leadership, teamwork, and competitiveness (Calvert 1992:118), those traits that would be useful in the public sphere, while girls' play was meant to impart fashion, etiquette, and a sense of style; indeed, the stereotypical tea party with stuffed animal and doll guests was, quite literally "womanhood in miniature" (Dawson 2003:68). In sum, play was meant to encourage socially desirable traits for each sex through play, that is to say, in highly structured contexts of gendered practice (Sofaer n.d.).

Finally, children's toys were the reflection of tensions resulting from a number of parental fears. As mentioned above, children were considered to be good and pure at birth, but were susceptible to evil and vice, which would lead them to the antithesis of the deeply held cultural values that Victorians so prized. Indeed, parental fear of the vices of the outside world sat uneasily next to the recognition of the child's need to play, which itself could be a source of idle amusement (Chudacoff 2007:68). Consequently, toys became a means of isolating children from the perils of modern society by structuring play such that children would be too preoccupied to consider other, less wholesome alternatives.

COMMERCIALIZATION OF CHILDREN

The transformation of the home into a unit of consumption rather than production adds yet another wrinkle to Victorian notions of childhood. Although Wilkie (2000:100) is correct when she states that oftentimes "children's artifacts are discussed as byproducts of parents' attempts to instill values into their children, not as statements made by children," up until the end of the nineteenth century it was the parents, specifically the mothers, who were marketed to on behalf of the children, not the children themselves (Cook 2004:71; Jacobson 2008:4), and therefore many of these toys are necessarily reflective of adult views and values.

As managers of the home, women were responsible for the bulk of the material purchasing decisions made by the household. This arrangement was not lost on advertisers and department stores, who lobbied extensively for the woman's dollar through advertising and cheap consumer goods, including children's items such as toys (Schlereth 1991). Toy manufacture quickly became a big business, and the number of American toy manufacturers grew from 47 in 1850 to 173 in 1880, and included such names as Milton Bradley, Parker Brothers, and Louis Marx. Toy manufacturing as big business was especially true for Germany, long one of the West's leading manufacturers of toys, particularly dolls. In 1890, Germany exported 27.8 million Marks' worth of toys, 40 million Marks in 1895, and 53 million Marks by 1901, supplying 60 percent of the world toy market (Ganaway 2008:372). The mass production of cheap material goods, including toys, enabled children of almost any social class to have material possessions in varying grades of quality. As Chudacoff (2007:74) points out, the role of technology is an often overlooked aspect of Victorian toys. New uses of textiles, wood, metal, ceramic, and glass combined with innovations such as sheet metal stamping, improved ceramic molding techniques, and paper printing machines, which enabled the cheap and efficient mass production of tin and iron toys, dolls, and board games and books, respectively, and enabled more parents to afford these kinds of toys for their children.

CHILDREN'S TOYS: A DISCUSSION OF DOLLS, CLOCKWORK TOYS, AND BOARD GAMES

Toys serve a social role, serving as a medium of symbolic communication between adult and child, and between the child and his or her peers (Wilkie 2000:105). As a medium of symbolic communication, toys are used to instill within children cultural values they will need when they enter the adult world, and suggest and reflect norms of behavior considered appropriate for children based on their age, gender, and socioeconomic class (Wilkie 2000:101). On the whole, Victorian-era toys served precisely these functions. Not only did they emphasize differing gender roles of men and women, they also reflected the Victorian belief that childhood was a pivotal period in the development of the orderly, moral adult.

As Calvert (1992:110–111) notes, almost all toys from the Victorian period were made for only one sex or the other and only a few toys, such as board games and educational toys, were approved for both sexes. Much archaeological research has been conducted on dolls as artifacts of female identity (i.e., Engmann 2007, Wilkie 2000, Yamin 2002). Although the doll was in fact known to be a plaything for nineteenth-century boys (Calvert 1992:116), it was still a strongly feminine object. Grober (1928:27) also notes that "a history of dolls is, of course, also a history of the fashions. . . . The doll . . . was always a lady dressed in the very latest fashion," such as the 1860–1880 French wood and bisque doll shown below (Figure 15.1). These types of dolls, known as "fashion dolls," "parisiennes," or "poupées," were made for wealthy children and were dressed in the latest French finery (Strong Museum 2010).

One such doll, "Miss Jewel" (Figure 15.1), from France, has a necklace of 30 glass lenses, each holding a miniature photograph. The doll has a cutout in its back that allows light to enter the doll's body, making the miniature photographs viewable. In addition, the doll has a kaleidoscope in her head, which the child/user could view through an opening in her mouth. This doll, and others like her, was therefore quite delicate and required exceedingly careful, feminine handling, and would encourage indoor play where the doll and her carefully stitched clothes, not to mention her unique accessories, would not be soiled or damaged.

For boys, one of the most popular toys of the late nineteenth century was the mechanical bank (Figure 15.2), which came in a variety of shapes and designs, almost always with male themes and characters, such as Uncle Sam and William Tell. This suggests that the mechanical bank was a distinctly masculine toy, since it was the duty of

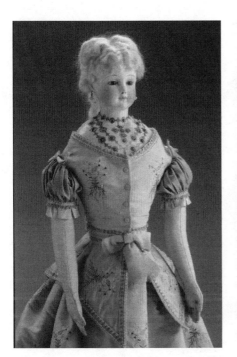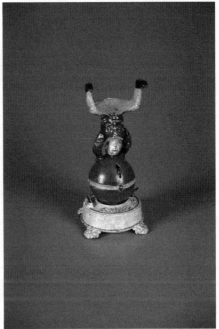

FIGURE 15.1 (left) Miss Jewel, 1860–1880 (ID# 74.1550; courtesy of Strong Museum of Play Online Collection).

FIGURE 15.2 (right) Clown Mechanical Bank, 1890 (ID# 73.1517; courtesy of Strong Museum of Play Online Collection).

the husband to go out and earn money for the household, without which it could not function. The premise behind the mechanical bank is relatively simple. Adding a coin to the bank would entertain the child, while also reinforcing the importance of saving money: in order to see the bank do a trick, a steady supply of coins was required. The mechanical bank, therefore, was meant to instill within the child the virtue of thrift while reducing the likelihood that money would be frittered away on frivolities and idle pastimes such as the penny arcade or dime novels, two perceived sources of childhood vice (Hill 1967[1873]).

An interesting development in children's' toys was the introduction of automatons and clockwork toys. The automaton (literally "acting by itself"), as a mechanical object, was not a new invention of the Victorian Age; indeed, the history of mechanical objects with the ability to move under their own power stretches far back into antiquity (Asimov 1984). The clockwork toy is one variety of the automaton, using clock gearing mechanisms to produce movement (Museum of American Heritage 1998). Though it is uncertain whether or not these toys were sold to specifically one gender or the other, Ganaway (2008) suggests that mechanical toys such as the clockwork tin train, shown below, (Figure 15.3), are generally associated with masculinity, although mechanical toys such as talking dolls were made for girls.

The clockwork toy is reflective of middle-class values in several ways. First, toys of this sort generally sold for a rather considerable amount and only middle- and upper-class families could afford them (Museum of American Heritage 1998). The ability to afford a clockwork toy, therefore, likely served as a reminder to the child that hard work, like that done by his father, would be enable him to buy those kinds of toys for his own children. On another level, the clockwork toy in general, and the motif of the toy train specifically, was a manifestation of the middle-class desire for order (Ganaway 2008:380). The clockwork toy, as a category of child's plaything, is very much a product of the Industrial Revolution, in which the mechanized toy mirrored the mechanization of the

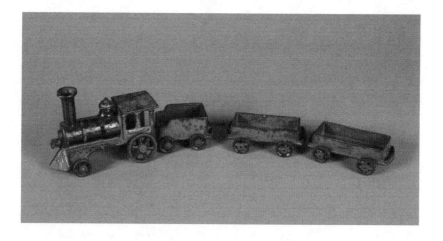

FIGURE 15.3 Tin Clockwork Train, 1890 (ID# 77.5279; courtesy of Strong Museum of Play Online Collection).

workplace. The parts for these toys required mass production of standardized, precision parts, which all fit together exactly right to produce the desired output, such as walking or talking. The toys were made for and sold to middle-class consumers, those who advocated mechanization in the workplace. In contrast, the working classes, such as the craftsmen who actually made and assembled the toys, saw an increasing decline in worker autonomy and the degradation of work through mechanization (Rice 1994). Toy trains also suggest order and mastery over the environment: they "could be made to run perfectly . . . they were never late. The workers did not strike, and the working class was not loud, noisy, or malodorous" (Ganaway 2008:380).

Lastly, the train was a symbol of the public sphere, of business, commerce, and travel; very masculine, middle-class endeavors. By the late 1800s, clockwork and other mechanical toys were made for children, but perhaps not with children in mind, illustrating what Baxter (2005:46) terms the "imperial practices of adults" and the "native practices of children." Clockwork toys are a reflection of both Victorian industrialization and "by means of which he attempted to simulate nature and domesticate natural forces . . . to imitate life by mechanical means" (Bedini 2002:1). These kinds of manufactured toys are made by adults to appeal to other adults, and the child is thusly marginalized (Mergen 1982:104).

BOARD GAMES AND EDUCATIONAL TOYS

As noted above, few toys were approved for use by both boys and girls, and those that were tended to be educational, intellectually and/or morally. One such game is *Mansion of Happiness*, (Figure 15.4) invented by the daughter of a New England minister in the 1840s, and the first mass-produced board game in the United States (Strong Museum 2010).

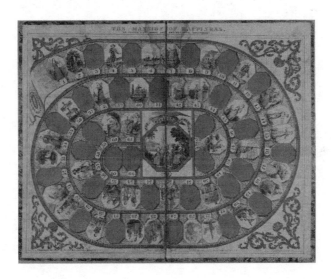

FIGURE 15.4 Mansion of Happiness, 1850 (ID# 78.412; courtesy of Strong Museum of Play Online Collection).

A player spins the spinner and moves a game piece along a path illustrated with various vices, including Audacity and Immodesty, and virtues such as Piety and Temperance (Jensen 2001). If a player landed on a virtue he or she would move forward one space, and if on a vice back one space, and sometimes, depending on the particular vice, all the way back to the starting position. The object of the game was to reach the Seat of Happiness (Heaven) in the center of the board. Other games, too, reflected both the Victorian notions of hard work, competitiveness, and self-improvement, especially for boys. For example, the goal of *The Game of District Messenger Boy* from 1890 (Figure 15.5) is to become President of the Telegraph Company (Board Game Geek 2010).

The board is divided up into a number of interconnected squares with arrows pointing the direction the player is to go. Like *Mansion of Happiness*, some of the squares have virtues and vices in which virtuous behavior is rewarded and evil behavior punished. However, the virtues, vices, punishments, and rewards are not the Christian-related ones of that earlier game. Instead, secular virtues such as Promptness, Discipline, and Affability earned players a promotion from lowly Messenger Boy to higher stations such as Clerk and Lineman, working one's way up the corporate ladder until he reaches the Office of President. However, landing on explicitly secular vices such as Impertinence, Stupidity, and Inattention sends players back to squares marked with Rebuke, Carelessness, and Discipline, respectively, which correct their deviant behaviors and enable them

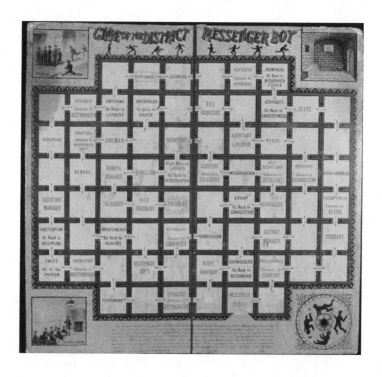

FIGURE 15.5 Game of the District Messenger Boy, 1890 (ID# 86.3001; courtesy of Strong Museum of Play Online Collection).

to continue their climb up the corporate ladder. The message of this game is clear: hard work, guided by the necessary virtues, will improve one's station in the corporate world, and ultimately, in life. It is also notable that spinners were used to determine the number of spaces a player moved, not dice, which were associated with gambling (Strong Museum 2010). Even games without an obvious moral message behind them, such as the tripartite board game package of *A Game of Cats and Mice, The Lost Diamond*, and *Gantalope* used spinners (or "Indicator," the "most desirable substitute for dice that has ever been devised" [McLoughlin Bros 1880]), for determining player movement (Board Game Geek, LLC 2010).

Other toys emphasized intellectual development. For example, the Kate Greenaway Educational wagon (Figure 15.6) has the letters A-M on one wheel, N-Z on the other, the numbers 1–12 on another wheel and the same numbers in Roman numerals on the other. The alphabet is printed around the base of the body with a picture of children dancing or playing together on it and a number of other scenes printed on it. This object is an excellent illustration of the Victorian parent's concern for teaching children through play. The wagon is rugged enough to go almost anywhere the child does, and the child can learn the building blocks of education wherever he or she travels.

Another early educational toy was the Magic Lantern (Figure 15.7 on page 286) an early image projector. Though this device was invented in the late seventeenth century, they reached their popularity in the nineteenth century and were fairly common by the end of that century (Strong Museum 2010). Slides showing a number of different subjects such as foreign lands, animals, plants, and natural wonders and reflected not only the opening up of the world by mass transportation and communication, but also middle-class notions of the importance of education for children.

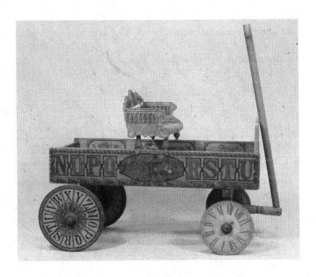

FIGURE 15.6 Kate Greenaway Educational Wagon, 1883–1893 (ID# 76.4585; courtesy of Strong Museum of Play Online Collection).

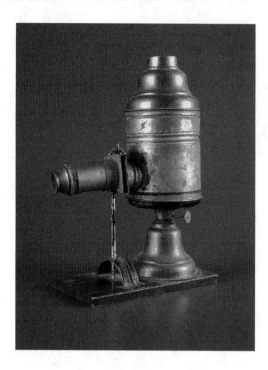

FIGURE 15.7 Magic Lantern, 1900 (ID# 78.11257; courtesy of Strong Museum of Play Online Collection).

NATIONALISTIC AND RACIAL TOYS

During the latter part of the nineteenth century, a number of nationalist movements emerged in several European countries as well as in the United States. These nationalistic sentiments subsequently found expression in all manner of children's toys. Significantly, patriotic toys were manufactured for girls as well as boys. The wax and cloth doll (Figure 15.8) appeals to civic pride, and suggests that such a pride begins at home, while toy soldiers enabled young boys to reenact the United States' most glorious victories in miniature scale. Patriotism also found itself in gender-neutral settings through educational toys. The 1900 *History of the United States* card game depicts the United States Navy at battle with a fleet of foreign ships, probably the Spanish Navy. The scene is reminiscent of the Spanish-American War, a conflict that fostered civic pride in the United States and showcased the country's entrance to its rightful place on the world stage. Glass slides depicting scenes from the conflict could also be purchased for the magic lantern, enabling the entire family to participate and share in nationalistic sentiments.

Toys with racial motifs also emerged during the Victorian period. Howe (1977:24) points out that Victorian racism was a "tragic contradiction," a jumbled mixture of an ethnocentrism characterized by the belief that some cultures were incapable of bettering

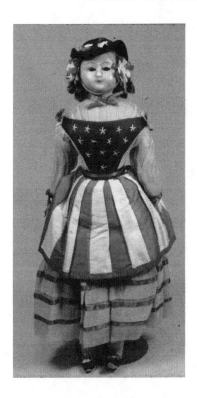
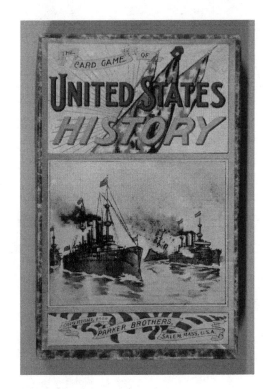

FIGURE 15.8 (left) Wax and Cloth Doll, 1850 (ID# 76.887; courtesy of Strong Museum of Play Online Collection).

FIGURE 15.9 (right) United States History Card Game, 1900 (ID# 107.2836; courtesy of Strong Museum of Play Online Collection).

themselves, at least when compared to Victorian conceptions of progress. Nationalism and biological racism, therefore, were manifested in hostility toward outsiders, those who could not be easily fit into the Victorian ordered cosmology. Consequently, racial toys, which Wilkinson (1974:100) defines as "symbolic artifacts created for children to play with to entertain themselves and learn racial attitudes and related social roles and racial dogma," provide an avenue into analysis of racial socialization and perceptions among the Victorian middle class, a group that would likely have relatively little contact with other racial groups. Toys of this sort generally appear on mechanical banks and figures, although dolls with dark-colored skin and other play objects were also manufactured and sold (Wilkinson 1974:101). Racial toys became much more common starting at the beginning of the twentieth century, although nineteenth-century examples such as the "Celebrated Negro Preacher" clockwork toy from 1882 are prevalent (Figure 15.10 on page 288).

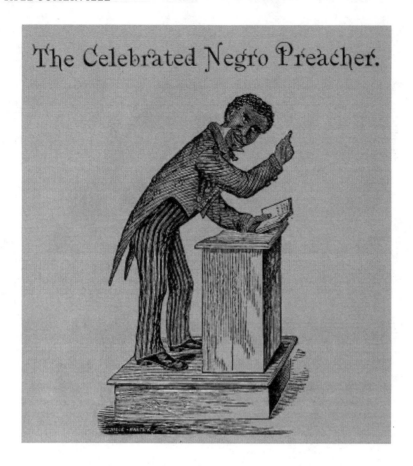

FIGURE 15.10 "Celebrated Negro Preacher" clockwork toy, 1882 (Automatic Toy Works Mechanical and Other Toys catalog).

Other toys of this type replicate nineteenth-century stereotypes of African Americans, portraying them as comical, musical, and jolly, often with grotesque physical features (Wilkinson 1974). Of the "Celebrated Negro Preacher, the toy is described in a catalog thus:

> He stands behind a desk, and slowly straightening himself up, turns his head from side to side and gestures vigorously with his arm. As he warms to his work, he leans forward over the pulpit, and shakes his head and hand at the audience, and vigorously thumps the desk. The motions are so life-like and comical that one almost believes that he is actually speaking. The face and dress alone provide irresistible laughter. He preaches as long as any preacher ought to, and stops when he gets through. (Automatic Toy Works 1882:4)

Importantly, although the vast majority of racialized toys depict African Americans, toys featuring other racial stereotypes such as gambling Chinese and dim-witted Irishmen were also sold. These objects, as the writer Bill Brown (2006:185) argues, "deanimate a stereotype, to arrest [it], to render it in three-dimensional stasis, [and] fix a demeaning and/or romanticizing racism with the fortitude of solid form" (for a more extensive examination of racialized toys and games and their roles in socializing children, see Barton and Somerville 2012).

Conclusion

The culture of middle-class Victorian America was defined by strongly delineated conceptions of gendered social roles infused within a set of motifs emphasizing an ordered, functionalist society that began with the ordered, functional individual socialized into his or her own prescribed gender roles and personal duties, all tinged with a unique sense of moral urgency. From an early age, boys and girls were nudged into their predetermined gender roles through the toys they were given and the forms of play that were enabled by these toys. Of course, children were not just passive consumers of adult values, as studies of the time noted (Croswell 1898). In large part, however, these efforts were successful, and our present conceptions of children, childhood, and acceptable toys for boys and girls, while modified somewhat, are still based on these older Victorian views.

Admittedly, the above remarks portray children as little more than pawns into which adult values were instilled through the toys they were given, and at the very least, "the extent to which children played with each toy . . . is impossible to discern" (Chudacoff 2007:85). In some regard, it is difficult to determine what children thought of mechanical banks, board games, dolls, and clockwork toys, yet some clues are apparent from journals and memoirs. Girls, in particular, were keenly aware of the differences between boys and girls and what was considered acceptable play behavior. One girl noticed that for boys, "their whole world was filled with doing, doing, doing, whereas [girls'] was made wholly of watching things get done," and many girls acted "unfeminine" by destroying their dolls or using them as weapons to attack boys (Chudacoff 2007:88). Indeed, many of these very ornate dolls were not played with at all. One woman recalled that while she had owned a very elegant, and very expensive, imported wax doll, her favorite toys were crude rag dolls she had made, due in no small part to the fact that the rag dolls were durable and more conducive to play in a number of different environments, as opposed to "the London doll that lay in waxen state in an upper drawer at home—the fine lady that did not wish to be played with, but only looked at and admired" (quoted in Calvert 1992:113). Nor were the possession of toys a barometer of a child's happiness. One man, the son of wealthy parents, mentioned that despite the fact that he had a large number of fantastic and expensive toys he did not have fond memories of his childhood, noting that he was often bored and "became blasé in the truest sense of the word" (quoted in Ganaway 2008:377).

In an 1898 survey of 2,000 boys and girls in Worcester, Massachusetts, the psychologist T. R. Croswell asked 1,000 boys and 1,000 girls to identify their favorite toys and games (Croswell 1898; Calvert 1992). Croswell found that, although 621 girls owned dolls, only 233 said playing with their dolls was their favorite activity, while only 27 boys named toy trains as their favorite pastime and only two children liked toy soldiers. In addition, only 87 boys and 34 girls listed board games as a favorite activity. Informal toys and games were most popular with children. Croswell's study identified more than 700 different kinds of amusements, all of which required very few, if any, manufactured materials to use. Toys were sometimes used in ways their creators never intended, and children were also quite inventive in making their own toys. One child created play money by punching out the tops of fruit and vegetable cans, while others used nature to make playthings such as the ubiquitous mud pie (Chudacoff 2007:84).

As the archaeologist Laurie Wilkie (2000:101) astutely notes, toys and children are recognizable and critical components of the material record, and the objects associated with them must be viewed as dialogues of control and resistance. These objects are no exception, and are an excellent illustration of the classic Victorian maxim, "A place for everything, and everything in its place." Victorian toys were attempts by parents to shape and control children's physical, mental, and moral bodies by instilling bodily and moral order within boys and girls, ensuring that they would become model, moral individuals who knew their respective roles in society. Yet it would be wrong to assume that Victorian children always, if ever, followed willingly the path shown to them by their parents. Consequently, these objects say much more about the adults giving the toys than the children who received them.

ACKNOWLEDGMENTS

Unless otherwise noted, the images in this paper are courtesy of the Margaret Woodbury Strong Museum of Play Online Collection, an excellent resource for the historical archaeologist interested in toys and children. Images are used under a Creative Commons Attribution—Noncommercial—No Derivative Works 3.0 United States License (http://creativecommons.org/licenses/by–nc–nd/3.0/us/). My sincere thanks to Dr. Güner Coşkunsu in providing guidance for this paper. Her boundless enthusiasm and interest in the archaeology of childhood is an inspiration. And as always, my deepest gratitude to Sissie Pipes, Robert L. Schuyler, Paul Powers, and Christopher P. Barton.

REFERENCES CITED

Asimov, I. 1984 *How Did We Find Out About Robots?* Walker, New York.

Automatic Toy Works 1882 *Mechanical and Other Toys.* New York City.

Barton, C. P., and K. Somerville 2012 Play Things: Children's Racialized Mechanical Banks and Toys 1870–1930. *International Journal of Historical Archaeology* 16:47–85.

Baxter, J. E. 2005 *The Archaeology of Childhood: Children, Gender, and Material Culture.* AltaMira Press, Walnut Creek, California.

Bedini, S. A. 2002 The Role of Automata in the History of Technology. Electronic document, web.mit.edu/lira/www/fall02_indStudy/b_edini_historyAutomata.pdf; accessed March 1, 2010. Massachusetts Institute of Technology.

Board Game Geek, LLC 2010 The Game of District Messenger Boy (1886). Electronic document, www.boardgamegeek.com/boardgame/14245/the–game–of–district–messenger–boy; accessed March 1, 2010.

Brown, B. 2006 Reification, Reanimation, and the American Uncanny. *Critical Inquiry* 32:175–207.

Calvert, K. L. F. 1992 *Children in the House: The Material Culture of Early Childhood, 1600–1900*. Northeastern University Press, Boston.

Chudacoff, H. 2007 *Children at Play: An American History*. New York University Press, New York City.

Cook, D. T. 2004 *The Commodification of Childhood*. Duke University Press, London.

Cross, G. S. 2004 *The Cute and the Cool: Wondrous Innocence and Modern American Children's Culture*. Oxford University Press, New York.

Croswell, T. R. 1898 Amusements of Worcester School Children. *Pedagogical Seminary* 6:314–371.

Dawson, M. 2003 The Miniaturizing of Girlhood: Nineteenth-Century Playtime and Gendered Theories of Development. In *The American Child: a Cultural Studies Reader*, edited by C. F. Levander and C. J. Singley, pp. 63–84. Rutgers University Press, New Brunswick, New Jersey.

Engmann, R. 2007 Ceramic Dolls and Figurines, Citizenship and Consumer Culture in Market Street Chinatown, San Jose. Unpublished archaeological report, Market Street China Town Archaeological Project, San Jose, California. Stanford University.

Ganaway, B. 2008 Engineers or Artists? Toys, Class, and Technology in Wilhemine Germany. *Journal of Social History* 42(2):371–401.

The Great Treasure Hunt 2010 Mechanical Banks. Electronic document, www.webuytreasure. com/gallery2/main.php/v/MechanicalBanks/boys_stealing_watermelons.gif.html; accessed March 9, 2010.

Grober, K. 1928 Children's Toys of Bygone Days: A History of Playthings of All Peoples from Prehistoric Times to the XIXth Century. Frederick A. Stokes, New York City.

Hill, T. E. 1967 [1873] *Never Give a Lady a Restive Horse: A Manual of Manners or, How to Do the Right Thing at the Right Time in the Various Important Positions of Life*. Diablo Press, Berkeley, California.

Howe, D. W. 1977 Victorian Culture in America. In *Victorian America*, edited by D. W. Howe, pp. 3–28. University of Pennsylvania Press, Philadelphia.

Jacobson, L. 2008 Advertising, Mass Merchandising and the Creation of Children's Consumer Culture. In *Children and Consumer Culture in American Society: a Historical Handbook and Guide*, edited by L. Jacobson, pp. 3–26. Praeger, Westport, Connecticut.

Jensen, J. 2001 Teaching Success Through Play: American Board And Table Games, 1840–1900. *Magazine Antiques* December:1–6.

McLoughlin Brothers 1880 *Directions for Playing the New Games of Cats and Mice, Gantalope, and Lost Diamond*. McLoughlin Brothers, New York. Electronic document, www.gamearchives. org/rules/McLoughlinBros_Cats+Mice.pdf; accessed March 1, 2010.

Mergen, B. 1982 *Play and Playthings: A Reference Guide*. Greenwood Press, Westport, Connecticut.

Museum of American Heritage 1998 Toys and More. Electronic Document, www.moah.org/ exhibits/archives/toysnmore/toys.html; accessed March 1, 2010.

Rice, S. P. 1994 Making Way for the Machine: Maelzel's Automaton Chess-Player and Antebellum American Culture. *Proceedings of the Massachusetts Historical Society* 106:1–16.

Ruskin, J. 1865 *Sesame and Lilies*. Henry Altemus, Philadelphia.

Schlereth, T. J. 1991 *Victorian America: Transformations in Everyday Life, 1876–1915*. Harper Collins, New York City.

Strong Museum of Play 2010 Online Collections. Electronic document, www.museumofplay.org/ collections/online; accessed March 1, 2010.

Wilkie, L. 2000 Not Merely Child's Play: Creating a Historical Archaeology of Children and Childhood. In *Children and Material Culture*, edited by J. Sofaer Derevenski, pp. 100–113. Routledge, New York.

Wilkinson, D. Y. 1974 Racial Socialization through Children's Toys: A Sociohistorical Examination. *Journal of Black Studies* 5(1):96–109.

Yamin, R. 2002 Children's Strikes, Parents' Rights: Paterson and Five Points. *International Journal of Historical Archaeology* 6(2):1–14.

PART IV

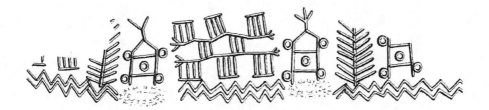

Commentaries

CHAPTER SIXTEEN

Theoretical Issues in Investigating Childhood

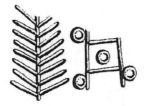

Frank Hole

As a traditional "dirt" archaeologist, I was exposed for the first time to the subject of children in archaeology, and I have learned a great deal from participating in the seminar and reading the contributions. This, of course, is the reason for holding such seminars: we learn from one another. The remarks that follow are from my distinctly personal perspective, yet I hope that there will be some ideas among them that spark further discussion and investigation.

There is general agreement that the study of children is closely related to attempts to recognize women, as well as various genders, ethnicities, and ages. All of these have, or achieve, identities through various passive and active processes, which may be discernible archaeologically when we know what to look for. The six theoretical papers in this session thoroughly discuss the enigma of searching for childhood, while the subsequent case studies provide examples of how we might see and understand childhood in the remote past. On the one hand, we recognize that individuals go through a developmental and social trajectory from birth through death. On the other hand, the way people conceptualize and actualize these biological and social changes varies considerably in different cultures today and no doubt in the archaeological past as well. Without children, it is obvious that there would be no human societies, but it remains a question, whether as archaeologists we should focus on discovery and interpretation of children, or on their developmental relationships to society at large With this latter perspective, children are part of the whole and are unremarkable except that adults had to create practices and institutions to enable them to develop to the age of reproduction, assume their social identities and economic roles, and thus ensure the viability of the family and society.

The very idea of family and society and, by extension, the role of children, is based on what we know from the modern world. As archaeologists, particularly those who work in the prehistoric ranges of time, we should question whether our modern notions have pertinence, although the biological fact of childhood is never in doubt. When even our conceptions of the role of children are not universal among today's cultures, it is hard to know even what we might look for archaeologically as evidence of children unless we keep the broader societal context in mind. There will be further similar observations in my discussion of the papers in this session.

Like others in this session, Baxter asks (and answers) the question of whether studies of children and childhood have a significant place in archaeology. She compares childhood studies to those of race, identity, and gender, all vying for legitimacy in the broad field of archaeology. All are concerned with personal identity. Many archaeologists treat children as incidental or irrelevant and are deterred by the idea that physical evidence of children, apart from burials, is likely to be scant, if not entirely absent. After reviewing a large corpus of literature on the subject of childhood in archaeology, Baxter sees some promising leads for investigation. However, the literature she cites is largely theoretical, referring only rarely to actual instances from ethnographic or historical literature.

Baxter reminds us that childhood is a concept that varies with context and she makes a good case for quite different concepts of childhood in Colonial America. The examples she uses, of the coral bell and family portraits, bespeak an elite status that may not have been typical of the common folk. She also raises the important point, also made by others in this session, that children are part of an integrated family and may be expected to grow into adult roles rather seamlessly within the family itself. We can contrast this with our world where children are removed from the family to attend school and lessons. In many societies, children play with one another away from direct parental supervision; in others, girls are kept at home, while boys roam. When the co-resident group is very small, there may be only one child. As these cases imply, there are very different potential ways that children might be recognized archaeologically or remain invisible.

It is somewhat easier to discuss concrete examples, and I return to the coral bell. It reminded me that in historic archaeology we often find clay pipes, fragments of porcelain dolls, bits of toy trucks, and other similar objects. These give insight into the family, its affluence, and role expectations, as well as to the structure of society and the ideology of its culture. Take dolls, for example. They depict babies, children, and adults, according to social norms. They say that children play, probably using dolls as actors in an imaginary world, which copies what they see in life. They also inform on gender roles, and many other aspects of their culture. In short, there is rich potential to reconstruct a vivid picture of people in the past. Unfortunately, these durable playthings which speak so eloquently in historic archaeology are absent from most archaeological sites, and perhaps their perishable analogs have been lost as well.

Scott Hutson's chapter is largely theoretical, examining the issue of the "visibility" of children in archaeology using direct "smoking gun" and indirect "relational" evidence. By way of illustration he considers figurines and architecture, and he employs a distinction between "children as active subjects or passive objects." In the former, children take an active role in creating their identities, whereas in the latter their growth as individuals is largely conditioned by the norms of their immediate society.

Archaeological evidence of children as active agents can be seen in productions that can be attributed to children, such as figurines indented with children's fingerprints, or "childlike" manipulation of the clay. In the making of figurines, children "reproduce a very particular theory of the body," which ultimately will contribute to the perpetuation of social norms. Toys, including figurines, made by children are a good example where children reproduce their version of a living context.

Hutson emphasizes the linkages among all age groups and suggests that children may have, in some cultures, been considered imbued with purity. Figurines made by them may thus have held some ritual significance and were used as magical amulets to protect the children from harm. Here the children were active agents and passive recipients. For an analogous situation, among modern cultures of the Near East, children may have amulets, blue beads, and capsules with verses of the Koran sewn into their clothing. In this case, however, children were the recipients, not the creators of the amulets; hence, they were passive.

While architecture seldom reveals evidence explicitly of children, we know that children lived in houses with other members of the co-resident group. The important point is that children learn spatial relations, uses of space, and norms of household behavior. Children are both passive recipients of common understandings, and active agents when they construct their own dwellings.

<hr />

Katherine Kamp has written a largely theoretical piece informed in part by her studies of Pueblo society. Like others, Kamp sees children's studies as similar to and part of age and gender studies, whose value is to enrich and enhance our understanding of past cultures. She argues that while studies of children must be an important part of archaeological interpretation, it is only through rigorous ethnoarchaeological studies of the relationship between children and material culture that archaeologists can advance the field, and she admonishes archaeologists to pay close attention to methodological rigor when conducting such studies.

Kamp reviews the kinds of archaeological evidence that may inform on children, but she raises cautions about each. For example, although text and art are rich sources of information they are inherently biased to show the point of view of the persons who created them. Other direct evidence, such as burials, can inform on the physical condition of the deceased, as well as on the ways ritual was employed on persons of different age and gender. Her pioneering of the use of fingerprints to identify the work of children is remarkable, but she cautions that just because children may have made an object, it does not follow that the uses and meanings of the objects can be inferred. One promising avenue of interpretation concerns the uses of space within the household, camp or village. She observes that children may have activity areas separate from those of adults and that close attention to the spatial distribution of these may lead to interpretations of children's activities.

Perhaps the most important part of her chapter is to consider how children participated in the trajectory of social and cultural development: individuals of different ages have different roles and responsibilities as they carry out their activities of daily living. Protection of the young, as well as the potential contributions of children to the economic and social well-being of the communities, should be considered. This leads to thinking about life expectancies, and reproducing viable families and communities. In other words, life is not just about the moment, but it needs to consider its future as well as its present needs. The remains we excavate are evidence of the success of this balancing act.

Nurit Bird-David's paper is an important corrective to those of us who normally use English (or another Western language) where social categories are based on the assumption that there is a separation between adults and children, where children have their own "worlds and cultures." Using her studies of a hunter-gatherer group in India, Bird-David explores the concept and term *children* and of the combine *parent-children*. She argues that the English terms create distinctions and implications that are not evident in hunter-gatherer (read very small group) societies. Such societies most likely represented nearly all human societies before the advent of agriculture, so her admonition is potentially applicable to most of human history. Nowhere in hunter-gatherer society is there a formal school where children are separated from the group and taught lessons. Rather we should think of adult-child communities as single and inseparable, but developing, entities.

She argues that, rather than distinguish between parent and child or to isolate childhood as a class by itself, in small societies children are part of, rather than separate from, the entirety of activity. She notes how in any small group there may be only one young person of a given age (child) and that perforce its interactions will always be with adults. In such circumstances the "child" participates in all activities, insofar as its physical abilities allow. Children are not "taught"; rather they learn by imitation and use the tools of adults. Children need not be overtly protected from danger since they are always "working" alongside adults. Children may play, often in imitation of adults, such as shooting arrows with tiny bows, but they are expected to pitch in when they can be useful.

In human history most groups must have been constituted somewhat along the lines outlined by Bird-David. In these communities, with very small populations, the distinctions between parent-child and adults-children may have been blurred, not least because life expectancies often were short and could break the biological connections unexpectedly. At some point in human history the idea of "family" became the dominant paradigm. It is possible that this occurred after the advent of agriculture, with residential stability and larger populations, but this is a matter for theorizing and investigation.

The paper by Joanna Sofaer delves into the seemingly intractable problem of identifying children when we have no bodies. For that matter we normally have few bodies of any age or sex, in relation to the potential population resident at a site. Even when we do find bodies, the information they yield is often confined to age, sex, pathology, or trauma. While such information can provide data on demographic profiles, it does little to inform on the kinds of lives the people led. Even when skeletons are found with beads, pots, sacrificed animals, and tools of various sorts, the lives of the people still remain largely conjectural. What do we make, for example of the few decorated skeletons among hundreds from the Epipaleolithic Natufian of the Levant? While most bodies were unadorned, a few, including children, women, and men, were richly adorned (Wyllie and Hole 2012). The social context that underlies these differences is entirely opaque. Clearly, the beaded bodies represent identities, but whose? Are they of the deceased or those who buried them? And what about the bodies without beads? Might they have been adorned with feathers and paint? Unfortunately even with modern advances in analysis, bodily adornment of individuals remains largely invisible. The point, however, is that the bodies with beads may have been the poor relations, not the elite. Sofaer maintains that archaeologists have been too preoccupied with bodies, and I agree. Except for biological markers, bones are mute.

There is, however, some potential for seeing "invisible" children in archaeology. As I interpret her argument, about how to make and use one's physical and social space, one can follow the *châine opératoire,* of both the making and using. Most explicitly, this can be seen in apprenticeship, but more broadly in the understanding that living, making, and using require periods of development before competence is achieved. Her arguments apply equally to all members of a society, not just children. Seeking evidence of tasks, variability in the ways they were achieved, and stages in the way individuals develop competence, may be a promising avenue for investigation.

Jack Meacham's chapter attempts to set out the ways we might conceive of children through the use of four metaphors: essence, organism, machine, and historical context. This chapter meshes in part with Sofaer's, particularly in regard to the instruction children are given and the ways they embrace or deviate from it. According to Meacham, society works toward developing a child and the child works toward establishing an identity. The specific ways these goals are accomplished varies according to the cultural milieu and the physical environments the child is exposed to.

In Meacham's terms, the *mechanistic* perspective (his metaphor) is one in which adults imbue children with social and cultural skills, as well as task-oriented skills. The former are taught in the context of society, and the latter through apprenticeship or education. From his *contextualist* perspective, the child learns not directly from adults, but from experience.

The relevance for archaeology and anthropology is that children teach themselves through interaction with their peers as well as adults. We see this all the time. Children learn from other children, and pass on to younger children, games, chants, and dances. Children create their own cultures with rules and ways of talking and behaving that are mysterious (perhaps deliberately so) to their parents. Beyond these, however, children play make-believe games in which they act out adult roles. Here, learning takes place through replicating behavior they have witnessed. Archaeologically, we may see evidence in the form of miniature vessels, figurines of livestock, and models of dwellings. In short, several forces act upon developing children, some are inherent or imposed, others created by children themselves.

While these ideas are both theoretical and empirical, there is another factor that must impact many, if not most, prehistoric societies. This is the composition of the co-resident group. In many hunter-gatherer groups there may be only one child, or children of different ages and sex. There is little opportunity for peer-to-peer interaction; rather, adult-child interaction, as Bird outlined, may be the norm. Moreover, among the simpler societies there may be little material culture that has survived. In such cases, there may be little physical evidence of children, hence "invisible."

One way to think about the notion of childhood in archaeology is to ask ourselves what archaeology is or what we would wish archaeology to be. By its nature, archaeology is mostly concerned with material things and the contexts in which they occur, both spatial and temporal. Archaeology has traditionally concerned itself with artifacts, which can be organized into a time-series—a kind of quasi-history in which the fates of individual "cultures" waxed and waned in response to social, political, technical, and environment changes. Many archaeologists see not people, but "cultures" subsisting, building, trading, and making artifacts. The traditional focus is on the collective rather than the individual. There is little room in these goals for ruminations about the roles of children. The principal actors in such scenarios were adults, and the effects on society of having to raise children have been ignored. This is traditional archaeology. What the scholars in this session want to do is to peer into the "cultures" and see the people, to see in their life histories a struggle to achieve personal identities. With this larger goal, it seems to me that, rather than focus narrowly on children, it would be better to consider the base unit of society, the family or co-resident group. Its social and biological composition differs among cultures and certainly has changed over human history. If we can get a handle on this it may speak more clearly about children than a focus exclusively on the latter.

References Cited

Wyllie, C., and F. Hole 2012 Personal Adornment in the Epi-Paleolithic of the Levant. In *7th International Conference on the Archaeology of the Ancient Near East*, Vol. 3, pp. 707–717. British Museum, London; Harrassowitz, Wiesbaden.

CHAPTER SEVENTEEN

Grubby Little Fingerprints

A Commentary on the Visibility of Childhood

Traci Ardren

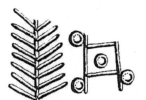

Güner Coşkunsu posed a fascinating question when she set out to organize the Third Annual Institute for European and Mediterranean Archaeology conference at the University of Buffalo. Coşkunsu challenged participants to address the question of whether children were visible or invisible in the archaeological record. At first glance, to someone deeply engaged with childhood studies like myself, this is a deceptively easy question to answer. Yes, children are visible everywhere in the archaeological record—in societies both recent and very ancient, children left an indelible mark on the material world around them which has been preserved for us to recover today.

But Coşkunsu was after something much deeper. Rather than debate the presence or absence of young people in the material record, she wanted us to explore why children remain such an enigma in archaeological theories and explanations of the past. Why, eight years after Jane Eva Baxter's landmark volume *The Archaeology of Childhood* (2005), and even longer since such foundational works as *Children and Material Culture* (Sofaer Derevenski 2000), *The Archaeology of Infancy and Infant Death* (Scott 1999), and *Invisible People and Processes: Writing Gender and Childhood into European Archaeology* (Moore and Scott 1997), and despite frequent conferences on the subject of childhood as a significant social identity, are so few archaeologists asking questions about how children and childhood structured the ancient societies we study (cf. Baxter 2008)? Participants in the conference were asked to literally materialize children in their studies of past cultures, not in the sense (only) of recovering the tangible remains of young people, but in the more profound sense of centering our perspective on the child and the unique social circumstances of this social identity. We should not underestimate how significant a shift this required, since traditional archaeological questions derive primarily from the values and concerns of modern Western society, and the Western gaze does not often come to rest upon children as cultural innovators or particularly meaningful components of social relations.

The title of this commentary is an allusion to familiar materializations that, like children in the ancient past, are everywhere, whether or not we are able to perceive them. Our self-imposed blinders are historically situated and not characteristic of all cultures, as much of the research presented in this volume demonstrates forcefully. All adults pass through the experiences of childhood, however a given society defines that period of life, and thus the nature of how childhood is understood and experienced, the cultural forms that are used to circulate what it means to be a child and to leave that status behind are part of everyone who survives to adulthood, whether we choose to acknowledge that experience or not. Returning to Coşkunsu's charge, that we explore why children are an archaeological enigma—the chapters in this volume make it abundantly clear, in a thoroughly current and overarching way, that data are present to explore the role of children in all ancient cultures and children are significant social actors in every culture. Thus, one answer to the question is simply that we, as a discipline, are still grappling with our own biases and cultural values, which continue to limit the questions we ask and the actors we deem of interest for sustained scholarly investigation.

The inquiries of contributors to this publication are both innovative and grounded in many of the most important and long-standing areas of archaeological inquiry. Themes that cross-cut the chapters include not only the construction of age-based identities such as childhood, but also such key arenas of cultural transmission as death and grieving, individual agency versus group membership, and gendered relations. My comments on the contributions will focus on each of these three themes.

Archaeologists have been studying the dead for as long as our field has existed, and we do so with both rigor and enthusiasm. But when we approach the burials of children, our usual scientific objectivity, with its expectation of emotionless description, flies out the window, despite decades of research into how children are treated in death. In our analyses, we comment on the "obvious" emotion conveyed by the miniature skeletal remains and grave goods, as one of the most significant characteristics of these funerary deposits. In point of fact, we do not know the emotional state of those who performed the funerary rituals we see materialized in the archaeological record, but we very often imagine that state to be similar to what is expected in modern Western culture where child death is automatically a tragedy. We turn our gaze upon those elements of the context that support this perspective on death, or alternatively comment on the (apparent) absence of emotion, often in a way that conveys how uncomfortable it is to us, that ancient societies of the past may not have been as sentimental or "caring" toward their young ones (Ardren 2011).

The very rich data provided on a Classical period infant cemetery in Lugano, Italy, by David Soren challenge us to understand how the rural inhabitants of Umbria understood and managed a widespread malarial epidemic that affected the very young members of the settlement. An abandoned villa was reutilized as an infant cemetery in which children were buried rapidly and with almost no grave goods. The presence of a large number of dogs buried in the same cemetery and the identification of the human remains as primarily fetuses and neonates are the distinguishing features of this special deposit. The fascinating analysis provided by Soren demonstrates that our anthropological understanding of infant death is an area in which much further research is required. Infants in particular have been conceptualized as liminal beings and not fully part of the human family, although the details of what this means vary in each culture (Gottlieb 2004; Hope 2009; Scott 1999). Paul Bahn provides a very useful summary of available data on Paleolithic child burials, some of which are at least 200,000 years old and thus establish that the deliberate burial of the young arose in concert with the origin of funerary treatments. From the site of La Ferrassie, France, Bahn shows that carefully made flint artifacts were placed frequently with the burials of infants and children during the Neanderthal period. The presence of grave goods such as flint or ochre with infant burials argues that the value of children to our earliest ancestors originated not in the work they could perform or their ability to accrue wealth for their families, but was rather inherent in their existence from birth or before, perhaps residing in the sense of potential an infant possesses. Children were not always as shielded from death and the dying as they are in our culture today, and Susan Langdon presents compelling data to demonstrate the presence of young people at the funerals of others within Iron Age Athens, Greece. Langdon identifies imperfectly made miniature ceramic vessels that are commonly found in graves of the period as a materialization of the connection between young potters and the deceased. An expectation that children were present and participated in funerals of the period is provided by iconography on elite status grave markers that show children as part of funerary ceremonies where they sit in the laps of women but also tend to, or interact with, the corpse. In addition to the very interesting contribution that children were present in mourning ceremonies, Langdon's study demonstrates clearly that they were not merely observers or passive participants in these socially charged exchanges, but were commemorated in image and object as key components of the mourning party.

Child burials are thus not only one of the strongest bodies of evidence for children in the past, they are an arena of cultural performance to which many modern scholars are drawn in order to evaluate childhood as similar or dissimilar to our own experiences today in the West. Burials seem to facilitate a connection with one of the strongest components of our own understanding of childhood—a deep emotional reaction and protectiveness that has been naturalized and essentialized to the degree that it is unquestioned. Grave goods in a juvenile burial are read as an effort to provide comfort to the deceased child, and an absence of grave goods is read as an absence of care or emotional connection. As a field we should acknowledge this pattern and the powerful hold child burials have over our imagination, either for their ability to connect us to the people of the past, or to materialize how differently childhood may have been experienced and understood in the past. But in either case our analyses could benefit from the greater utilization of theories of emotion, commemoration, memory, and ancestral construction in order to more clearly identify what was actually being materialized in child burials. Rather than relying primarily upon our instinctive and emotive reactions to child remains, an attempt to discuss infant or child remains as part of the continuum of ancestor creation or as one of many ways memory is manifested, for example, could open up new ways of seeing children as connected and constituent parts of broader cultural phenomena.

Another theme that bridges many of the contributions and which holds the promise of significantly changing our current understanding of children in the past is the active role of children as autonomous and effectual agents. Traditional archaeological models of ancient cultures barely acknowledge the presence of children, and many of the contributors to this volume have dedicated themselves to addressing this erasure of what was often one-half or more of the ancient populace. As with other previously "invisible populations," studies of childhood in the past began with efforts to locate material evidence of young people and later proceeded to more complex questions about how and if childhood existed within the many cultures of human history. Today we discuss how childhood is experienced as a social identity and the actions of different populations or cohorts of children. The field of Childhood Studies, broadly defined, has abundant examples to support a perspective that individual children can be innovators, prophets, kings, or criminals—in short, there is little use in essentializing the social category of children into a single entity that obscures the variation inherent in this large population as well as the important intersections of age and other social identities such as race or class. Many of the chapters in this volume elaborate on this perspective by providing compelling case studies of how individual children can not only be seen in the past, their contributions to the material record reflect important phenomena and beliefs that differ greatly from our own. While children are often described as "little sponges" in the modern West (i.e., as passive receivers of culture without significant agency), this is hardly the case in all cultures where youth is not an inherent barrier to power, holiness, or eroticism. Authors who explore these data are to be commended for setting aside, or attempting to expand, many of the deeply ingrained and biologically justified notions of children as incomplete humans, incapable of agency or self-interested action.

Sharon Moses presents new data on the micromorphology of domestic structures at Çatalhöyük that make a significant contribution not only to methodological innovations that allow us to capture a greater range of activities but also to our ability to link activities to learning and enculturation. Exploring domestic rituals at Neolithic Çatalhöyük, Turkey, Moses argues convincingly that children would have participated in normal plastering and whitewashing activities, and she finds evidence for a distinctive form of figurine fragment in these contexts that may be evidence of children's material culture. In this thoughtful analysis, Moses centers her study around the participation of children in a common activity but also shows how that participation was likely a key arena for socialization through sacred narratives or storytelling. Domestic arenas are powerful locations for the circulation of knowledge and practice, and Moses shows how children were both contributors to, and beneficiaries of, those cultural circulations. Children were likely participants in repetitious rituals of plastering that purposefully hid small meaningful objects within the walls and plaster surfaces of these homes, and thus were brought into group membership through this specific arena of learning and memory.

The study of adult height dimorphism as an indicator of childhood health by Eva Rosenstock takes a very different methodological approach but still arrives at conclusions that reflect the actions and agency of children. Rosenstock asserts that adult height at death can be read as an indication of childhood health and diet, with the added feature that sex determination of an adult skeleton is much more reliable than of a juvenile. The analyses of this chapter rely upon large datasets but provide a compelling window into the actions and outcomes of individual children. Given that diet is so closely tied to power differentials such as gender, age, and class, the examination of individual health circumstances viewed against a broader temporal or regional pattern illuminates how certain families or even persons were impacted by cultural habits but also how they may have manipulated and challenged such norms. This study shows that even in the realm of subsistence, something we tend to assume was not under the control of young people, children had their own role in provisioning themselves, with lifelong consequences.

Questions of children as agents of desire have confounded scholars for centuries, and debates about the role of pederasty within the Classical world continue to be highly polarized and contentious. While young boys are acknowledged to have been the subject of sexual interest for Athenian men, the role of young boys in sexual encounters within Rome is less well understood or explored. Jeannine Diddle Uzzi contributes a new analysis of the Clementia Sarcophagus and shows that non-Roman young boys are depicted on the sarcophagus in a sexualized manner because iconographic conventions of the Roman Empire eroticized the state of captivity. Military and sexual conquest were conflated, Uzzi argues, and the young (both male and female) were regular objects of sexual interest. By exploring the power of a young body to inspire longing within ancient Roman society, this compelling case study also reveals certain young individuals as agents of desire. Youth, or the age status of preadulthood, was acknowledged to possess a particular kind of influence and power in this society, a unique characteristic that shaped social relations. When coupled with the visual aspects of non-Romaness and the Roman eroticism of captivity, certain children were clearly both the object and agents of desire. The rich data provided by Uzzi also allow her to consider the age of consent, and how such transitional periods varied for different populations within the Roman Empire, thus helping us to see childhood as hardly a consistent set of experiences, even within a single culture.

This same sense of childhood or youth as defined by a unique character manifests in a very different manner in the study of American Victorian toys by Kyle Somerville. While exploring playthings considered appropriate for the same age range as Uzzi's sexually active captives, the data available to Somerville in the form of middle-class American board games, steel trains, and dolls materialize a very different conceptualization of this cohort. Both Roman sarcophagi and Victorian toys are objects manufactured by adults with children in mind, and as such reinforce dominant cultural values and conceptualizations of children. As Somerville explains, Victorian toys reflect a growing desire for an ordered society, and thus instructed young people in a highly gendered world in which travel and education were increasingly accessible. Yet they also can be read as an indication that childhood was perceived as a time of innocence, with a sacred nature that would erode as the young grew to adulthood. Victorian society strove to protect this unique state of childhood purity and prolong the period before children succumbed to immorality and bad habits, impulses that may have been fostered in part by declining birthrates and increasing amounts of parental time for interaction with children. Somerville, like many of the other contributors to this section, does an excellent job of illustrating how even when it is not acknowledged explicitly, childhood can be understood as a period or experience filled with power and even moral authority.

Through these varied studies of the specific nature of young people we can see how the social identity of child or youth was constructed and performed in radically different ways. Identities are formed through repeated behaviors and the circulation of information about what those behaviors mean to a given social imaginary or collectivity. Decades of research has shown that very little if any aspect of gendered identity truly derives from a biological imperative—culture constructs ways to understand biological difference and, likewise, the field of Childhood Studies shows that cultures manage the biological differences of age in vastly different ways. Adolescence seems to be a time that is particularly susceptible to a wide range of cultural values, and youth of twelve years of age are ascribed everything from adult responsibilities to child-like toys, depending upon the cultural framework used to make sense of the dramatic biological changes that occur during this period of life. With the acknowledgment that biology alone does not drive the understanding of childhood or adolescence comes a renewed attention to the practices that constitute experiential learning as a means of identity formation. The performance of age-appropriate behaviors is as deliberate a choice as the performance of gender-specific behaviors, and while our archaeological studies have done an increasingly convincing job of exploring how tasks and activities relegated to children, such as plastering walls or playing with toys, solidified an age-based identity through the manipulation of material objects, we must also keep in mind that individual children will have chosen not to perform in culturally appropriate ways or to maneuver around such norms to achieve a different end. Childhood Studies today is conceptually free to identify such individual agents and capture their unique contribution to the material record of history.

The contributions to this important conference reinforce the well-established principle that in many cultures gendered practices are a fundamental way in which we can observe difference within the age-based identity of a child. There appear to be very few times and places in which all children shared the same sets of chores or opportunities, as the case studies presented here demonstrate in detail. Thus, the intersection of gender and age is a powerful nexus for expanding our understanding of childhood in the past, and as our work in this area progresses we should expand deeper into the variations that exist within the younger population of the cultures under study. Perhaps gender is a uniquely salient component of childhood and especially the transition to adolescence and adulthood, given that sexual differentiation surfaces as a visually significant feature of social interactions, often at what is considered the end of childhood and the beginning of adolescence. Or perhaps it is the materialization of processes of socialization that we can read solidified in gendered toys, tools, and ornaments, but there is ample evidence that one of the most significant reasons to study children in ancient cultures—as a means to understand cultural reproduction—is a social process which by its nature circulates ideas about, and is in turn constituted by, the gendered nature of the world.

The contribution by Keri Brown on the promising new developments in the use of ancient DNA testing to reveal children and family groups in the archaeological record clearly demonstrates not only a new methodological technique that will, hopefully, become more common in archaeological analyses but also how powerful our interpretations can become if and when we are able to insert gendered identities into all analyses. The potential for this new avenue of research to benefit studies of age- and gender-based identities is immense, as patterns of artifact associations with human materials subjected to DNA analysis can then be used by those unable to extract or recover DNA. The application to studies of sex-selective infanticide are particularly apt—long assumed to have been practiced predominantly on female infants, studies of DNA recovered from infants buried near a Roman bathhouse at Ashkelon and in Roman Britain produced contrasting results for Brown. In Ashkelon, the majority of infants were male, and in Roman Britain the population was mixed, although males were more common. Obviously, the practice of selective female infanticide was not supported in either case, a conclusion with wide-reaching implications for our understanding of childhood, parenting, gender-based identities, and reproductive choices within the Roman Empire.

The juncture between gender and age is visible in many of the other case studies in this section; from the nutritional differences that led to gender disparities in height in the chapter by Rosenstock, to the eroticization of non-Roman youth in the iconographic study by Uzzi, to the materialization of adult ideas about appropriate gender roles conveyed through Victorian toys, much of the material record of childhood has a gendered component that structured and differentiated the lives of young men and women from a very early age. Of course, the use of these artifacts helped perpetuate gender roles as well as the expectations of childhood through their deployment in appropriate performances.

Societies share a social imaginary of childhood that interprets and constructs the ways in which the biological and cultural aspects of young lives will converse. As Heather Montgomery has noted, the term *child* is a relational one, and is used as often to describe interactions between people as to describe a group of individuals at a particular stage of life (Montgomery 2009:55). Often we are described as the "child of" throughout our lives, to reflect ongoing relationships of support and affection within families, and in some societies everyone is considered a "child of" god, the king, a forest, etc. Montgomery cites Nurit Bird-David, who in her study of the Nayaka hunter-gatherers of South India found that the Nayaka use the word *child* to describe themselves in relation to their surroundings. "[They] use the word makalo (children) to describe themselves vis-à-vis the forest and vis-à-vis all invisible and previous dwellers in their area, whom they call respectively 'big parents,' or in some cases 'grandparents.' 'Children' is a concept that is central to their sense of themselves, their place in the world, and their relationship with their surroundings; it recurs in their moral and ritual discourse" (Bird-David 2005:93).

Obviously, for the Nayaka the interactions of parent and child are a powerful metaphor for human interactions generally, and they share a social imaginary in which the social identity of child is a model for human behavior rather than a transitory status of incompleteness. When Nayaka state they are children of the forest, they are circulating an idea that life within the forest is relational and experienced as a series of interactions based on dependence and reciprocity. Colonial-era Maya mythological texts, such as the Popul Vuh, from the Quiche people of highland Guatemala, also utilize the terms *children* and *grandparents* to frame the relations between humanity and the creator gods. After the first humans are made of corn dough, they thank the Makers and say, "Truly now, double thanks, triple thanks, that we've been formed, we've been given our mouths, our faces . . . thanks to you we've been formed, we've come to be made and modeled, our grandmother, our grandfather" (Tedlock 1985:166). The two main avatars of this mythological cycle known as the Hero Twins, who through their cunning and skill model correct human behavior, are referred to as "boys" throughout the story, while the Makers tell the animals they made, "Now name our names, praise us. We are your mother, we are your father," (Tedlock 1985:78). Nearly all the relationships described in the Popul Vuh are described in familial terms, and the dependencies of children and adults upon one another are used as a familiar metaphor for the interdependencies of humanity and the gods.

The investigation of age-based social identities such as childhood is crucial to modern social archaeology for many reasons. It is an expedient way almost anyone can connect with the lives and experiences of ancient people, thereby dissolving the arbitrary line we have erected between past and present. But perhaps more importantly, identity construction is a fundamental human process of great interest to anthropology and many other social sciences because it reflects one of the basic ways in which cultures reproduce themselves, as well as how they change. The ideas a culture holds about how young people are made into adults involve a set of interlocking identities we choose to call gender, age, and even nation, etc. that have to be reproduced through a shared understanding of mutual participation (Taylor 2004). Identities, as a form of social community building, are one of the primary mechanisms by which cultures reproduce themselves through instruction and performance of values, goals, behaviors, etc. While such behaviors and beliefs leave a material residue available to archaeologists, these data are reflections of common understandings, worked out through dialogue and interaction (Taylor 2002:106). As Sorensen (2000) has explained, archaeology may best be able to look at how social identities such as gender or childhood are constructed and lived, as these practices involve material things and physical arrangements or practices. But we should never lose sight of the fact that what we recover are materializations of shared ideas, or more accurately, the materialization of individual negotiation or dialogue around shared ideas. As the contributors to this volume demonstrate, there are rich data available to approach questions about how the experiences of death and grieving, individual autonomy, and gendered relations were constructed to pivot around the understanding of age. Children, and specific cultural understandings of childhood, must be at the center of our investigations of social identities and how societies grow, change, and reproduce themselves. Like fingerprints, which are present everywhere even though they are difficult to perceive, age-specific social groups, especially children, have a central role to play in our understanding of ancient society.

REFERENCES CITED

Ardren, T. 2011 Empowered Children in Classic Maya Sacrificial Rites. *Childhood in the Past* 4:133–145.

Baxter, J. E. 2005 The Archaeology of Childhood: Children, Gender, and Material Culture. AltaMira Press, Walnut Creek, California.

Baxter, J. E. 2008 The Archaeology of Childhood. *Annual Review of Anthropology* 37:159–175.

Bird-David, N. 2005 Studying Children in Hunter-Gatherer Societies: Reflections from a Nayaka Perspective. In *Hunter-Gatherer Childhoods: Evolutionary, Developmental, and Cultural Perspectives*, edited by B. Hewlett and M. Lamb, pp. 92–101. Aldine, New York.

Gottlieb, A. 2004 *The Afterlife is Where We Come From: The Culture of Infancy in West Africa.* University of Chicago Press, Chicago.

Hope, V. M. 2009 *Roman Death: The Dying and the Dead in Ancient Rome.* Continuum, London.

Montgomery, H. 2009 *An Introduction to Childhood: Anthropological Perspectives on Children's Lives.* Wiley–Blackwell, Malden, Massachusetts.

Moore, J., and E. Scott (editors) 1997 *Invisible People and Processes: Writing Gender and Childhood in European Archaeology.* Leicester University Press, London.

Scott, E. 1999 *The Archaeology of Infancy and Infant Death.* British Archaeological Reports 819. Archaeopress, Oxford.

Sofaer Derevenski, Joanna (editor) 2000 *Children and Material Culture.* Routledge, New York.

Sorensen, M. L. 2000 *Gender Archaeology.* Polity Press, Cambridge.

Taylor, C. 2004 *Modern Social Imaginaries.* Duke University Press, Durham.

Tedlock, D. 1985 *Popul Vuh: The Mayan Book of the Dawn of Life.* Simon and Schuster, New York.

Contributors

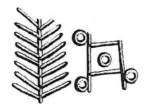

Traci Ardren, Professor and Chair, Department of Anthropology, University of Miami

Paul Bahn, Independent

Jane Eva Baxter, Professor and Chair, Department of Anthropology, DePaul University

Peter F. Biehl, Professor and Chair, Department of Anthropology, State University of New York at Buffalo

Nurit Bird-David, Department of Sociology and Anthropology, University of Haifa

Keri Brown, Manchester Interdisciplinary Biocentre, University of Manchester

Güner Coşkunsu, Arkeoloji Bölüm Başkanı, Edebiyat Fakültesi, Archaeology Department, Mardin Artuklu Üniversitesi Yenişehir Yerleşkesi

Frank Hole, Professor Emeritus, Department of Anthropology, Yale University

Scott Hutson, Associate Professor, Department of Anthropology, University of Kentucky

Kathryn Kamp, Earl D. Strong Professor of Social Studies, Department of Anthropology, Grinnell College

Susan Langdon, Professor and Chair, Department of Art History and Archaeology, University of Missouri

Jack A. Meacham, Retired

Sharon Moses, Assistant Professor, Department of Anthropology, Northern Arizona University

Eva Rosenstock, Group Leader Emmy Noether Junior Research Group, Institute of Prehistoric Archaeology, Free University Berlin

Joanna Sofaer, Senior Lecturer in Archaeology, Department of Archaeology, University of Southampton

Kyle Somerville, Archaeologist/Principal Investigator, Powers and Teremy, LLC
David Soren, Regents Professor, Department of Classics, The University of Arizona
Jeannine Diddle Uzzi, Associate Professor, Department of Modern and Classical Languages and Literatures, University of Southern Maine

Index

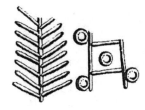